AF734607

KJ Lee Essential Medicine Series

nova
Medicine & Health
New York

KJ Lee Essential Medicine Series

K. J. Lee, MD, FACS - Series Editor-in-Chief
Yale University School of Medicine
New Haven, Connecticut, USA
Quinnipiac University
Netter School of Medicine
Hamden, Connecticut, USA
Hofstra University
Zucker School of Medicine
Hempstead, New York, USA

Essential Facial Plastic and Reconstructive Surgery. Volume 1: General Principles, Reconstruction of Defects, Congenital Anomalies, Trauma, and Facial Nerve Rehabilitation
Yan Ho Lee, MD and Ira Papel, MD (Editors)
2024. ISBN: 979-8-89113-306-8 (Hardcover)
2024. ISBN: 979-8-89113-749-3 (eBook)

Essential Rational Healthcare Economics: Past, Present and Future
Mark E. Lee, MBA and K. J. Lee, MD, FACS (Editors)
2024. ISBN: 979-8-89113-315-0 (Hardcover)
2024. ISBN: 979-8-89113-499-7 (eBook)

Essential Otology and Neurotology
William H. Slattery III, MD and Andrea Vambutas, MD (Editors)
Helena Wichova, MD (Associate Editor)
2023. ISBN: 979-8-88697-645-8 (Hardcover)
2023. ISBN: 979-8-88697-822-3 (eBook)

Essential Head and Neck Oncology and Surgery
Maie A. St. John, MD, PhD, FACS and Benjamin L. Judson, MD, MBA (Editors)
Josephine H. Nguyen, MD (Assistant Editor)
2023. ISBN: 979-8-88697-438-6 (Hardcover)
2023. ISBN: 979-8-88697-746-2 (eBook)

Essential Sleep Medicine and Surgery
Maria V. Suurna, MD, FACS and Stacey L. Ishman, MD (Editors)
Josephine H. Nguyen, MD (Assistant Editor)
2021. ISBN: 978-1-68507-220-9 (Hardcover)
2021. ISBN: 978-1-68507-389-3 (eBook)

More information about this series can be found at https://novapublishers.com/product-category/series/kj-lee-essential-medicine-series/

Yan Ho Lee, MD
Ira Papel, MD
Editors

Essential Facial Plastic and Reconstructive Surgery

Volume 1: General Principles, Reconstruction of Defects, Congenital Anomalies, Trauma, and Facial Nerve Rehabilitation

nova
Medicine & Health
New York

Copyright © 2024 by Nova Science Publishers, Inc.
DOI: https://doi.org/10.52305/ICQT2648

All rights reserved. No part of this book may be reproduced, stored in a retrieval system or transmitted in any form or by any means: electronic, electrostatic, magnetic, tape, mechanical photocopying, recording or otherwise without the written permission of the Publisher.

We have partnered with Copyright Clearance Center to make it easy for you to obtain permissions to reuse content from this publication. Please visit copyright.com and search by Title, ISBN, or ISSN.

For further questions about using the service on copyright.com, please contact:

Copyright Clearance Center
Phone: +1-(978) 750-8400 Fax: +1-(978) 750-4470 E-mail: info@copyright.com

NOTICE TO THE READER

The Publisher has taken reasonable care in the preparation of this book but makes no expressed or implied warranty of any kind and assumes no responsibility for any errors or omissions. No liability is assumed for incidental or consequential damages in connection with or arising out of information contained in this book. The Publisher shall not be liable for any special, consequential, or exemplary damages resulting, in whole or in part, from the readers' use of, or reliance upon, this material. Any parts of this book based on government reports are so indicated and copyright is claimed for those parts to the extent applicable to compilations of such works.

Independent verification should be sought for any data, advice or recommendations contained in this book. In addition, no responsibility is assumed by the Publisher for any injury and/or damage to persons or property arising from any methods, products, instructions, ideas or otherwise contained in this publication.

This publication is designed to provide accurate and authoritative information with regards to the subject matter covered herein. It is sold with the clear understanding that the Publisher is not engaged in rendering legal or any other professional services. If legal or any other expert assistance is required, the services of a competent person should be sought. FROM A DECLARATION OF PARTICIPANTS JOINTLY ADOPTED BY A COMMITTEE OF THE AMERICAN BAR ASSOCIATION AND A COMMITTEE OF PUBLISHERS.

Library of Congress Cataloging-in-Publication Data

Names: Lee, Yan Ho, editor. | Papel, Ira D., editor.
Title: Essential facial plastic and reconstructive surgery / Yan Ho Lee, MD, Ira D. Papel, MD, editors.
Description: New York : Nova Medicine & Health, [2024]- | Series: KJ Lee essential medicine series | Includes bibliographical references and index. | Contents: v. 1 General principles, reconstruction of defects, congenital anomalies, trauma, and facial nerve rehabilitation -- |
Identifiers: LCCN 2024020055 (print) | LCCN 2024020056 (ebook) | ISBN 9798891133068 (hardcover) | ISBN 9798891137493 (ebook)
Subjects: LCSH: Surgery, Plastic--Textbooks.
Classification: LCC RD118 .E78 2024 (print) | LCC RD118 (ebook) | DDC 617.9/5--dc23
LC record available at https://lccn.loc.gov/2024020055
LC ebook record available at https://lccn.loc.gov/2024020056

Published by Nova Science Publishers, Inc. † New York

To my husband Jonathan Y Lee for your unwavering support in life. Somehow you always know when I need you to help me solve an issue and when I need you to just listen to my grievances.

To my daughter Evie SY Lee who brightens up my day no matter what.

To my family Patrick Ho, Pauline Ho, and Lam Ho for believing in me, and reminding me that I am capable of so many things.

To my co-editor I.P. for being my mentor. Your insight has always amazed me, and your ability to collaborate across disciplines is inspiring.

YHL

To Leslie, Jillian and Haley for putting up with my sometimes-crazy evening work hours.

To the residents, fellows and surgeons who will study this text and make the efforts meaningful.

To Dr. Yan Lee for her tireless work in seeing this project to completion. It would have not happened without her.

Ira D. Papel, M.D.

Contents

Foreword and Acknowledgements

As the knowledge of medicine has grown exponentially, it is necessary to have books each encompassing one subspecialty. I had the vision of creating a book for each subspecialty building from the formula and on the success of *Essential Otolaryngology-Head and Neck Surgery*, the inceptive book, which is in its 12th Edition, 50th year, and has been translated into several languages. It was cited as one of the most read texts in the field worldwide. Working with President Nadya S. Gotsiridze-Columbus, CEO of Nova Science Publishers, Inc., we developed K. J. Lee Essential Medicine Series to launch the subspecialty books. After a national search, we were fortunate to have Dr. Yan Lee and Dr. Ira Papel to be Editors of this book. We commend the scholarly contents of the chapter contributing authors. It is with great pleasure and honor for me to say they all worked very hard and have done a superb job. I thank them all and kudos to them.

Like the inceptive book, I have no doubt this book will find its way to libraries, to the reference sections of emergency rooms, urgent care centers, as well as the dorm rooms, apartments, and homes of medical students, residents, fellows, young attendings, physician assistants, nurse practitioners and others.

This book is not only a great text and reference for medical professionals, but it can also be of value for people outside the medical field to understand key concepts in order to better communicate with providers.

K. J. Lee, MD, FACS, Editor-in-Chief
KJ Lee Essential Medicine Series

Acknowledgements

We would like to thank Dr. K.J. Lee for his mentorship and sponsorship. Dr. Lee has been pivotal in the training and education of otolaryngology head and neck surgeons for decades. We are honored he has entrusted us with the task of editing this book.

To the authors who contributed to this book: We are so fortunate to have colleagues from various specialties and subspecialties who are collectively experts in our field. Your experience and knowledge truly enrich the content of this book. We could not ask for contributors who are more dedicated to the field of Facial Plastic and Reconstructive Surgery.

Part 1. Basic Principles

Chapter 1

Anatomy and Embryology

Benjamin M. Laitman, MD, PhD
and Mingyang Gray, MD

Introduction

Branchial Arches, Clefts, Pouches

Table 1.1. Branchial Arches.

Arch	Nerve	Artery	Muscles/Ligaments	Cartilage/Bone
1	Semilunar ganglion, V3	Internal maxillary	• Anterior malleal ligament • Sphenomandibular ligament • Tensor tympani muscle • Mastication muscles, mylohyoid muscle • Anterior belly of digastric muscle • Tensor palatini muscle	• Meckel's cartilage: o Mandible o Head, neck, manubrium of malleus o Body and short process of incusi
2	Geniculate ganglion, VII	Stapedial artery* (*usually degenerates)	• Stylohyoid ligament • Stapedius muscle • Facial muscles, posterior belly of digastric muscle	• Reichert cartilage: o Manubrium of malleus o Long process of incus o All of stapes superstructure except footplate and annular ligament (vestibular portion) o Part of pyramidal eminence o Lower part of facial canal o Styloid process • Lesser cornu of hyoid • Part of body of hyoid
3	IX	Common carotid	• Stylopharyngeus muscle • Superior and middle constrictor muscles	• Greater cornu of hyoid and rest of hyoid
4	Superior Laryngeal nerve (SLN)	Left: arch of the aorta Right: proximal subclavian	• Thyroid cartilage • Cuneiform cartilage	• Stylopharyngeus muscle • Superior and middle constrictor muscles
6	Recurrent laryngeal nerve (RLN)	Left: Pulmonary artery, ductus arteriosus Right: degenerates	• Cricoid cartilage • Arytenoid cartilages • Corniculate cartilage • Upper Trachea	• Intrinsic laryngeal muscles • Inferior constrictor muscle

In: Essential Facial Plastic and Reconstructive Surgery. Volume 1 ISBN: 979-8-89113-306-8
Editors: Yan Ho Lee and Ira Papel
© 2024 Nova Science Publishers, Inc.

1. There are five branchial/pharyngeal *arches,* each with an associated *cleft/groove* and *pouch.*
   a. Arch derivatives: *mesoderm.*
   b. Cleft/groove: *ectoderm.*
   c. Pouch: *endoderm.*
2. Each arch has an associated nerve, artery and cartilage bar
3. Nerves
   a. Nerves are *anterior* to their respective arteries (exception: fifth arch nerve is posterior to artery)
   b. Hypoglossal nerve lies caudal to all arches
      i. First: Semilunar ganglion, V_3
      ii. Second: Geniculate ganglion, VII
      iii. Third: IX
      iv. Fourth: Superior laryngeal nerve (SLN)
      v. Fifth/Sixth: Recurrent laryngeal nerve (RLN)
4. Arteries
   a. Two ventral (fuse completely) and two dorsal aortas (fuse caudally) in early embryonic life
      i. First and second arch arteries degenerate during embryonic life
         - The second arch artery (stapedial artery) has an upper branch that passes through a mass of mesoderm, which later chondrifies and ossifies as the stapes
         - Generally degenerates but has the potential to persist postnatally.
      ii. Third: precursor to the common carotid artery bilaterally.
      iii. Fourth: *Left* - arch of the aorta; *Right* - proximal subclavian
      iv. Fifth/sixth: *Left* - pulmonary artery and ductus arteriosus; *Right* - degenerates
         - Fifth/sixth arch nerve (RLN) is posterior and caudal to the artery
         - On the left, nerve loops around ductus arteriosus and aortic arch
         - On the right, as aortic precursor degenerates, RLN loops around proximal subclavian

Arch Derivatives

First

1. Meckel cartilage:
   a. Mandible
   b. Head, neck, manubrium of malleus
   c. Body and short process of incus
   d. Anterior malleal ligament
   e. Sphenomandibular ligament

2. Tensor tympani muscle
3. Mastication muscles, mylohyoid
4. Anterior belly of digastric muscle
5. Tensor palatini muscle

Second

1. Reichert cartilage:
    a. Manubrium of malleus
    b. Long process of incus
    c. All of stapes superstructure except footplate and annular ligament (vestibular portion)
    d. Part of pyramidal eminence
    e. Lower part of facial canal
    f. Styloid process
    g. Stylohyoid ligament
    h. Lesser cornu of hyoid
    i. Part of body of hyoid
2. Stapedius muscle
3. Facial muscles, posterior belly of digastric muscle

Third

1. Greater cornu of hyoid and rest of hyoid
2. Stylopharyngeus muscle
3. Superior and middle constrictor

Fourth

1. Thyroid cartilage
2. Cuneiform cartilage
3. Inferior pharyngeal constrictor muscle
4. Cricopharyngeus muscle
5. Cricothyroid muscle

Fifth/Sixth

1. Cricoid
2. Arytenoids
3. Corniculate
4. Trachea
5. Intrinsic laryngeal muscles
6. Inferior constrictor muscle

*The sternocleidomastoid muscles are derived from the cervical somites posterior and inferior to the arches

Pouch Derivatives

1. First: Middle ear cavity

2. Second: Tonsillar fossa, palatine tonsil
3. Third: Inferior parathyroids (2), thymus
4. Fourth: Superior parathyroids (2)

Fascial Layers[3, 4]

1. Superficial Cervical Fascia
2. Envelopes Platysma and muscles of facial expression
3. Boundaries:
    a. Superior: zygomatic process
    b. Inferior: clavicle
4. Fascial planes overlying platysma are confluent with superficial musculoaponeurotic system (SMAS) and the superficial temporalis fascia/temporoparietal fascia (TPF)
5. Main plane of resistance to deep neck spread of cellulitis
6. Allows mobility of skin over deep neck structures
7. Deep Cervical Fascia
8. **Superficial layer (investing fascia)**
    a. Envelopes: trapezius, sternocleidomastoid, strap muscles (sternohyoid, sternothyroid, thyrohyoid, omohyoid), submandibular and parotid glands, muscles of mastication: masseter, pterygoids, temporalis
9. **Middle Layer (visceral fascia)**
    a. Envelopes: strap muscles, pharynx, larynx, trachea, esophagus, thyroid, parathyroid, buccinators, pharyngeal constrictors
    b. Forms buccopharyngeal fascia which overlies pharyngeal wall (anterior border of retropharyngeal space)
10. **Deep Layer (prevertebral fascia)**
    a. Envelopes: paraspinous muscles, cervical vertebrae
    b. Two layers: prevertebral and alar layers
    c. "Danger space" is between these two fascial components
11. **Masticator Space**
    a. Contents: masseter muscle, lateral and medial pterygoid muscles, ramus and posterior body of mandible, temporalis muscle tendon, inferior alveolar nerve (V3), internal maxillary artery
12. **Temporal Fossa**
    a. Contents: Temporalis muscle, temporal fat pad

Facial Bones (Figure 1.1)

1. Face includes an underlying bony skeletal support structure; contributes to:
2. Facial shape important for both function and cosmesis
3. Support and protection for viscera
4. Paranasal sinuses are mucosal-lined cavities within the facial skeleton
    a. Lightens the face/head

b. Protective "crumple zone" for nearby viscera

5. Upper and lower jaws contain teeth
6. Lower jaw is mobile and suspended by temporomandibular joints
7. Bony skeleton is covered by soft tissues of various thicknesses, including periosteum, muscles, fat, and skin
8. Viscera of facial area include brain, eyes, oral structures, major and minor salivary glands, nerves, blood vessels, and lymphatics
9. Facial bones
10. Frontal bone
11. Maxilla
12. Zygoma (2)
13. Nasal bones (2)
14. Mandible
15. Orbit (7 bones)
16. Medial wall: ethmoid bone, lacrimal bone, nasal process of maxilla
17. Floor: orbital process of maxilla, orbital process of palatine bone, sphenoid
18. Lateral wall: zygomatic bone, frontal bone, greater wing of the sphenoid
19. Roof: frontal bone

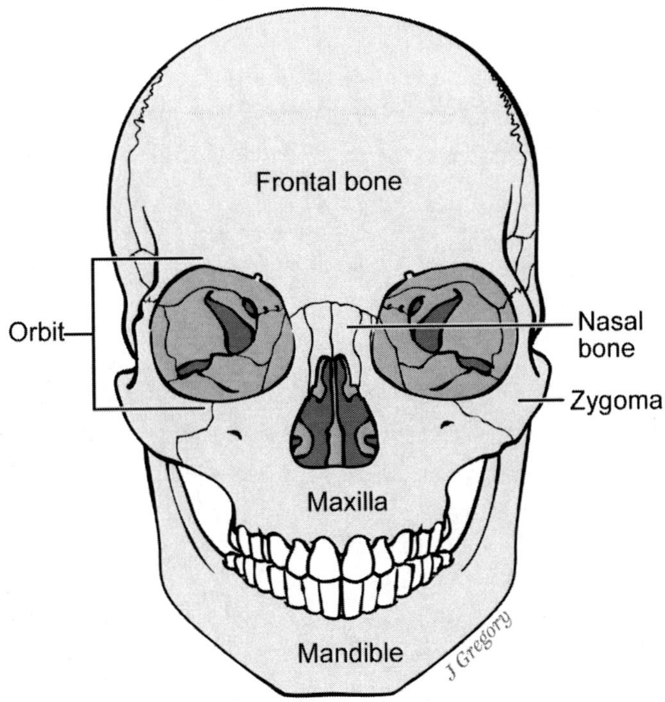

Figure 1.1. Facial bones. Printed with permission from ©Mount Sinai Health System.

Dental Anatomy and Occlusion (Figure 1.2)

1. Adult dentition: 32 teeth in total

   a. 16 maxillary teeth: 1-16 from upper right third molar to upper left third molar
   b. 16 mandibular teeth: 17-32 from lower left third molar to lower right third molar
2. Pediatric dentition (deciduous teeth): 20 teeth in total
   a. 10 maxillary teeth: A-J from upper right second molar to upper left second molar
   b. 10 mandibular teeth: K-T from lower left second molar to lower right second molar
3. Teeth have external enamel, and underlying dentin
4. Pulp is central where nerve roots enter
5. Cementum overlies dentin within tooth root; attached to periodontal ligament which anchors tooth in socket
6. Angle Classification System
   a. **Class I occlusion**: Mesial buccal cusp of the first maxillary molar sits within mesobuccal groove of first mandibular molar
   b. **Class II malocclusion**: Mesial buccal cusp of the first maxillary molar is anterior to the first mandibular molar (retrognathism, overjet, overbite)
   c. **Class III malocclusion**: Mesial buccal cusp of the first maxillary molar is posterior to the first mandibular molar (prognathism, anterior crossbite, negative overjet, underbite)
7. **Overjet:** is the extent of horizontal (anterior-posterior) overlap of the maxillary central incisors over the mandibular central incisors
8. **Overbite**: vertical (superior-inferior) overlap of the maxillary central incisors over the mandibular central incisors

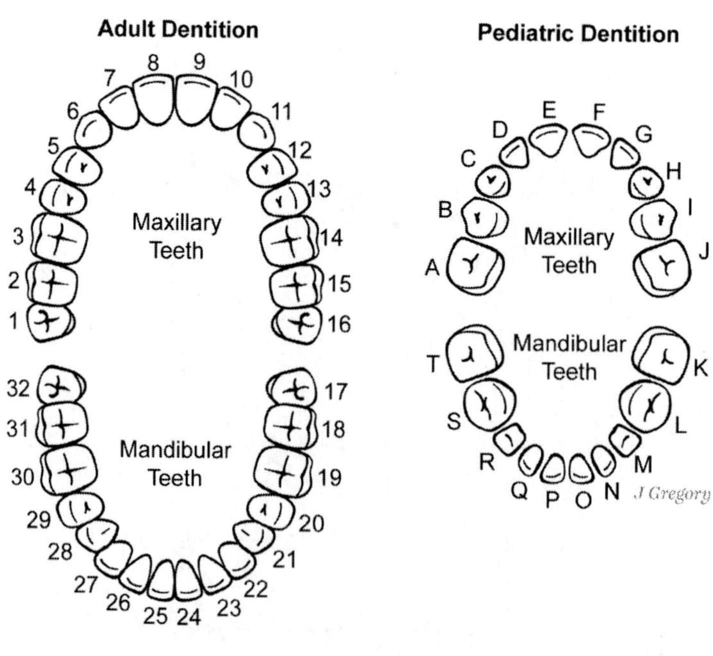

Figure 1.2. Dental anatomy and occlusion. Printed with permission from ©Mount Sinai Health System.

Facial Musculature (Figure 1.3)

1. Innervated by cranial nerve VII
2. Innervation occurs from the underside of the muscles with the exception of the *mentalis, levator anguli oris, buccinator,* which are innervated superficially
3. **Occipitofrontalis**: consists of two parts: frontal and occipital bellies, each inserts on galeal aponeurosis
    a. Frontalis has no bony attachments; fibers are continuous with procerus, corrugators, and orbicularis oculi; attached to the skin of the eyebrows
    b. Function: raises eyebrows
4. **Procerus**: arises from tendinous fibers over lower nasal bones and upper lateral cartilage, inserting onto skin of lower forehead between eyebrows at midline; fibers merge with frontalis
    a. Causes horizontal rhytids at the level of the brow at midline
    b. Function: pulls skin in between eyebrows downward, assists in nostril flaring
5. **Corrugator supercilii**: pyramidal muscle arising from superciliary arch and inserting on eyebrow skin
    a. Causes vertical rhytids on forehead
    b. Function: Draws eyebrows down and medially producing a frown
6. **Nasalis:** sphincter-like muscle of nose
    a. Function: compresses nasal cartilages and flares nostrils
7. **Depressor septi nasi:** connects maxilla and orbicularis oris muscle to nasal septum
    a. Function: draws nasal alae downwards, reducing nostril size
8. **Orbicularis oculi:** arises from nasal part of frontal bone, frontal process of maxilla, and medial palpebral ligament
    a. *orbital* portion forms a complete ellipse
    b. *palpebral* portion arises from medial palpebral ligament, forms a series of concentric curves and inserts into lateral canthus.
    c. Consists of preseptal and pretarsal muscles
    d. Function: closes the eyelids
9. **Auricular muscles (anterior, superior, posterior):** not readily functional in humans
    a. Functions: auricularis anterior draws ear forward and upward; auricularis superior raises it; auricularis posterior draws it backward
10. **Orbicularis oris:** composed of four quadrants of muscles that interact and give appearance of a circular sphincter muscle; has fibers from adjacent muscles that insert into lips, such as those from buccinator
    a. Function: closes mouth and puckers lips
11. **Risorius**: arises from parotid fascia and inserts into angle of mouth
    a. Function: retracts mouth during smiling
12. **Buccinator:** forms lateral wall of oral cavity, anterior cheek
    a. Pierced by parotid duct
    b. Function: pulls back angle of the mouth, flattens cheek area; holds cheek to teeth during chewing (forces food to occlusal surface of posterior teeth)

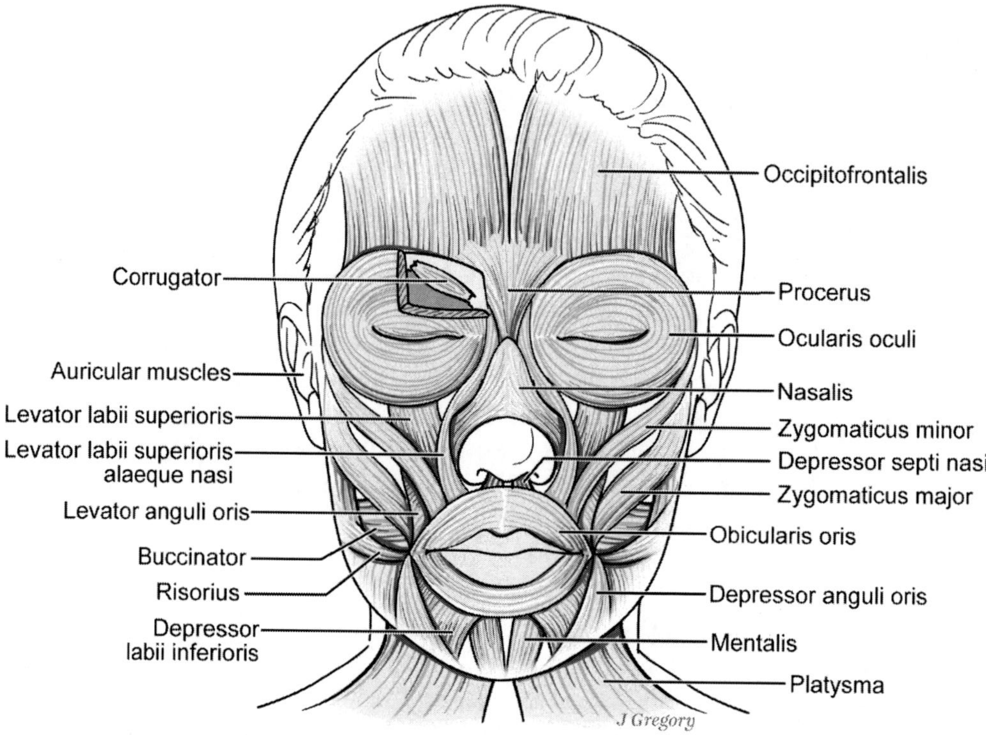

Figure 1.3. Facial musculature. Printed with permission from ©Mount Sinai Health System.

13. **Zygomaticus major:** muscle arises on zygoma to corner of mouth
    a. Bifid zygomaticus major muscles are a variant that is responsible for cheek dimpling
    b. Function: draws angle of mouth superiorly and posteriorly; involved in smiling
14. **Zygomaticus minor:** synergistic with zygomaticus minor
    a. Function: draws angle of mouth superiorly and posteriorly; involved in smiling
15. **Levator anguli oris:** originates at canine fossa of maxilla, under infraorbital foramen, inserts at angle of mouth
    a. Function: elevates angle of mouth medially
16. **Levator labii superioris:** broad sheet of muscle fibers underneath orbicularis, extending medially to side of nose and laterally to zygoma; inserts in alar cartilage and upper lip
    a. Function: elevates upper lip
17. **Levator labii superioris alaeque nasi:** attaches from frontal process of maxilla and inserts into skin of lateral nostril and upper lip
    a. Function: dilates nostril and elevates upper lip (snarling, gummy smile)
    b. Referred to as "Elvis Muscle" because of his signature snarl
18. **Depressor anguli oris:** also known as triangularis muscle; connects mandible to angle of mouth

a. Supplied by buccal branches of facial nerve in addition some marginal mandibular nerve branches
b. Function: depresses corner of the mouth, involved in frowning

19. **Depressor labii inferioris:** originates on lateral mandible and inserts on skin of lower lip
    a. Primarily innervated by marginal mandibular branch of facial nerve
    b. Function: depresses and everts lower lip, exposing lower teeth, involved in smiling
20. **Mentalis:** originates at mental protuberance and inserts into soft tissue and skin of chin and lip
    a. Causes chin wrinkles
    b. Function: upward and inward movement of chin soft tissue; raises central lower lip; involved in pouting
21. **Platysma:** broad muscle sheet, originates on upper clavicle, pectoralis and deltoid muscles; travels obliquely to mandible; platysma deficient in midline
    a. Innervated by cervical branch of facial nerve
    b. Responsible for neck wrinkles and banding
    c. Function: creates bowstring effect on side of neck, fibers move away from midline; has role in depressing lower lip

Skin

1. Cross sectional anatomy of skin
2. Made of three major layers:
    a. Epidermis
    b. Dermis
    c. Subcutaneous tissue "hypodermis"
3. **Epidermis**
    a. Embryologically arises from a combination of ectoderm and neural crest cells
    b. Vast majority of cells are *keratinocytes*; much smaller percentage of Merkel cells, melanocytes, and Langerhans cells
    c. Epidermis itself has no blood vessels; nutrients arise from blood capillaries in upper dermis via diffusion
    d. Epidermis can be histologically subdivided (from superficial to deep) into:
        i. Stratum corneum
        ii. Stratum granulosum
        iii. Stratum lucidum (not in head and neck skin)
        iv. Stratum spinosum
        v. Stratum basale: contain basal progenitor cells of epidermis that proliferate, and daughter cells of this layer differentiate and change shape into more superficial skin layers
4. **Dermis**
    a. Embryologically derives from mesoderm

   b. Comprised of connective tissue, collagen, elastin, hyaluronic acid, proteoglycans
   c. Has many fibroblasts that produce this connective tissue
   d. Contains mechanoreceptors, nocioceptors, thermoceptors that participate in the sensation of touch, pain, and temperature respectively
   e. Has hair follicles, sweat and sebaceous glands, apocrine glands
   f. Has blood and lymphatic vessels
   g. Divided into two main layers:
      i. Papillary dermis: named for finger-like papillary projections that extend into epidermis; comprised of loose areolar connective tissue
      ii. Reticular dermis: contains thick compact collagen, elastin, and reticular fibers; contains hair roots, sweat and sebaceous glands, sensory receptors, and blood vessels
5. **Subcutaneous layer "hypodermis"**
   a. Attaches skin to underling bone, muscle
   b. Supplies overlying skin with blood
   c. Composed of loose connective tissue, elastin
   d. Cellular components: fibroblasts, macrophages, and adipocytes (fat cells)
6. **Langer's lines**: topographical lines on the body, parallel to the natural orientation of collagen fibers within the dermis
   a. Incisions parallel to these lines may heal better with less scaring because of reduced tension on the wound
7. **Relaxed skin tension lines**: tension line/furrow created when the skin is pinched/relaxed in the absence of local tension
   a. often runs in parallel to Langer's lines, however there are areas in which these run in different directions
   b. RSTLs are perpendicular to Lines of Maximal Extensibility.
8. **Lines of Maximal Extensibility**: areas where the skin can lengthen more under tension due to stretching of elastic fibers. Skin extensibility is also known as mechanical creep. This will result in reduction in wound closure tension over time because the tensions will be reduced when skin is under continuous strain. To reduce tension on wound it is thus beneficial to recruit skin in a line of maximal extensibility.

Scalp

1. Useful mnemonic for layers: SCALP
   a. S: Skin, containing hair follicles and sebaceous glands
   b. C: (Subcutaneous) connective tissue
   c. A: Aponeurosis (epicranial or galeal aponeurotica) - fibrous tissue that connects frontalis and occipitalis.
   d. L: Loose areolar tissue
   e. P: Periosteum/Pericranium - adherent to underlying bone to which it provides nutrition
2. Blood supply: supraorbital artery, supratrochlear artery, superficial temporal artery, occipital artery

3. Scalp innervated by:
    a. Supratrocheal nerve, supratrocheal nerve: from the ophthalmic (V1) division of CN V; provides sensation to scalp to around level of vertex
    b. Greater occipital nerve: C2; provides sensation posteriorly up to vertex
    c. Lesser occipital nerve: C2; provides sensation behind ear
    d. Zygomaticotemporal nerve: from V2 of CN V; provides sensation to temple
    e. Auriculotempral nerve: from V3 of CN V; provides sensation to hair-bearing temple

Hair

1. 100,000-150,000 hair follicles in scalp
2. Stages of hair growth:
    a. Anagen: growth phase; 90% follicles in this phase
    b. Catagen: involutional/transition phase; hair follicle detaches from underlying blood supply
    c. Telogen: resting phase; without nourishment from blood supply, hair eventually falls out; 5-10% follicles in this phase
    d. Exogen: shedding phase
3. Hair follicle consists of:
    a. Papilla: base of hair follicle, made of connective tissue and capillaries
    b. Hair matrix
    c. Root sheath
    d. Bulge: on outer root sheath, insertion point for arrector pili muscles; houses stem cells that supply follicle with new cells; may have a role in epidermal wound healing by providing cells for re-epithelialization

Changes with Aging

1. Epidermal thickening
2. Decrease in epidermal cell variety (reduction in melanocytes, Langerhan cells)
3. Dermal atrophy
4. Thinning of papillary dermis: approximately 1% per year in adult life
5. Decreased collagen production with shorter, more coarse bundles
6. Reduction in production of elastin and increased fragmentation of elastin chains resulting in disordered collection of fibers
7. Increase in ground substance of dermis, hyperplastic fibroblasts, degranulated mast cells (inflammatory state)
8. Increased skin laxity and wrinkling (rhytidosis)
9. Photo-damage
10. Soft tissue ptosis
11. Bone resorption of facial skeleton: particularly involving maxilla (medial and pyri-form region), orbital rim (superomedial, inferolateral), and mandible (pre-jowl)

Facial Nerve

1. Development of the Extratemporal Facial Nerve
    a. Gestational Week 8: extratemporal branches of facial nerve are formed
    b. Gestational Week 12: peripheral branches of facial nerve are developed and interconnected
    c. Term: facial nerve branches are all present; nerve is more superficial in nature than adult facial nerve as mastoid process is not fully developed
    d. Age 1-3: mastoid process develops which displaces extratemporal facial nerve more medially and inferiorly
    e. Development of external ear correlates with that of facial nerve
        i. Because facial nerve is nerve of second branchial arch, any malformations in second arch derivatives may alter facial nerve structure or course
2. Facial nerve function: mixed nerve that contains multiple fiber types
    a. *Special visceral efferents:* fibers to muscles of facial expression, stapedius, posterior digastric, stylohyoid
        i. There is bilateral innervation to upper facial musculature (upper motor neuron tracts in brain cross/re-cross before reaching pontine facial nerve nucleus)
        ii. Tracts to lower face only cross once; therefore, lesions proximal to facial nerve nucleus spare upper face of involved side, allowing forehead movement and eyelid closure, whereas distal lesions produce complete paralysis of affected side
    b. *General visceral efferents:* parasympathetic activity via nervus intermedius to geniculate ganglion and then lacrimal glands, nasal mucosa, and submandibular, sublingual glands
    c. *Special sensory afferents:* taste from anterior 2/3 tongue via chorda tympani to solitary nucleus (chorda tympani to lingual nerve to nervus intermedius to solitary nucleus
    d. *Somatic sensory afferents:* sensation from posterior external auditory canal, concha
    e. *General visceral afferents:* signals from nasal mucosa
3. Facial nerve branches: exits via stylomastoid foramen, lateral to styloid process
    a. Branches to posterior digastric, stylohyoid
    b. Once the nerve enters parotid gland it splits at pes anserinus into an upper (temporozygomatic) and lower (cervicofacial) divisions
    c. Five branches are identifiable upon exiting parotid gland substance
        i. Temporal
        ii. Zygomatic
        iii. Buccal
        iv. Marginal Mandibular
        v. Cervical
    d. There are anastomotic networks in buccal branches

   e. Nerves can be identified superficially underneath superficial musculoaponeurotic system after exiting parotid at imaginary line from lateral canthus to angle of mandible
4. Landmarks for identification of extratemporal facial nerve:
   a. Tragal pointer: nerve identified 1 to 1.5 cm deep to and just anterior and inferior to lateral edge of external canal cartilage
   b. Tympanomastoid fissure: nerve can be identified 6 to 8 mm below inferior "drop-off" of fissure
   c. Posterior belly of digastric muscle at its insertion to the mastoid process: nerve exits stylomastoid foramen just anterior to this
   d. Retrograde dissection from distal branches

Ear

1. Topographical features (Figure 1.4)

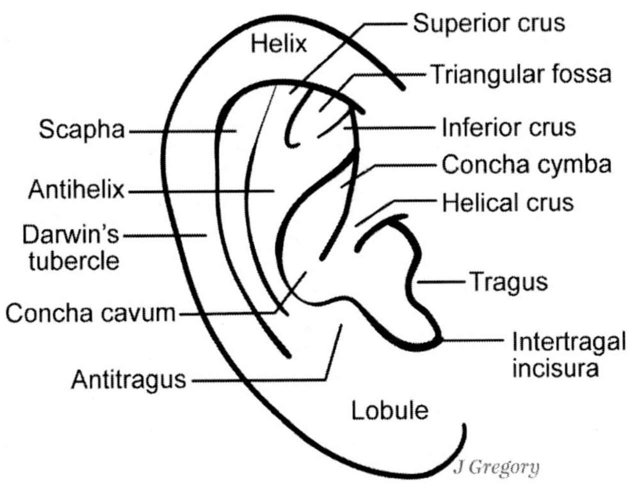

Figure 1.4. Ear anatomy. Printed with permission from ©Mount Sinai Health System.

   a. **Helix**
      i. Darwin's tubercle: thickening of the helix at junction between upper and middle thirds
   b. **Helical crus**: divides concha into *concha cymba* and *concha cavum*
   c. **Antihelix**
      i. Has two antihelical crura: superior and inferior
      ii. Two crura serve as boundaries of the *triangular fossa*
   d. **Tragus**
   e. **Antitragus**
   f. **Intertragal incisura**: divides tragus and antitragus
   g. **Scapha**

h. **Concha Cymba**: superior to helical crus
i. **Concha Cavum**: inferior to helical crus and continuous with external auditory canal (EAC) meatus
j. **Lobule**

Auricle

1. Made of fibroelastic cartilage
2. Has more memory in curved portions of auricle
3. Skin is closely adherent anteriorly and more loosely adherent posteriorly
4. Auricle is attached to head by:
    a. Skin
    b. Cartilaginous extensions into EAC
    c. Ligaments
    d. Auricular muscles
5. Circulation, contribution of perichondrium
    a. External carotid artery, posterior auricular artery, superficial temporal artery
6. External ear innervation (relevant for blocks)
    a. Preauricular: V3
    b. Concha: VII, X
    c. Posterior helix/lobule: great auricular nerve (C3) and lesser occipital nerve (C2,3)
    d. Post auricular surface: great auricular nerve (C3) and lesser occipital nerve (C2,3), VII, X
7. Embryology
    a. External ear is from both first and second branchial arches
    b. Gestational week 6: condensation of mesoderm of first and second arches gives rise to six hillocks **(hillocks of His)**
        i. First Arch:
            - First hillock: tragus
            - Second hillock: helical crus
            - Third hillock: helix
        ii. Second Arch:
            - Fourth hillock: antihelix
            - Fifth hillock: antitragus
            - Sixth hillock: lobule and lower helix
    c. Gestational week 7: cartilage formed
    d. Gestational week 12: hillocks fuse to form auricle
    e. Gestational week 20: auricle reaches adult shape
    f. Age 5: auricle is 80% adult size
    g. Age 9: auricle reaches adult size
    h. Concha is formed by first cleft/groove (ectoderm)
        i. Concha cymba: upper part
        ii. Concha cavum: middle part

iii. Intertrag incisura: lower part

Eyelid

1. Anatomy
    a. Blood supply: angular branch of facial artery
    b. Innervation:
        i. CNIII: levator palpebrae superioris
        ii. CNVII: orbicularis oculi, lacrimal gland (parasympathetic)
        iii. Sympathetic innervation: Mueller muscle
    c. Upper eyelid (superficial to deep) (Figure 1.5)

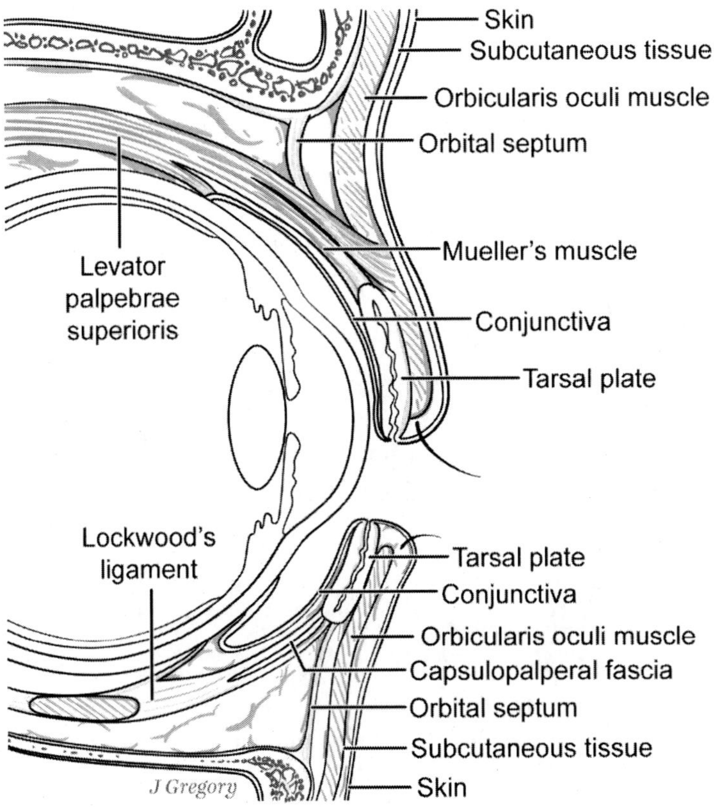

Figure 1.5. Eyelid anatomy. Printed with permission from ©Mount Sinai Health System.

i. **Skin**
ii. **Subcutaneous tissue**
iii. **Orbicularis oculi**: forms transition between brow and eyelid, surrounds eye
    - Orbital portion: surrounds bony orbit
    - Levator portion: overlies eyelid
iv. **Levator palpebrae superioris**: retracts upper eyelid

- Levator supported by *Whitnall's ligament* at orbital aperture
- Levator splits into levator aponeurosis anteriorly and Mueller's muscle posteriorly
- Laterally and medially it inserts into canthal tendons
- Fuses with orbital septum and skin dermis at upper eyelid crease
- Attaches to orbicularis and anterior tarsal plate more inferiorly in upper eyelid
- **Mueller's muscle** (superior tarsal muscle): closely adherent to conjunctiva and inserts onto tarsal plate; sympathetically activated and raises eyelid 1-2mm

v. **Orbital septum** (continuous with orbital periosteum, originates at *arcus marginalis*)
- Divides eyelid into anterior lamella (skin, orbicularis oculi) and posterior lamella (conjunctiva, tarsal plate)
- **Tarsal plate** is in same plane, closer to eyelid margin; provides rigidity and support to upper eyelid
  - 8-10mm tall
  - Meibomian glands: sebaceous glands within the tarsal plate, secrete lipid component of tear film, meibum
- Does not extend over upper surface of tarsal plate.

vi. Conjunctiva
- **Wolfring glands**: small tubular accessory lacrimal glands found in lacrimal caruncle of eyelid
- *Plica semilunaris*: fold of conjunctiva in medial aspect of eye; vestigial remnant of nictitating membrane or third eyelid

vii. Distance from lash line to upper eyelid crease is ~8-10 mm

viii. Lid crease should be at the level of the nasion

d. Lower eyelid (superficial to deep):

i. **Skin**

ii. **Subcutaneous tissue**

iii. **Orbicularis oculi**

iv. Lower lid retractors
- **Capsulopalpebral fascia** (analog of levator palpebrae)
- Extension of inferior rectus muscle that depresses lower eyelid with downward gaze
- Adherent to underlying conjunctiva

v. **Orbital Septum**
- Tarsal plate: 4-5mm
- Meibomian glands

vi. **Conjunctiva**
- Wolfring glands

e. **Lockwood's ligament (Suspensory ligament of Lockwood):**

i. Continuous band of fibrous tissue slung beneath eyeball from side to side

ii. Ends of suspensory ligament blend with cheek ligaments and with medial and lateral horns of aponeurosis of levator palpebrae superioris

2. Preaponeuotic fat:
   a. Deep to septum, superficial to levator palpebrae
      i. Upper lid fat pads: medial, central
         - Lacrimal gland is on lateral aspect of upper orbit (divided from fat pads by lateral horn of levator palpebrae aponeurosis)
      ii. Lower lid fat pads: medial, central, lateral
         - Inferior oblique separates medial and central compartments
      iii. Medial compartment fat is whiter and denser
   b. Retro-orbicularis oculi fat (ROOF): fat pad deep to orbicularis oculi above orbit
   c. Sub-orbicularis oculi fat (SOOF): deep part of malar fat pad under eye, anterior to zygomaticus major and levator labii superioris muscles
3. Effects of aging:
   a. Festoons: redundant folds of lax skin or orbicularis muscle that hang from canthus to canthus
   b. Malar bags: Areas of soft tissue fullness and edema on lateral edge of infraorbital ridge and zygomatic prominence; difficult to improve with lower blepharoplasty
4. Asian eyelid anatomy variations (Figure 1.6)
   a. Usually, upper eyelid crease made at junction of levator palpebrae superioris aponeurosis and orbital septum; the muscle inserts on tarsus inferiorly and interdigitate with skin and orbicularis complex
      i. Superior to this point on orbital septum, preaponeurotic fat pads form a barrier between levator and the skin/orbicularis.

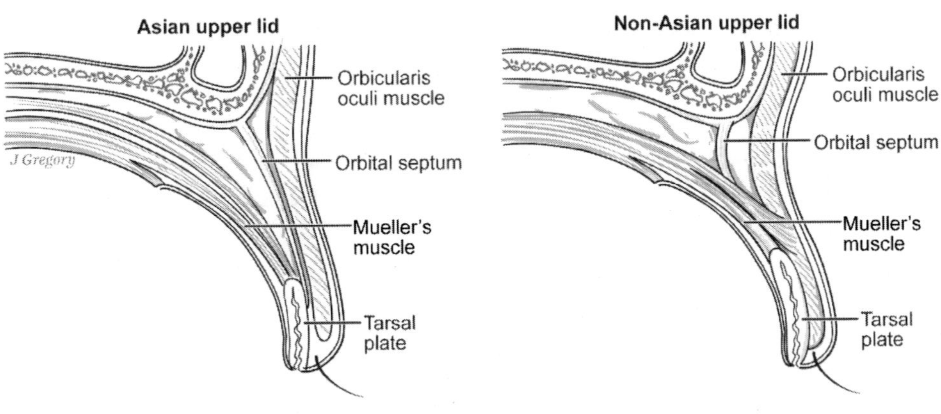

Figure 1.6. Asian eyelid anatomy variations. Printed with permission from ©Mount Sinai Health System.

   b. In some eyelids, upper crease is not as apparent, and can look fuller Possible anatomic causes:
      i. Tarsal plate is shorter
      ii. Orbital septum insertion is diffuse, not well defined and can be more inferior

iii. Preaponeurotic fat pad subsequently extends farther inferiorly
iv. Preseptal fat pat can also extend more inferiorly
v. More inferior fat pad extension limits fusion of levator aponeurosis with skin/orbicularis

c. Some Asian eyelids also have more prominent epicanthal folds formed by horizontal redundancy of skin and orbicularis in medial canthal region

Nose (Figure 1.7)

1. Embryology
   a. Gestational week 3-4: nasal placode (derived from ectoderm) appears
   b. Gestational week 5: Placodes become depressed below surface and appear as invaginated pits; nasal pit extends backward into oral cavity but is separated from it by bucconasal membrane

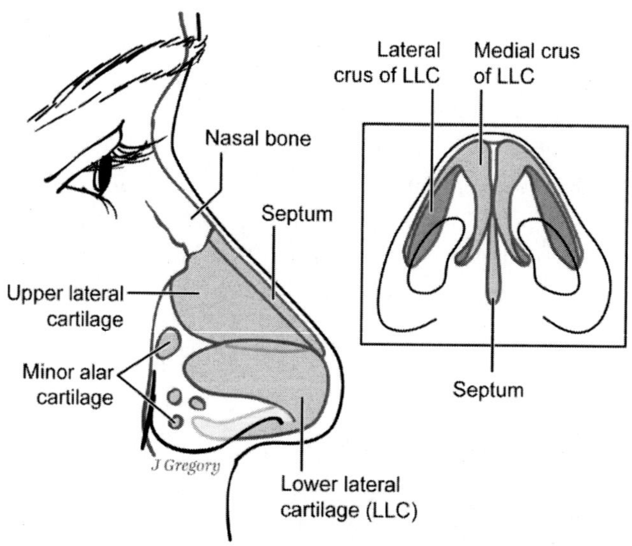

Figure 1.7. Nasal anatomy. Printed with permission from ©Mount Sinai Health System.

   c. Gestational week 7-8: bucconasal membrane ruptures to form posterior nares (failure here can lead to choanal atresia)
      i. Nasal pit extends up to forebrain, and the epithelium in this region thickens to become specialized olfactory sensory cells.
      ii. Anteriorly: Maxillary process fuses with lateral and medial nasal process to form anterior nares. Fusion here creates the *nasolacrimal groove* in which will reside the nasolacrimal duct.
      iii. Frontonasal process (mesoderm): gives rise to nasal septum and premaxilla.
      iv. Gestational week 9: the posterior septum overlies the oral cavity until maxillary palatal shelves grow medially and fuse with the septum to

form the secondary palate. Hard palate completes formation by 9th week.

v. Gestational week 8-24: nostrils are covered with an epithelial plug that eventually resorbs.

2. Anatomy
   a. Lower lateral cartilage
      i. Medial crus
      ii. Intermediate/middle crus
      iii. Lateral crus
   b. Upper lateral cartilage
   c. Minor alar cartilages: 3-4 sesamoid cartilages that sit in dorsal ala between/behind upper lateral and lower lateral cartilages
   d. Nasal bones
   e. Septum
3. Skin thickness contribution to anatomic feature
   a. Critical factor in determining final results
   b. Moderate skin thickness: generally has best outcomes
   c. Thick sebaceous skin: more postoperative edema, also may have poorer results even when underlying structures are appropriately contoured
   d. Thin skin: can reveal minor irregularities
   e. Nasal skin is thicker at nasion, thinner over the rhinion
   f. From rhinion to supratip, skin becomes thick again
4. Components of nasal thirds
   a. Upper third: nasal bone, skin
   b. Middle third: upper lateral cartilages, septum, skin
   c. Lower third: lower lateral cartilages, septum, skin
5. Nasal tip support
   a. Major
      i. Size, shape, and resilience of medial and lower lateral crura
      ii. Medial crural footplate attachment to caudal border of quandrangular/cartilaginous septum
      iii. Scroll region: attachment of caudal border of upper lateral cartilage to cephalic border of alar cartilage
   b. Minor
      i. Interdomal ligaments
      ii. Dorsal cartilaginous septum
      iii. Membranous septum
      iv. Sesamoid complex extending support of lateral crura to piriform aperture
      v. Attachment of alar cartilages to overlying skin and musculature
      vi. Nasal spine
   c. Tripod model of support: 3 legs supporting nasal tip
      i. Each lower lateral crura is one leg
      ii. Conjoined lower medial crura act as central leg
6. Nasal valve:
   a. Borders:

i. Nasal septum
ii. Caudal margin of upper lateral cartilages
iii. Inferior turbinate

b. Ideal angle is 15°

Palate/Lips

1. Embryology (Figure 1.8)
   a. Lip
      i. Gestational week 4: paired maxillary prominences begin to appear (first arch) and frontonasal prominence from mesenchyme ventral to forebrain
      ii. Gestational week 5: nasal placodes invaginate forming medial and lateral nasal prominences
      iii. Gestational weeks 6-7: medial growth of maxillary prominences meets paired medial nasal prominences and frontonasal prominence to form upper lip
   b. Palate
      i. Gestational weeks 5-12:
         - Maxillary prominences fuse and push medial nasal prominences more medially by 12 weeks
         - Intermaxillary segment (with incisor teeth buds) formed by fusion of paired medial nasal prominences
      ii. Gestational weeks 5-6: soft palate muscles migrate towards midline from both sides of developing oropharynx

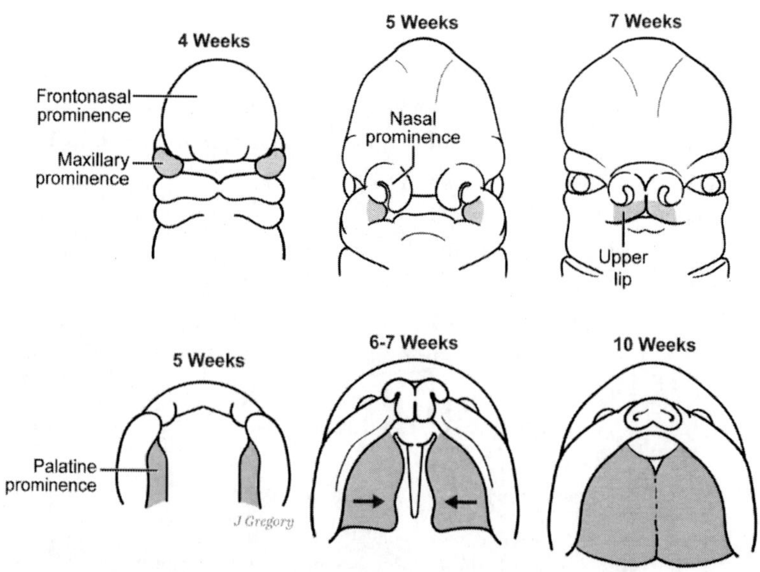

Figure 1.8. Embryology. Printed with permission from ©Mount Sinai Health System.

iii. Gestational weeks 6-7: palatal shelves grow medially from maxillary prominences

iv. Gestational weeks 9-10: soft palate muscles move into a horizontal orientation, paralleling palatal shelves

v. Gestational weeks 8-12:
- Fusion of palatal shelves form secondary palate; secondary palatal fusion occurs from anterior at incisive foramen to posterior at uvula
- Soft palate tissue and muscles fuse by 12th gestational week

2. Anatomy

a. Lip

i. Muscles:
- Orbicularis oris: creates sphincter around mouth
- Lip elevators: zygomaticus major, zygomaticus minor, levator labii superioris, levator labii superioris alaeque nasi, levator anguli oris
- Lip depressors: Depressor anguli oris, depressor labii inferioris, mentalis

ii. Blood supply: superior labial artery (off facial artery)
- Deep to orbicularis oris muscle

iii. Primary innervation: buccal and marginal mandibular branches of CNVII

iv. Vermillion border (white roll): mucoepithelial junction between cutaneous lip and mucosal lip (red-white junction)

v. Dry lip: portion of mucosal lip exposed to air

vi. Wet lip: portion of the mucosal lip that is exposed to saliva, separated from dry lip by wet-dry junction

vii. Philtrum: extends from nasal septum to tubercle of lip
- Median dimple: midline dimple above central portion of cupid's bow formed by decussation of muscles to contralateral philtral column and attachment of orbicularis oris to dermis
- Ridges: paramedian columns formed at embryonic fusion plane between maxillary and frontonasal prominences; elevation of vermillion at junction with philtrum forms peak of **cupid's bow**

b. Palate

i. **Primary palate**: anterior to incisive foramen

ii. **Secondary palate**: posterior to incisive foramen

iii. **Hard palate**: posterior to incisive foramen but anterior to soft palate musculature at levator veli palatini muscle
- Premaxilla (anteriorly) and vertical segments of the palatine bone (posteriorly) which contain greater palatine foramina and lesser palatine foramina
  - Greater palatine foramen: greater palatine vessels and greater palatine nerve

- Lesser palatine foramen: lesser palatine nerves
- Blood supply: greater palatine artery

iv. **Soft palate**: posterior to hard palate

- Muscles:
  - **Levator veli palatini**
  - **Tensor veli palatini**
  - **Musculus uvula**
  - Palatal arches: border palatine tonsil
    - Palatoglossus: more anterior in the mouth
    - Palatopharyngeus: more posterior towards the pharyngeal wall
  - All innervated by CN X except tensor veli palatini (innervated by CN V3)
- Blood supply: descending palatine branch of facial artery, palatine branch of ascending pharyngeal artery, and lesser palatine artery

Summary Points

1. Understanding the embryology and development of facial anatomy is critical for evaluation and treatment of head and neck concerns or pathology.
2. Detailed knowledge about neurovascular structures can decrease risk of bleeding complication and facilitate appropriate anesthesia for procedures and surgeries.
3. Understanding key landmarks and structures enables surgeons to communicate effectively about patient concerns and surgical techniques.

References

[1] Chen EY, Sie KCY: Cummings otolaryngology--head & neck surgery. In: *Otolaryngology--head & neck surgery.* 6th ed. edn. Edited by Flint PW, Haughey BH, Lund V, Niparko JK, Robbins KT, Thomas JR, Lesperance MM. Philadelphia, PA: Elsevier/Saunders; 2015.

[2] Moore KL: *The developing human : clinically oriented embryology,* Eleventh edition. edn. Edinburgh ; New York: Elsevier; 2020.

[3] Maves MD: Bailey's head and neck surgery : otolaryngology. In., *Fifth edition. edn.* Edited by Johnson JT, Rosen CA. Philadelphia: Wolters Kluwer Health /Lippincott Williams & Wilkins; 2014.

[4] Netter FH: *Atlas of human anatomy*, Sixth edition. edn. Philadelphia, PA: Saunders/Elsevier; 2014.

Chapter 2

Facial Proportions and Subunits

Sarah Kidwai, MD
and Wayne F. Larrabee Jr., MD, MSH, FACS

Introduction

An intimate understanding of facial anatomy, its subunits and proportions, is crucial in facial plastic surgery. In this chapter, we review the basic principles of facial proportions and subunits that guide interventions in facial plastic surgery.

Facial Analysis

In order to establish a surgical or non-surgical plan, a thorough examination of facial proportions and skin quality is necessary. The surgeon's understanding of a patient's goals and desires is important for optimal results.

1. Facial width (Figure 2.1) – The face can be divided into five equal fifths in the vertical direction. The lateral-most fifths are measured by the distance between the lateral-most point of the helix to the lateral canthus. The next two fifths is measured by the distance between the lateral and medial canthi. The final fifth is the distance between the two medial canthi (which is equivalent to the distance between the right and left alar bases). [1]
2. Facial length (Figure 2.2) – The face can be divided into three equal thirds in the horizontal direction. From superior to inferior, this is divided into:
    a. Upper third: forehead (including frontal bone, supraorbital rims, and glabella); trichion to glabella [1]
    b. Middle third: zygomas, maxilla, nasal bones, and orbits, vertical rami of mandible; glabella to subnasale [1]
    c. Lower third: mandible, anterior to vertical rami; subnasale to the menton [1]
3. Frankfort line – a line drawn from the superior portion of the cartilaginous external auditory canal through the infraorbital rim. In photography of the lateral view, this line should be parallel to the floor. [2]
4. Facial landmarks (Figure 2.3) [3]
    a. Trichion – where hairline and forehead meet at midline (midsagittal plane)
    b. Glabella – most prominent portion of forehead (midsagittal plane), above root of nose

In: Essential Facial Plastic and Reconstructive Surgery. Volume 1 ISBN: 979-8-89113-306-8
Editors: Yan Ho Lee and Ira Papel © 2024 Nova Science Publishers, Inc.

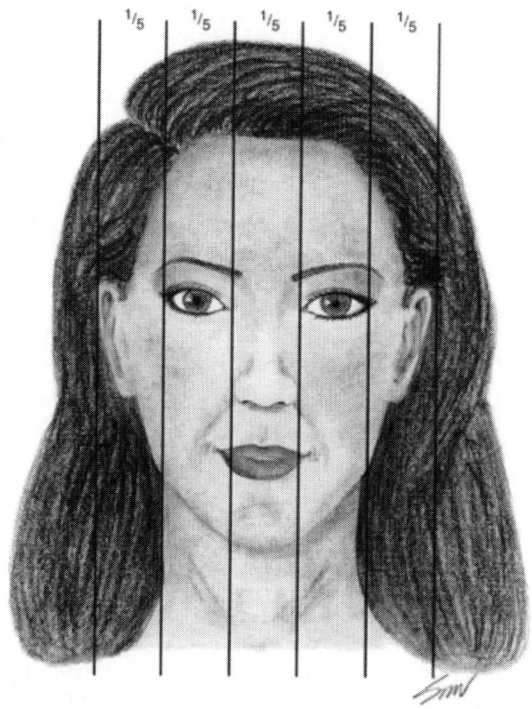

Figure 2.1. Facial width divided into equal fifths.

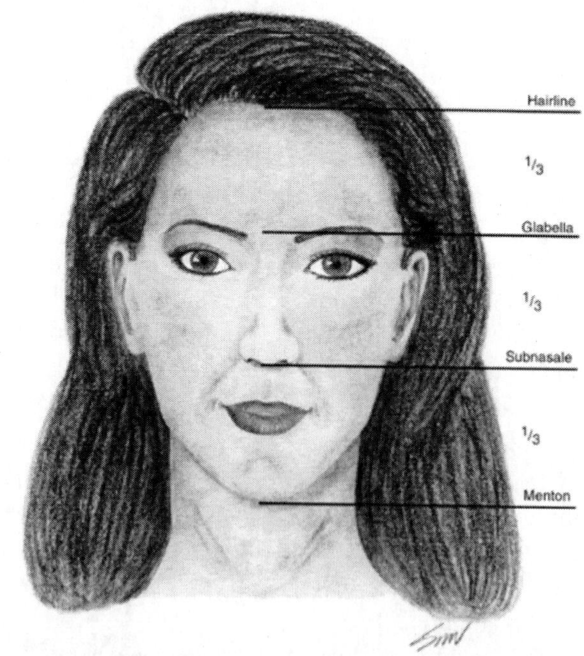

Figure 2.2. Facial length divided into equal thirds.

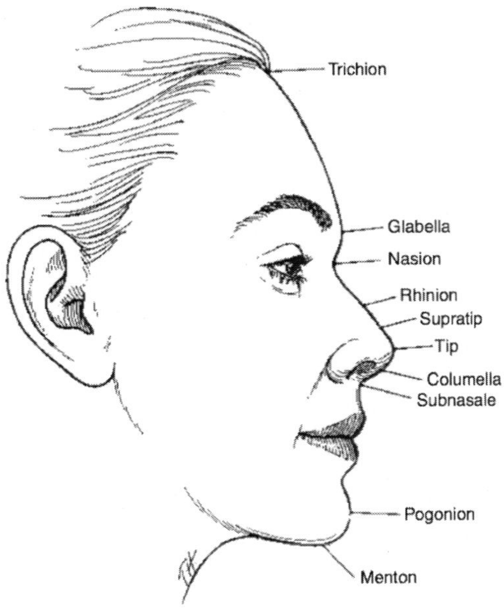

Figure 2.3. Facial landmarks.

c. Nasion – deepest point in nasofrontal angle, corresponds to nasofrontal suture line
d. Radix – root of nose, point at which nose originates from glabella
e. Rhinion – junction of bony and cartilaginous nasal dorsum where skin is the thinnest
f. Supratip – area of depression above the tip
g. Pronasale - nasal tip; anterior-most point of nose
h. Tip defining point – most anterior projection of nasal tip; corresponds to apex of lobular arch of lower lateral cartilage
i. Nasal base – inferior portion of nose composed of the lateral crural of the lower lateral cartilages and their medial crura
j. Subnasale – point at which columella meets upper cutaneous lip
k. Stomion – contact point of the upper and lower lips in midsagittal plane when mouth is closed
l. Pogonion – anterior-most point on chin
m. Menton – soft tissue point at inferior-most point of chin at midline
n. Gnathion – lowest point at midpoint of mandible
o. Cervical point – area between submental area and neck
p. Gonion – the point of the angle of mandible

5. Facial Angles (Figure 2.4)
   a. Nasofacial angle—angle between the plane of the face (glabella to pogonion) and the nasal dorsum; normally 30-60° (average 36°) [4]
   b. Nasolabial angle—angle between a line from the upper lip mucocutaneous border to the subnasale and a line from the subnasale to the most anterior point on the columella; ideal range is 90° to 95° (up to 105°) in men, and 95° to 110° (can be 90° to 120°) in women [4]

c. Nasofrontal angle—angle between the nasal dorsum and a tangent passing through the nasion and the glabella; ideal range is 115° to 135° [4]
d. Nasomental angle—angle between the nasal dorsum and the nasomental line (nasal tip to pogonion); ideal range 120° to 132° [4]
e. Cervicomental angle – angle between a line from glabella to pogonion and a line from menton to cervical point; ideal range 80° to 95° [4]

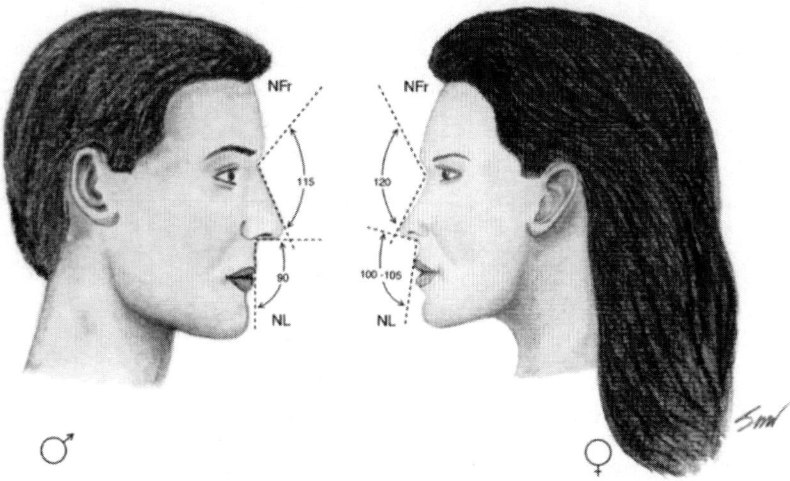

Figure 2.4. Facial angles. Nasofrontal angle and nasolabial angles shown.

Skin

1. Fitzpatrick Scale [5]
    a. Class I: very white, always burns, never tans
    b. Class II: white, usually burns, tans minimally
    c. Class III: white to olive, sometimes burns, tans
    d. Class IV: brown, rarely burns, always tans
    e. Class V: dark brown, very rarely burns, tans profusely
    f. Class VI: black, never burns, tans profusely
2. Glogau classification of photoaging [6]
    a. Class I: mild – no wrinkles
    b. Class II: moderate – wrinkles in motion
    c. Class III: advanced – wrinkles at rest
    d. Class IV: severe – only wrinkles

Upper Third of Face

1. Layers of scalp and forehead
    a. Skin
    b. Subcutaneous tissue

   c. Galea aponeurotica
   d. Loose areolar tissue
   e. Pericranium
2. Hairline
   a. Female – 5- 6 cm above the eyebrows
   b. Male - >6 cm above the eyebrow
   c. Norwood classification of male pattern baldness [7]
      i. Type I – minimal or no recession of hair line
      ii. Type II – areas of recession at frontotemporal hair line
      iii. Type III – deep symmetrical recession at temples
      iv. Type IV – hair loss from vertex, limited recession of frontotemporal hair line
      v. Type V – vertex hair loss separated from frontotemporal region by a band of hair
      vi. Type VI – Frontotemporal and vertex regions are joined together
      vii. Type VII – A narrow band of hair in horseshoe shape remains
3. Muscles
   a. Brow elevators
      i. Frontalis – horizontal rhytids of forehead
   b. Brow depressors
      i. Corrugators – vertical "11" lines in glabella
      ii. Procerus – horizontal lines in glabella
      iii. Orbicularis oculi – Periocular lines or "crow's feet"
4. Ideal brow position
   a. Female (Figure 2.5)
      i. Begins medially at a vertical line drawn perpendicular through alar base
      ii. Terminates laterally at an oblique line drawn through the lateral canthus of the eye and the alar base

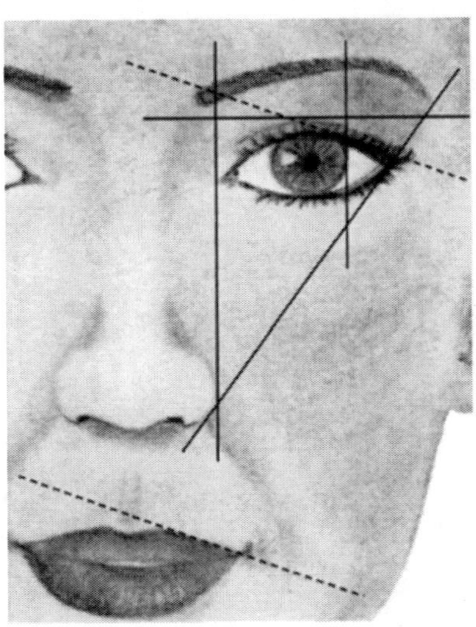

Figure 2.5. Ideal female brow position.

iii. Medial and lateral ends of the brow are approximately at the same level
iv. Medial end of club shaped and tapers out laterally
v. Apex of brow at a vertical line through lateral canthus

b. Male
i. Similar to above
ii. Apex of brow at a vertical line through lateral limbus
iii. Minimal arching and positioned at or just above the supraorbital rim

5. Periorbital region
   a. Intercanthal distance equal to width of one eye
   b. Intercanthal axis slightly upward from medial to lateral producing upward lateral canthal tilt
   c. Anterior lamella – skin and orbicularis oculi
   d. Middle lamella – orbital septum
   e. Posterior lamella – lower lid retractors and conjunctiva
   f. Upper lid covers iris by 1-2 mm
   g. Upper lid crease parallels the lash line
   h. Minimal to no scleral show between lower lid and iris

Middle Third of Face

1. Nasal analysis
   a. Subunits (Figure 2.6)
      i. Dorsum
      ii. Paired sidewalls
      iii. Tip
      iv. Paired ala
      v. Paired soft tissue triangle
      vi. Columella

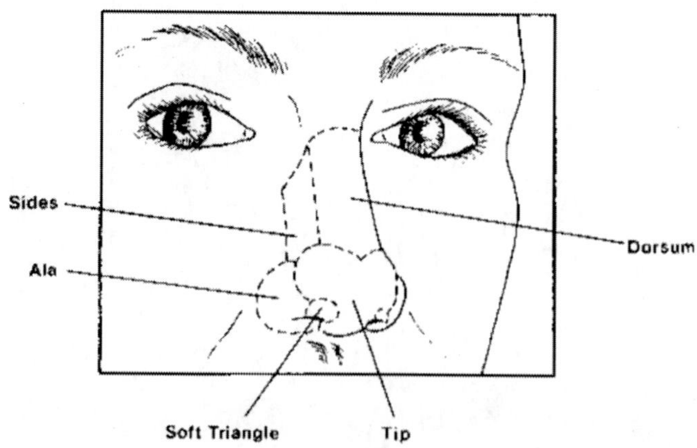

Figure 2.6. Nasal subunits.

b. Structural Support of the Nose
    i. Upper third – nasal bones
    ii. Middle third – upper lateral cartilages, cartilaginous dorsum and septum
    iii. Lower third – lower lateral cartilage, septum
c. Nasal projection
    i. Tip to lip ratio - distance from vermillion border to subnasale is equal to distance from subnasale to tip [8]
    ii. 50-60% of nasal projection should be anterior to upper lip [8]
d. Nasal length
    i. Crumley's method – 3:4:5 triangle where the hypotenuse is nasal length [9]
    ii. Goode's method – projection defined by a line drawn perpendicularly from a line drawn from nasion to alar groove. Ratio of nasal projection to nasal length is 0.50-0.60 [10]
e. Nasal base – should be an equilateral triangle; columella to lobule ratio 2:1
f. Columellar show – ideally 2-4 mm of columellar show

2. Malar region
    a. Hinderer analysis – line from lateral commissure of lip to lateral canthus and line from inferior aspect of ala to tragus. [11]
    b. Area posterior and superior to the junction of the two lines should be most prominent part of malar eminence

Lower Third of Face

1. Dentition
    a. Angle Class I occlusion - The mesiobuccal cusp of the first maxillary molar fits in the mesiobuccal groove of the first mandibular molar.
    b. Angle Class II malocclusion—Mesiobuccal cusp of the first maxillary molar is anterior to the first mandibular molar.
    c. Angle Class III malocclusion—Mesiobuccal cusp of the first maxillary molar is posterior to the first mandibular molar. [12]
2. Chin
    a. Microgenia "small chin" - in a patient with class 1 occlusion, if a vertical line drawn from vermillion border of lower lip to chin is anterior to pogonion
    b. Micrognathia "hypoplastic mandible" – can be associated with chromosomal abnormalities and syndromes
    c. Retrognathia – the position of mandible is recessed compared to the maxilla
3. Neck
    a. Dedo classification of the neck [13]
        i. Class I – minimal laxity
        ii. Class II – skin laxity
        iii. Class III – submental jowling and excess fat
        iv. Class IV – anterior platysmal banding

v. Class V – congenital or acquired micrognathia
vi. Class VI – low-lying hyoid bone

Ears

1. Average width of ear is 55% of length
2. Average height is 6-6.5cm
3. Long axis is parallel to dorsum of nose
4. Long axis is tilted 15-20 degrees from vertical
5. Conchomastoid angle: angle which conchal bowl makes with mastoid cortex - 90°
6. Auriculocephalic angle: angle between plane of mastoid and line extending from the helical root to the most lateral border of the helix - 20-35° [4]
7. Scaphoconchal angle: angle defining antihelix - 90°
8. Distance from helical rim to mastoid skin [1]
    a. 10 mm to 12 mm at superior pole
    b. 16 mm to 18 mm at middle third
    c. 20 mm to 22 mm at level of cauda helix

Summary Points

1. Dividing the face into upper, middle, and lower thirds is helpful for comprehensive facial analysis
2. Overall facial analysis should include Fitzpatrick classification, Glogau classification
3. The upper third includes analysis of the hairline, eyebrows, periorbital region
4. The middle third includes analysis of the nose and malar region
5. The lower third includes analysis of the lip, chin, and neck
6. There are male and female differences in facial anatomy that should be considered in surgical planning

References

[1] Hadlock T, Lindsay R, Cheney M. "Chapter 34: Facial Plastic Surgery." *Essential Otolaryngology*, edited by Lee KJ. New York, N; The McGraw-Hill; 2012.

[2] Larrabee Jr, WF. "Preoperative Facial Analysis." *Aesthetic Facial Surgery*, edited by Krause CJ, Mangat DS, Patorek N. Lippincott Williams & Wilkins; 1991.

[3] Koch JR, Hanasono MM. "Chapter 13: Aesthetic Facial Analysis." *Facial Plastic and Reconstructive Surgery*, edited by Papel ID, Nachlas NE. St. Louis, MO: Thieme Medical Publisher; 2002.

[4] Meneghini F. "Chapter 5: Basic Facial Analysis." *Clinical Facial Analysis*, edited by Schroder G. Springer; 2005.

[5] Fitzpatrick TB. "The validity and practicality of sun-reactive skin types I through VI." *Arch Dermatol*. 1988 Jun;124(6):869-71.

[6] Glogau RG. "Aesthetic and anatomic analysis of the aging skin." *Semin Cuban Med Surg*. 1996 Sep;15(3):134-8.

[7] Norwood OT. "Male pattern baldness: Classification and incidence." *South Med J.* 1975;68:1359-65.

[8] Sheen JH, Sheen AP. *Aesthetic Rhinoplasty*. St. Louis, MO: Mosby Year Book; 1987.

[9] Crumley RL, Lanser M. "Quantitative analysis of nasal tip projection." *Laryngoscope*. 1998;98:202-208.

[10] Goode RL. "A method of tip projection measurement." *Proportions of the esthetic face,* edited by Powell HB. Thieme-Stratton;1984.

[11] Hinderer UT. "Malar implants for improvement of the facial appearance." *Last Reconstr Surg*. 1975;56:157-65.

[12] Angle EH. "Classification of malocclusion." *Dental Cosmos.* 1899;41:248-264.

[13] Dedo DD. "How I do it: Practical suggestions on facial plastic surgery. A preoperative classification of the neck for cervicofacial rhytidectomy." *Laryngoscope*. 1980;90:1894-6.

Chapter 3

Wound Healing and Wound Care

Rohini Bahethi, MD
Philip J. Miller, MD
and Boris Paskhover, MD

Introduction

1. Understanding the phases of wound healing helps to elucidate the various challenges against proper wound healing
2. Local and systemic factors play a role in wound healing and scar maturation; interventions on any of these factors can help to improve outcomes
3. Scar appearance (including hypertrophic scar and keloid) is a major concern for many patients, and it is important to offer strategies to minimize scar appearance

Phases of Wound Healing (4 Phases)

1. Hemostasis
    a. Primary Hemostasis
        i. Begins immediately after tissue injury
        ii. Two components:
            - Vascular
                - Reflex vasoconstriction of capillaries which prevents further blood effluent
                - Severed arteries retract into surrounding tissue
                - Hematoma formation around site of injury provides extravascular pressure to further collapse surrounding capillary beds, slowing bleeding and diverting blood flow from area of injury
            - Platelet
                - Exposure of subendothelial collagen and Von Willebrand factor allows platelets to adhere to site of injury and aggregate to form a soft platelet plug
                - This plug is easily disrupted by outside forces and requires stabilization via secondary hemostasis
    b. Secondary Hemostasis

In: Essential Facial Plastic and Reconstructive Surgery. Volume 1 ISBN: 979-8-89113-306-8
Editors: Yan Ho Lee and Ira Papel © 2024 Nova Science Publishers, Inc.

i. Waterfall Cascade Model of Clotting [1] (Figure 3.1)
   - Most widely accepted model for cascade of events leading to a stable fibrin clot
   - Involves two pathways that merge into one common pathway to generate a stable fibrin clot

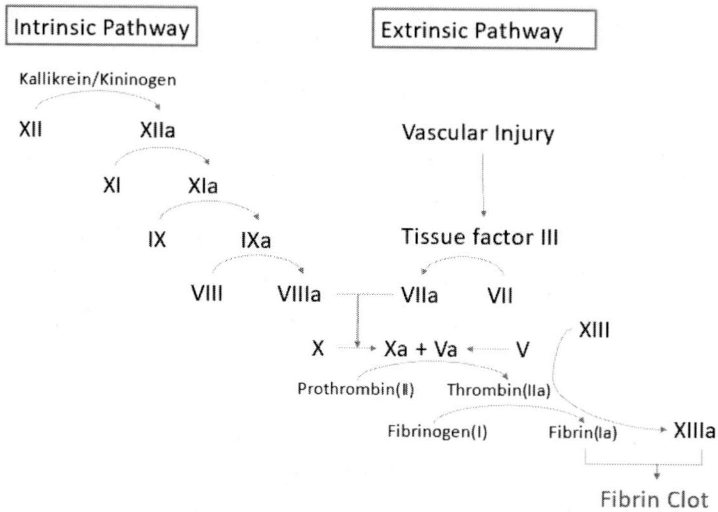

Figure 3.1. The Waterfall Cascade Model of coagulation developed by MacFarlane, Davie and Ratnoff.

ii. Extrinsic Pathway
   - Tissue factor needed to activate extrinsic pathway; named because tissue factor is contained in extraluminal space and must be exposed via injury
   - TF activates factor VII to VIIa; together, activate factor X to Xa

iii. Intrinsic Pathway
   - All components exist in circulation but require activated platelets to start this process
   - A complex (containing high molecular weight kininogen, factor XII, kallikrein) creates activated factor XIIa (FXIIa)
   - Complex of FXIIa and high molecular weight kininogen forms factor XIa, which in turn forms factor IXa
   - A complex (containing factor IXa, factor Xa, thrombin and calcium) cleaves factor VIII to factor VIIIa which forms a feedback loop to create more activated factor Xa

iv. Common Pathway
   - Factor Xa is formed via intrinsic or extrinsic pathways as listed above. FXa, FVa and calcium assemble to form the prothrombinase complex which creates thrombin from prothrombin

- Thrombin cleaves soluble fibrinogen into insoluble fibrin which is cross-linked by factor XIIIa

2. Inflammation
   a. Innate response
      i. Mast cells are activated and immediately degranulate
         - Release of pro-inflammatory mediators including histamine, leukotrienes and cytokines that trigger vasodilation after initial vasoconstrictive phase (Table 3.1)
         - Increased vascular permeability allows ease of access of intravascular inflammatory components and cells to wound site
      ii. Complement cascade and activated platelets release chemoattractive factors

Table 3.1. Key cytokines involved in wound healing

Cytokine	Role
Transforming Growth Factor Beta-1(TGF-β-1)	Neutrophil and monocyte chemotaxis to wound site Fibroblast and epithelial cell proliferation Activates proteolytic activity
Tumor Necrosis Factor Alpha (TNF-α)	Promotes epithelial and fibroblast proliferation Activates proteolytic activity
Interleukin-1 (IL-1)	Activates proteolytic activity Attracts neutrophils
Interleukin-6 (IL-6)	Epithelial cell recruitment Granulation tissue formation
Epidermal growth factor (EGF)	Fibroblast and epithelial cell recruitment
Keratinocyte Growth Factor (KGF)	Promotes epithelial cell proliferation
Vascular endothelial growth factor (VEGF)	Promotes neovascularization, increases endothelial proliferation and vascular permeability
Fibroblast Growth Factor-2 (FGF)	Neovascularization and fibroblast proliferation Granulation tissue formation Production of matrix metalloproteinaseis Epithelium and collagen formation
Platelet Derived Growth Factor (PDGF)	Fibroblast and smooth muscle proliferation and migration Protein formation Angiogenesis Neutrophil and monocyte chemotaxis

b. Neutrophilic Stage
    i. First 24-36 hours after initial injury
    ii. Neutrophils perform initial phagocytosis to eliminate microbes and foreign bodies as well as debride nonviable tissue
        - Interestingly, neutrophils may be detrimental to wound repair in non-contaminated settings
        - Neutrophils produce reactive oxygen species, elastase and other substances that are toxic to microbes but also may affect healthy surrounding cells and extracellular matrix
        - Neutrophils are eliminated via apoptosis

c. Monocytic Stage
    i. 48-72 hours after initial injury
    ii. Monocytes
        - Differentiate to become tissue macrophages
        - Continue phagocytosis and release critical growth factors (TGF-alpha, fibroblast growth factor (FGF), collagenase) to attract and differentiate fibroblasts
        - Clear initial neutrophilic infiltrate from wound
        - Stimulate angiogenesis by releasing vascular endothelial growth-factor

d. Lymphocytic Stage
    i. After 72 hours
    ii. Primarily differentiated T-lymphocytes (attracted by IL-1, complement components and IgG breakdown products)
    iii. Assist in the regulation of collagen production and breakdown as well as other extracellular matrix components

e. Length of the inflammatory phase often dictates the time course for healing and maturation
    i. Oral mucosal wounds often heal faster and with less scar formation compared to dermal wounds
    ii. Prior studies showing that oral wounds tend to have less inflammatory infiltrate (of all 4 phases) which may contribute to these findings

3. Proliferation
    a. Day 3 to about two weeks after initial injury
    b. Fibroblasts
        i. Synthesize a new extracellular matrix
        ii. Differentiate into myofibroblasts that assist in wound contraction
    c. Granulation Tissue
        i. Healing tissue contains a higher proportion of type III collagen than unwounded tissue or mature scars
        ii. Has less tensile strength than type I collagen
    d. Angiogenesis
        i. Allows for continued oxygenation and nutrient delivery through all wound healing phases

   ii. Local hypoxia triggers production of vascular endothelial growth factor (VEGF) which triggers proliferation of endothelial cells
      - Cytokines produced by tissue macrophages
      - Other cellular signaling molecules involved in angiogenesis include FGF, PDGF, TGF-alpha and TGF-beta

4. Remodeling (Maturation)
   a. Type 1 Collagen
      i. Mature scars contain a higher proportion of type I collagen compared to type III collagen, which is predominant in granulation tissue
      ii. Type 1 collagen is remodeled and organized into cross-linked bundles (Matrix metalloproteinases and TGF-beta are key to this step)
      iii. This contributes to increased tensile strength of new scar, however matured scars reach only a maximum of 80% of original tensile strength
      iv. Apoptosis reduces number of fibroblasts, macrophages and newly-vascularized capillaries from a maturing wound, and non-essential extracellular matrix is degraded to increase tensile strength
   b. Re-epithelialization
      i. Initially, a single layer of epithelial cells forms a cover over wound bed, growing in an advancing front from periphery to center
      ii. Continued contraction of wound and maturation leads to epithelial proliferation and eventually a near-full or full-thickness epithelial layer

Aspects Influencing Wound Healing

1. Many factors may influence wound healing from temporality to integrity of final fully-healed wound **[2]**
2. Local Factors
   a. Wound edema in an enclosed space may increase pressure on tissues in wound
      i. Must happen in a wound that has reached some level of epithelialization or has been closed surgically
      ii. Increased hydrostatic pressure outside local capillaries minimizes outward flow of nutrients and may lead to capillary collapse
      iii. Decreased blood flow leads to decreased oxygenation of wound which may predispose to tissue hypoxia
   b. Infection
      i. Contamination of surgical wounds from extrinsically introduced bacteria and/or normal skin flora may contribute to wound infection
      ii. Robust inflammatory response combats and removes bacteria (Disorders affecting neutrophil and macrophage function may limit inflammatory response)
      iii. Biofilm formation

- Bacteria may produce an extra cellular polysaccharide matrix which protects colonies from antibiotic penetrance
- Limits penetrance of neutrophils
- Staphylococcus species and Pseudomonas species heavily implicated
- May result in chronic wounds

3. Systemic Factors
    a. Stress
        i. Physiologic stress associated with upregulation of pro inflammatory cytokines including IL-1, IL-6 and TNF-alpha which may prolong inflammatory phase
        ii. Endogenously produced glucocorticoids suppress immune response required to progress through stages of wound healing
        iii. Exogenous glucocorticoid intake suppresses inflammatory and proliferative stages
        iv. Psychological stress may also impact wound healing
    b. Diabetes
        i. In diabetic patients, wounds associated with hypoxic environment
            - May increase number of free oxygen radicals
            - Decreased levels of VEGF contribute to disordered angiogenesis
        ii. High glycemic content may also add to oxidative stress and create a favorable environment for bacterial growth and biofilm formation
        iii. Dysregulated immunity of both humoral and innate immune systems may inhibit body's ability to remove infection
        iv. Diabetic neuropathy
    c. Smoking
        i. Smoking associated with worse outcomes and adversely affects inflammatory phase by reducing neutrophil function as well as decreased IL-1 production
        ii. Proliferative phase prolonged by decreased fibroblast and myofibroblast proliferation, and decreased re-epithelialization
        iii. Other associated complications include wound dehiscence, anastomotic leaks, necrosis and decreased wound strength
        iv. Ideally should wait at least 4-6 weeks after smoking cessation to perform elective surgical interventions
    d. Alcohol use
        i. Alcohol primarily decreases wound angiogenesis by decreasing VEGF
        ii. Decreased level of collagen production and remodeling
    e. Nutritional factors
        i. Malnutrition associated with poorer surgical outcomes and longer, less efficacious wound healing **[3]**
        ii. Protein deficiency

- Collagen is primary protein involved in scar formation; global protein deficiency and deficiencies in specific amino acids may impair appropriate collagen production and wound healing
- May result in decreased wound strength

iii. Vitamin C deficiency
- Along with iron, a required cofactor for hydroxylation of collagen at lysine and proline residues allowing for cross-linking
- Facilitates neutrophil function
- Decreases fibroblast proliferation
- Decreases angiogenesis
- Increases wound infection rates

iv. Vitamins A and E
- Have antioxidant functions
- Vitamin A is also required for epithelial development and immune system function

v. Arginine
- Nonessential amino acid
- May stimulate T-lymphocytes
- Decreases wound infections

Radiation and Wound Healing

1. Primary effect on cancer cells is during G2 through M phases
2. Effects targeted towards rapidly dividing cells
3. Ionizing radiation results in permanent damage to tissue and vascular endothelium, preventing angiogenesis in wounded, previously irradiated tissue
4. Dysfunctional granulation tissue formation and epithelialization
5. Early effects of radiation may disrupt the inflammatory and proliferative phases of wound healing [4]
   a. Overaccumulation of proinflammatory cytokines including TGF-beta, VEGF, TNF-alpha, INF-gamma and IL-1 and IL-8 lead to matrix overproduction and fibrosis
   b. Disruption of granulation tissue formation and vascularization, which leads to disorganized collagen deposition causing low tensile strength in healed areas
      i. Matrix metalloproteinases are dysregulated

Surgical Scar Formation and Management

1. Optimal surgical scar outcomes are thin, flat and closely color-matched to surrounding skin
2. Surgical incisions in head and neck most commonly closed by primary intention

   a. Different techniques exist to maximize closure strength while maintaining aesthetic and functional capacity (Dependent on surgeon preference)
   b. One study examining tissue glue use vs subcuticular suture with and without adjuvant scar management techniques of non-ablative fractional laser and intralesional triamcinolone injection found optimal aesthetic outcome with a subcuticular suture and scar management techniques, though the latter may be less feasible in a routine setting **[5]**
      i. Monocryl is a good choice for superficial subcuticular techniques; low risk of foreign body reaction, absorbable
      ii. Prolene is another strong option for interrupted superficial closures, though care must be taken to use this material in patients that are able to follow up for suture removal
   c. Use of adhesive strips (Steri-strips) do not seem to impact scar healing **[6]**
   d. Ultimately, aesthetic outcome of surgical incision closure is surgeon dependent and surgeons should choose closure techniques that are best suited to their style
3. Hypertrophic Scar and Keloid formation
   a. Hypertrophic Scar: thickening of scar tissue NOT beyond original margins of scar
   b. Keloid: growth of scar tissue beyond original margins of scar; has propensity for recurrence
   c. Certain subgroups of patients, predominantly patients of African descent may demonstrate a propensity to form hypertrophic scars or keloids even with controlled surgical incisions
   d. Upregulation of cytokines, particularly IL-6 may contribute to keloid formation (TGF-beta may also contribute)
   e. Use of silicone-based products and paper tape can help prevent the formation of hypertrophic scars and keloids
   f. Intralesional steroid injection with triamcinolone (i.e., Kenalog) and 5-fluorouracil is a favored option for treating severe keloids and hypertrophic scars [7]
   g. Pulsed dye laser: generally second-line treatments to above but may demonstrate some efficacy
   h. Botulinum toxin is gaining traction as a possible method to reduce hypertrophic scars but mechanism is unclear
   i. Low-dose fractionated radiotherapy is another option, though it is less common given the theoretical risk of malignancy at radiated sites
   j. Surgical excision/revision is less ideal in keloid-forming patients given the propensity of recurrence
   k. No consistent single treatment has been proven to be effective in keloids
   l. In known keloid-forming patients, early intervention with methods above as well as minimizing incisions are critical in generating optimal results
4. Depressed scars - can be treated with fillers, laser- and non-laser resurfacing and further surgical procedures to revise scars
5. Other Treatments to Enhance Wound Healing
   a. Hyperbaric oxygen

    i. "Pushes" more oxygen into tissue
    ii. Benefit of increased oxygen radicals in infected wounds may also carry anti-microbial effects
    iii. Commonly used in treatment of osteoradionecrosis and other radiated wounds as well as diabetic ulcers

b. Rapamycin
    i. Mammalion target of rapamycin (mTOR) inhibitor
    ii. MTOR upregulated in injured stratified squamous epithelia; serves to upregulate proliferation, but in certain phenotypes, tends to be overreactive
    iii. May prevent hypertrophic or keloid scarring

c. Special dressings/delivery systems [8]
    i. Hydrogel membranes - may enhance re-epithelialization by maintaining a moist environment over wound bed
    ii. Hydrogels and scaffolds
        - May be useful to allow for continuous exposure to key elements of wound healing by acting as a carrier for key growth factors that normally, in-vivo have short half life
        - Enhance critical regenerative pathways
    iii. Silver nanoparticle impregnated materials - may enhance re-epithelialization and fibroblast differentiation

Summary Points

1. The 4 phases of wound healing include: hemostasis, inflammation, proliferation, and remodeling
2. Many local and external factors influence wound healing, and those who take care of head and neck concerns need to understand these factors and their role in wound healing
3. Various treatment options are available to minimize appearance of scars and to treat hypertrophic/keloid scars

References

[1] Bailey, B., Johnson, J. and Rosen, C., 2014. *Bailey's head and neck surgery - otolaryngology*. Philadelphia: Wolters Kluwer, Lippincott Williams et Wilkins.

[2] Larjava, H., 2012. *Oral wound healing*. Chichester, West Sussex, UK: Wiley-Blackwell.

[3] Laliberté F, Bloom I, Alexander AJ. The Critical Role of Nutrition in Facial Plastic Surgery. *Facial Plast Surg Clin North Am*. 2019 Aug;27(3):399-404. doi: 10.1016/j.fsc.2019.04.005. PMID: 31280854.

[4] Haubner F, Ohmann E, Pohl F, Strutz J, Gassner HG. Wound healing after radiation therapy: review of the literature. *Radiat Oncol*. 2012 Sep 24;7:162. doi: 10.1186/1748-717X-7-162. PMID: 23006548; PMCID: PMC3504517.

[5] Chung JH, Kim DS, Cheon JH, Yoon JM, Baek SK, Jung KY, Yoon ES, Park SH. Current Protocol for Aesthetic Scar Management in Thyroid Surgery. *Laryngoscope*. 2021 Jul;131(7):E2188-E2195. doi: 10.1002/lary.29441. Epub 2021 Feb 10. PMID: 33567135.

[6] Custis T, Armstrong AW, King TH, Sharon VR, Eisen DB. Effect of Adhesive Strips and Dermal Sutures vs Dermal Sutures Only on Wound Closure: A Randomized Clinical Trial. *JAMA Dermatol*. 2015 Aug;151(8):862-7. doi: 10.1001/jamadermatol.2015.0174. PMID: 25875131; PMCID: PMC4982140.

[7] Lee Peng G, Kerolus JL. Management of Surgical Scars. *Facial Plast Surg Clin North Am*. 2019 Nov;27(4):513-517. doi: 10.1016/j.fsc.2019.07.013. PMID: 31587770.

[8] Park JW, Hwang SR, Yoon IS. Advanced Growth Factor Delivery Systems in Wound Management and Skin Regeneration. *Molecules*. 2017 Jul 27;22(8):1259. doi: 10.3390/molecules22081259. PMID: 28749427; PMCID: PMC6152378.

Chapter 4

Tissue Expansion

Tareq Sawan, MD
and Yan Ho Lee, MD

Introduction

Tissue expansion was first reported in 1957 for reconstruction of a traumatic auricular deformity [1]. Tissue expansion is a reconstructive option that takes advantage of the natural response of tissue to continuous mechanical stress load to allow local tissue advancement or rotation into a defect, as well as increasing surface area of tissue in preparation for regional or free tissue transfer. It provides donor tissue with the similar color, texture, thickness and sensation and, when used for local reconstruction, minimizes donor site morbidity seen in autologous grafting and free-tissue transfer.

Histological Properties of Skin

1. Collagen
    a. Triple helix configuration
    b. Types I and III: predominant component of dermis
    c. Collagen filaments → collagen fibrils → collagen fibers
    d. Relaxed skin: collagen fibers are convoluted
    e. Stretched skin: collagen fibers re-align in parallel configuration
2. Elastic Fibers
    a. Composed of elastin and microfibrillar protein
    b. Recoil causes collagen fibers to return to relaxed, waxy configuration
    c. Excess stretch → elastic fibers fragment → loss of ability to recoil
3. Ground Substance
    a. Proteoglycans occupying the interstitial space between collagen and elastic fibers
    b. Acts as a lubricant

Mechanics of Stretch

1. Elastic material (e.g., coil spring)
    a. Hooke's Law: Linear relationship between stress and elongation

In: Essential Facial Plastic and Reconstructive Surgery. Volume 1 ISBN: 979-8-89113-306-8
Editors: Yan Ho Lee and Ira Papel © 2024 Nova Science Publishers, Inc.

   b. Not a function of time: a constant load over time does not result in progressive elongation.
   c. Returns to original shape after release of load
2. Viscous material (e.g., bubble gum)
   a. Nonlinear relationship between stress and elongation.
   b. Function of time: a constant load over time leads to progressive elongation.
   c. Does not spontaneously recover after release of load.

Skin Properties

1. Combines both viscous and elastic properties (i.e., viscoelastic).
2. Lower stress loads: skin exhibits elastic properties (Figure 4.1)
3. Higher stress loads: collagen fibers maximally aligned → skin exhibits viscous properties → loses its recoil elastic properties (Figure 4.1) → elongation becomes a function of load AND time
4. Creep: stretch of a material under a constant load over time.
   a. Mechanical creep: elongation of skin beyond its inherent stretch when constant tension is applied
      i. Attributed to straightening of collagen fibers to lie in a parallel configuration, micro-fragmentation of elastic fibers and displacement of interstitial fluid, resulting in increased skin viscosity.
      ii. *Stress Relaxation* is the progressive reduction in force required to maintain the stretched skin's length
   b. Biologic creep: increased mitotic activity secondary to sustained forces on tissue.

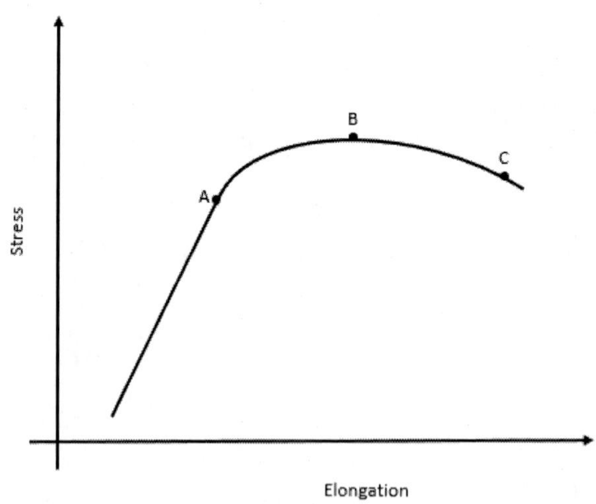

Figure 4.1. Response of skin to stress. Skin exhibits linear elongation secondary to stress until the collagen fibers are maximally aligned (Elastic limit; point A). The skin exhibits viscous properties and loses its elastic properties past point A, achieving maximal tensile strength at point B. Past point B, the skin exhibits accelerated elongation as a result of rupture of collagen fibers (point C).

Tissue Changes During Expansion

Skin is a multilayered structure consisting of epidermis, dermis, and hypodermis (subcutaneous tissue). Each component responds differently to long term tissue expansion:

1. Epidermis [2]
    a. Increases in surface area
    b. Thickness increases or remains the same
    c. Stretch → increases intercellular spaces → Increased mitotic activity, mainly in stratum basale
2. Dermis [2]
    a. Papillary layer: finer collagen fibers and elastic tissue
    b. Reticular layer: dense collagen fibers
    c. Thins with expansion. Amount of thinning depends on rate of expansion
    d. Fibroblasts activated →increases collagen production. Collagen fibers re-orient to lie in parallel positions
    e. Melanocytes activated → increases melanin production → transient hyperpigmentation with expansion lasting up to several months
    f. Thickness returns to pre-expansion levels within 2 years
3. Hypodermis (Subcutaneous layer) [2]
    a. Consists of fat, collagen, neurovascular structures, lymphatics, hair follicles, sebaceous glands and connective tissue
    b. Thins by up to 50% with expansion → returns to normal thickness within 2 years
    c. Expansion induces fat necrosis and increases interlobular space → filling of these spaces with collagen
    d. Hair follicles move further apart but number of follicles is unchanged. Stress of expansion induces Telogen phase → transient alopecia lasting several months
4. Muscle [3]
    a. Muscle atrophies and thins with expansion
    b. Hyalinization occurs followed by calcification in some cases
    c. Caution when expanding muscle of facial expression (i.e., frontalis)
5. Blood Vessels [4]
    a. Local tissue hypoxia related to expansion induces angiogenesis
    b. Arteries and veins elongate with no change in vessel wall diameter
    c. Clinically, has enhanced survival rate similar to delayed flaps
6. Nerves: [5]
    a. Elongation of peripheral nerves
    b. No significant changes in nerve conduction velocities when expander pressure <40mm Hg
    c. Expansion >40-60 mmHg induces nerve ischemia leading to edema and demyelination
7. Bone (from compression of the expander) [6]

a. Reversible cranial and long bone resorption (decreased thickness and volume due to osteoclastic activity; bone density is unchanged)
b. Greater effect on cranial bone vs long bones
c. Inner table of skull is unchanged and no evidence of increased intracranial pressure observed
d. Following expander removal, bone remodeling begins within 5 days and is back at baseline by 2 months

Capsule Formation [6]

1. A dense fibrous, vascularized capsule develops around the expander as early as 7 days after placement
2. Vascularity of capsule increases overall vascularity of flap
3. Consists of myofibroblasts → can result in contracture and reduced elasticity of flap post-expansion.
4. Grossly disappears within several weeks of expander removal

Indications for Tissue Expansion in Head and Neck Reconstruction

Tissue expansion is best suited in areas with robust vascular supply and thick skin with underlying bone to support the expander device (i.e., scalp and forehead). Cheek region may not tolerate expansion due to relatively thin skin and risk of damage to facial mimetic muscles and facial nerve. Neck expansion potential is limited by underlying neurovascular structures. It is a valuable reconstructive option in burns, alopecia, trauma, and defects secondary to skin cancer or congenital lesion excisions when used to expand:

1. Local tissue prior to local transfer
2. Regional tissue (e.g., pre-expansion of myocutaneous pectoralis flap or supraclavicular island flap prior to regional tissue transfer)
3. Distant tissue (e.g., expansion of radial forearm or scapular tissue prior to free tissue transfer.

Technical Considerations

1. Types of tissue expansion:
   a. Conventional internal soft tissue expander: silicone rubber with remote or integrated injection port to inject saline
   b. Self-inflating internal soft tissue expander: osmotically active hydrogel enclosed in silicone membrane with small pores allowing slow absorption of body fluids; reaches maximal expansion over 4-6 weeks
   c. Carbon dioxide driven tissue expanders

d. External tissue expanders: devices that apply continuous tension to wound edges to allow primary closure or smaller wound; can be used in acute wounds due to trauma or cancer resection requiring timely resection
e. Serial excisions allow for sequential tissue stretch without the use of an implant

2. Expander considerations
   a. Circular, oval, rectangular or crescentic in shape. Rectangular expanders provide greatest surface area gain (Rectangle: up to 38% increase; Crescent: up to 28% increase; Round: up to 25% increase) [7]
   b. Expander base should be 2.5-3 times of the area to be reconstructed to account for flap contracture (goal expansion can be approximated using circumference of the expander subtracted by the base width)
   c. Maximize potential by using more than 1 expander adjacent to defect (Figure 4.2)

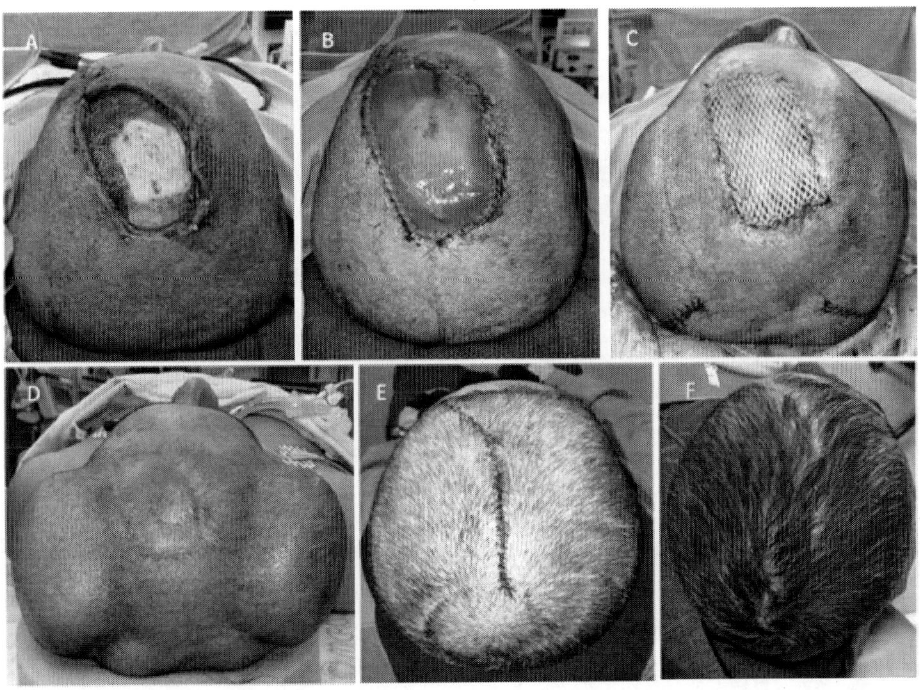

Figure 4.2. Tissue expansion for scalp defect reconstruction. Patient with full thickness soft tissue loss of the scalp; B. Application of bi-layered skin substitute for granulation tissue; C. Meshed STSG with placement of bilateral rectangular tissue expanders with ports; D. Tissue expanders expanded over 8 weeks; E. Closure of the wound with hair bearing skin; F. 4 weeks post-operative visit.

3. Insertion of expander
   a. Incision should ideally be planned to act as the leading edge during advancement of expanded skin. If adjacent tissue is unfavorable (i.e., increased risk of wound dehiscence), may use a remote incision (plan this to avoid compromising future local flap options)
   b. Characteristic of skin determines dissection plane

i. In thick-skin areas or structures prone to stretch injury (i.e., facial nerve in the face), a superficial plane (e.g., supra-SMAS) is preferable
ii. If overlying skin is thin (e.g., forehead) or unstable, a deeper plane is preferable to ensure skin integrity and vascularity

c. A separate tunnel, preferably over a bony prominence, is created bluntly to accommodate the injection valve
d. Once a pocket is created, it is thoroughly irrigated and the sterile expander is placed with all edges rolled out
e. The injection valve is placed through the previously created tunnel and may be secured with a non-absorbable suture
f. The expander is inflated by injecting 10-20ml of saline into the injection valve to ensure continuity of the system from the valve to the balloon (may use methylene blue in the initial expansion fluid to ensure future injections are in the appropriate space)
g. Incision is closed in multiple layers with interrupted 3-0 PDS sutures in deep layers and interrupted non-absorbable (Prolene or Nylon) sutures on the skin; Skin sutures may be removed at 10 days
h. The balloon is inflated enough to obliterate dead space without placing undue tension on incision

4. Expansion process
   a. No expansion is done during the initial two weeks until healing of the incision site
   b. In the case of traditional tissue expanders, topical 1% lidocaine is applied to the skin. A 21g needle attached to a 20cc Luer-lock syringe is pierced through skin into the injection valve. Withdraw to ensure needle is in correct space.
   c. Inject approximately 10% of the expander volume each time
      i. Other end points for each session: discomfort or blanching of the overlying skin.
      ii. Space injections 1 week apart
      iii. Expanders can sometimes be "overfilled" to 10-50% depending on the manufacturer's guidelines
      iv. Allow 2-4weeks after final expansion before removal of implant and local flap; allows completion of biologic creep to minimize contracture of the expanded tissue
   d. Intraoperative expansion: rapid cyclical expansion of skin surrounding defect by
      i. mechanical creep
      ii. enhanced undermining and tissue recruitment during rapid expansion

Complications

1. Cheek and neck areas are associated with increased complications; scalp has the lowest complication rate

2. Dehiscence of skin overlying the expander due to:
    a. Incisional dehiscence if incision is placed too close to area of expansion or if fast absorbing sutures used for closure of deeper layers of incision
    b. Progressive thinning of overlying skin with over-inflation of the expander (>40mm Hg) or when expanding tenuous skin (inherently thin or previously irradiated skin); in case of mild dehiscence, can continue expansion process
3. Implant infection: rare due to excellent blood supply of head and neck area
4. Hematomas and seromas: may necessitate serial aspirations
5. Bone erosion: full thickness erosion rare in adults; expansion of scalp in pediatric patients is not recommended until closure of anterior and posterior fontanelles
6. Alopecia: secondary to hair follicle 'shock' (usually transient). Common guideline is that >40% expansion of hair bearing area (scalp) will result in noticeable alopecia
7. Intractable pain: primarily in forehead expansion due to compression of supraorbital and supratrochlear nerves

Summary Points

1. Tissue expansion is a reconstructive option that utilizes inherent soft tissue mechanical and biological properties to achieve tissue gain in preparation for local, regional or free tissue transfer.
2. Mechanical creep is achieved when tissue is acutely stretched beyond its inherent elasticity.
3. Biologic creep is achieved when slow tissue stretching induces tissue regeneration.
4. Histologic changes include epidermal thickening, dermal thinning, subcutaneous atrophy, muscle atrophy and neurovascular elongation.
5. Tissue expanders come in various sizes and shapes. For circular expanders, the base diameter should be at least 2.5x the anticipated defect to allow closure.
6. Meticulous planning of tissue expansion is key to a successful result. Skin color, texture, thickness and hair bearing qualities should be taken into account when planning for expander placement
7. Expansion may require at least 8 weeks of serial inflations to achieve optimal results.

References

[1] Neumann, C.G., The Expansion of an Area of Skin by Progressive Distention of a Subcutaneous Balloon: Use of the Method for Securing Skin for Subtotal Reconstruction of the Ear. *Plastic and Reconstructive Surgery*, 1957. **19**(2): p. 124-130.

[2] Pasyk, K.A., L.C. Argenta, and C. Hassett, Quantitative analysis of the thickness of human skin and subcutaneous tissue following controlled expansion with a silicone implant. *Plastic and reconstructive surgery*, 1988. **81**(4): p. 516-523.

[3] Gur, E., Hanna, W., Andrighetti, L., and Semple, J.L. Light and Electron Microscopic Evaluation of the Pectoralis Major Muscle following Tissue Expansion for Breast Reconstruction. *Plastic and Reconstructive Surgery,* 1998. **102**(4): p. 1046-1051.

[4] Cherry, G.W., Austad, E., Pasyk, K., McClatchey, K., and Rohrich, R.J. Increased Survival and Vascularity of Random-Pattern Skin Flaps Elevated in Controlled, Expanded Skin. *Plastic and Reconstructive Surgery*, 1983. **72**(5): p. 680-685.

[5] Hall, G.D., Van Way, C.W., Kung, F.T., and Compton-Allen, M. Peripheral nerve elongation with tissue expansion techniques. *The Journal of trauma*, 1993. **34**(3): p. 401-405.

[6] Johnson, T.M., Lowe, L., Brown, M.D., Sullivan, M.J., and Nelson, B.R. Histology and physiology of tissue expansion. *The Journal of dermatologic surgery and oncology*, 1993. **19**(12): p. 1074-1078.

[7] van Rappard, J.H., G. Sonneveld, and J. Borghouts, Geometric planning and the shape of the expander. *Facial plastic surgery*, 1988. **5**(04): p. 287-290.

Chapter 5

Grafts: Skin, Cartilage, and Bone

Julia Toman, MD

Introduction

The goal of the reconstructive surgeon is to restore form and function. At times defects cannot be addressed with tissue that is immediately adjacent to the defect or there is loss of multiple types of tissue. This situation then requires the use of various grafted materials. These materials can include skin, cartilage, and bone and be obtained from a variety of sources including the patient, other humans, or animals. With the wide variety of grafting materials available, it is important that the surgeon understand the nuances of each of these grafting materials to choose the appropriate material for a given defect.

The ideal grafting material has the following biologic properties:

1. Has no immune or carcinogenic effects
2. Is structural and mechanical similarity to missing tissue
3. Is easy to sculpt
4. Is mechanically and chemically stable
5. Has predictable integration

The ideal graft is:

1. Readily available
2. Has low cost
3. Has the ability for sterility and purity

Skin

Layers

1. Epidermis (superficial): consisting of keratinizing stratified squamous epithelium
2. Dermis (deep): made up of fibrous connective tissue matrix containing collagen, elastic tissue fibers, and ground substance; contains various structures including epidermal appendages, blood vessels, nerves, and the pilosebaceous units

In: Essential Facial Plastic and Reconstructive Surgery. Volume 1 ISBN: 979-8-89113-306-8
Editors: Yan Ho Lee and Ira Papel © 2024 Nova Science Publishers, Inc.

Skin Grafts

1. History can be traced to ancient India over 2500 years ago (skin grafted over amputated nose)
2. In modern medicine, skin grafting continues to play a large role in resurfacing of a variety of defects [1]
3. The goal in skin grafting is to transfer the healing burden to an area of less aesthetic importance.
4. Skin grafts are utilized in areas where local tissue flaps cannot be reasonably used and removes the need for additional scars on the face
5. Unfortunately, skin graft can leave a patch-like appearance due to color and thickness differences (which might be improved with dermabrasion)
6. Three main types:
    a. Full-thickness
    b. Split thickness
    c. Composite
7. Graft viability
    a. Depends on the vascularity and microcirculation of the surface of the recipient site, vascularity of the donor tissue, contact between the graft and the recipient site, and a variety of systemic patient factors
    b. Avascular areas larger than 1 cm are not likely to support a skin graft since they rely solely on vascular supply from the wound edges
    c. For bony defects without periosteum, the bony cortex can be drilled to the level of punctate bleeding to improve the vascular bed for the skin graft
    d. For deep wounds, a period of granulation for 2-3 weeks is allowed prior to placing a skin graft
8. Healing of skin graft follows a series of 3 stages (Table 5.1)

Table 5.1. The 3 Stages of Skin Graft Healing

1. Imbibition	Passive diffusion of nutrients to the graft from the underlying recipient bed and lasts for the first 24-48 hours. Separation of the graft from the wound bed such as with a hematoma, will prevent the diffusion of nutrients and lead to graft failure necessitating bolstering/closure of dead space between the graft and the recipient area
2. Inosculation	Occurs during the first 24-48 hours and after 48-72 hours, capillaries in the recipient site begin to grow into the graft
3. Neovascularization	Final stage of neovascularization with new complete vascular supply to the graft occurs over 3-5 days

9. Full Thickness Skin Graft
    a. Consists of both epidermis and dermis
    b. Benefit of having dermis is that the graft is more resistant to contracture and maintains the texture and pigment of normal skin
    c. Initially may have a blanched appearance but develop a pink coloration over 3-7 days indicating neovascularization
    d. Erythema can persist for 4-6 weeks

e. Provides better tissue match as well as ease of harvest
f. Lower rate of survival than split thickness skin grafts, especially in larger grafts
g. Longer healing times
h. Applications
    i. Best on areas of the face with thinner skin or areas of natural concavity (eyelids, nasal side wall, columella, temple and medial canthus)
    ii. In recipient sites with thicker skin (with greater sebaceous content), there is more likely to be a contour step off (can be addressed with a dermal fat graft post operatively)
    iii. Avoid in margin of the nostril, eyelid and vermillion; scar contracture in these areas will result in distortion of the surrounding structures
    iv. Defects that are superficial (involving loss of skin only with preservation of underlying muscle and subcutaneous tissues) are better suited to full thickness skin grafting
i. Common Donor Sites:
    i. Upper eyelid, forehead, melolabial fold, pre-auricular, post-auricular, and supraclavicular regions
    ii. Choice depends on the needs of the defect regarding skin thickness and color match
    iii. Chosen for their good tissue match and ability to allow for primary closure

10. Split Thickness Skin Graft
    a. Composed of epidermis and varying amounts of the superficial dermis
    b. Benefit of increased survival since they have greater exposure of capillaries and overall less tissue which requires neovascularization
    c. Disadvantages of poor color and texture match and propensity for contraction
    d. Range in thickness from 0.012-0.030 inches thick; the thicker the graft, the better the color and quality match
    e. Applications:
        i. Temporary coverage prior to definitive repair
        ii. Covering large defects when cosmesis is not a concern
        iii. In the very elderly or high-risk patients where larger flaps are not an option
        iv. Facilitate monitoring for cancer recurrence
    f. Common Donor Sites:
        i. Hip/thigh
        ii. Buttock
        iii. Upper inner arm
11. Composite Graft
    a. Contains 2 or more tissue layers
    b. Most common are skin-cartilage grafts but their use is limited by their high metabolic demands and thus high failure rate. [2]

   c. Should not be larger than 1 cm to decrease the metabolic demands, however, larger grafts can be successful if placed in areas with a reliable vascular supply with no portion of the graft further than 1 cm from the wound edge. [3]
   d. Commonly employed for thickness defects of the nose, specifically the nostril margin, columella, and the nasal facet with the donor site being various parts of the auricle
12. Dermal Graft
   a. Can be used for filling defects or serving as barriers
   b. Commonly harvested from abdomen, buttock, hip, groin, or thigh
   c. Allografts available (Discussed in Chapter 6)

Cartilage

Cartilage makes an ideal grafting material in that it is easily shaped while maintaining structural integrity. There are three types of cartilage in the human body: fibrous, articular, and elastic hyaline. [4] Cartilage is made up of chondrocytes, matrix (secreted by the chondrocyte), and water and is avascular in nature receiving nutrients from the overlying perichondrium. [4] Cartilage can be harvested from both humans and animals with various methods for preservation for allografting including storage in chemical fixatives, freezing and radiation. Sources of cartilage include septal cartilage, auricular/conchal cartilage, and costal cartilage (autologous or allograft).

Autologous Cartilage

Autologous sources have historically been preferred due to beliefs that autologous sources have lower rates of complications. A benefit of non-autologous cartilage is that there is essentially a limitless supply compared with autologous. Regardless of the cartilage source, important principles of grafting include care with handling and carving of the graft and use of snug pockets or fixation to prevent migration of the grafted material.

1. Sources of Cartilage
   a. Septal Cartilage
      i. Hyaline cartilage
      ii. Low donor site morbidity and may already be within the surgical field (rhinoplasty)
      iii. Can be used for larynx, orbital floor and small auricular reconstructions for stabilization
   b. Auricular Cartilage
      i. Elastic cartilage; more resilient than septal cartilage
      ii. Conchal bowl is a common source with minimal donor site morbidity
      iii. Can also be harvested as a composite graft with skin lining although a flap or graft will be needed for donor site repair

    iv. Helical root can be harvested up to 1.5 cm for cartilage alone or in combination with skin.
c. Costal Cartilage (Figure 5.1 a)
    i. Can provide for larger volume of cartilage and is more structurally robust
    ii. Has decreased pliability
    iii. Warping and resorption of costal cartilage are common concerns
    iv. Resorption is thought to be mediated via an immune response to chondrocytes which are more extensively exposed with diced or carved cartilage [5]

Homograft Cartilage

1. Kridel and Konior (1993) showed a low level of graft warping with irradiated homograft costal cartilage [6] in nasal cases.
2. Kridel et al found no increased risk of complication with the use of irradiated homologous cartilage compared to autologous cartilage sources; homologous rib was more cost effective and time effective compared to autologous cartilage [7]
3. Saadi et al (2019) found no significant difference between autograft and allograft with regard to graft resorption, warping, infection, or need for revision surgery [8]
4. Can be used for auricular reconstruction, laryngotracheal reconstruction, nasal reconstruction, and facial augmentation

Xenograft Cartilage

1. Provides another source of grafting material
2. Ryu et al. investigated the use of porcine ear cartilage and found that similar to human cartilage, the porcine ear cartilage was covered in perichondrium and composed of chondrocytes and chondroblasts. When transplanted into rats, they noted no inflammatory reaction. [9]
3. While this has not yet been translated to human use, xenografting provides a potential source of grafting material

Applications of Cartilage Grafts

1. Most commonly used for nasal cosmetic and reconstructive surgeries and auricular reconstruction
2. Ortiz-Monasterio et al. summarized uses of cartilage in primary aesthetic rhinoplasty: 1) increased and defined the dorsum in thick skin, 2) add projection and angularity to the tip, 3) project the columella, 4) and correct the acute nasolabial angle [10]

3. In functional rhinoplasty, cartilage used to address dynamic collapse with batten grafts or alar rim grafts, and to widen a narrowed airway via spreader grafts, septal replacement/reconstruction, or septal extension grafts. [8] (Figure 5.1 b)
4. Used in contouring and supporting the nose in ethnic rhinoplasty, reconstruction in cleft lip/palate noses, correction of the over-resected nose and saddle nose deformities. [11-15]
5. In rhinoplasty, septal cartilage is the preferred source of grafting cartilage due to its ease of accessibility, carving and low rates of complications
6. Auricular cartilage and rib cartilage are also used in nasal surgery especially in the complex revision nose or in noses which require significant augmentation/structural support
7. Auricular reconstruction of microtia defects has traditionally utilized a large costal cartilage framework. The contralateral cartilage of ribs 6-7 form a natural curve which help in the carving and shaping of the ear construct. [16]

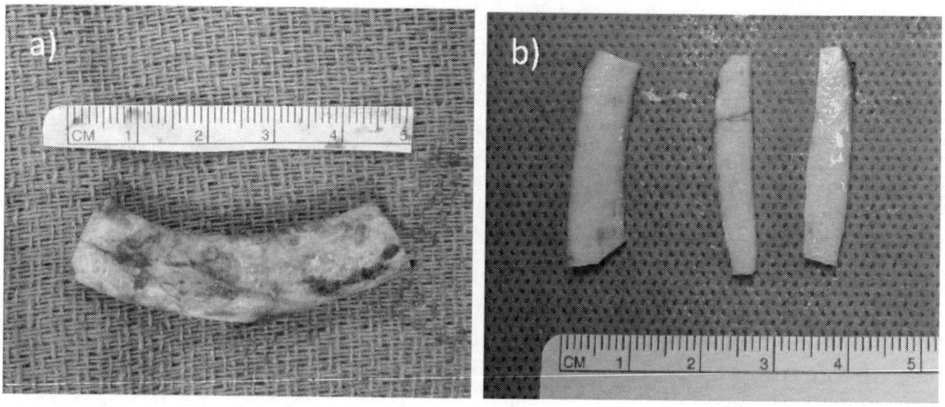

Figure 5.1. a) Costal cartilage harvested from patient; b) costal cartilage carved into columella strut and bilateral spreader grafts.

Bone

Bony defects in the head and neck can range from small to large resulting from a variety of etiologies including trauma, malignancy, or surgical excision. The bony skeleton of the head and facial structures has unique combination of functional and aesthetic requirements. Bone grafting plays an integral role in restoration of form and function. Bone grafts can also be used for augmentation in the facial skeleton such as over the cheeks to restore or expand facial contour. The earliest recorded bone graft was use in 1670 by Van Meekren who utilized canine calvarial bone graft for reconstruction of a Russian soldier skull defect. [17]

1. Characteristics
   a. Made up of osteocytes that occupy lacunar cavities in a matrix of tightly condensed collagen and a ground substance composed of calcium hydroxyapatite

b. Two types of bone used for grafting: endochondrial bone and membranous bone (defined by embryologic origin and anatomic location)
c. Membranous bones of the face, calvarium and ribs are formed via the direct deposit of bone within the vascularized mesenchyme
d. Endochondrial bones include the long bones and the iliac crest which are from endochondrial ossification of cartilage precursors. [18] Endochondrial bone contains greater proportion of cancellous bone and have increased rates of resorption with grafting. [19]
e. All bone have 2 types of tissue – cortical outer layer and inner cancellous area.
    i. Cortical bone - contains densely packed organic matrix combined with a mostly hydroxyapatite in organic component which is covered by 2 layers of periosteum, an external layer of fibrocytes and an internal layer of endothelial-like cells. The cortical bone contains the haversian canals which contains capillaries connecting with large tubules of the nutritive canal system. It is around these haversian canals that bone is deposited in concentric circles
    ii. Cancellous bone - has a trabeculated network which surrounds bone marrow, and contains osteocytes/bone progenitor cells
f. Cortical or cancellous bone are used in grafting independently or in combination
g. Ideal bone graft has provision of a template for the bone growth, induction of bone formation, differentiation of bone forming cells, and supplies the bone forming cells to the site of the defect [20]
h. Success dictated by the type of graft used, the site of implantation, vascularity in the area, immunogenicity potential of the graft, as well as local and systemic factors [21]

2. Bone Healing - involves one or more of 4 processes: incorporation, osteoconduction, osteoinduction, osteogenesis. (Table 5.2)

Table 5.2. Bone Healing Processes

Incorporation	Occurs when bone graft adheres to host tissues; requires immobilization with tight contact between the bone graft recipient bone/surrounding soft tissue and a well vascularized recipient bed
Osteoconduction	The predominant mechanism; involves capillary and osteoprogenitor cell ingrowth from the recipient site utilizing the vascular channels within the grafted bone. [22, 23] Graft acts as a scaffold for the cellular ingrowth. Grafted old bone is eventually resorbed. [24]
Osteoinduction	The stimulation of undifferentiated mesenchymal cells in bone graft to differentiate into pre-osteoblasts which go on to become bone producing cells. The inductive agent is bone morphogenic protein (BMP) along with a cascade of other enzymes and inhibitors. [22-24]
Osteogenesis	The process of new bone formation by surviving osteoblasts within the bone graft. Most common mechanism of bone growth in a vascularized bone graft but occurs to a lesser extent in the non-vascularized bone graft. Cortical bone grafts are especially dense therefore slowing early revascularization and major role of osteogenesis [22]

3. Different bone grafts: autografts, allografts, xenografts, and synthetic materials.
    a. *Bone Autografts*
        i. Bone is transferred from one part of the body to another part of the body in the same individual
        ii. Gold standard in bone grafting
        iii. Combines all three of the bony healing principles including transfer of osteogenic cells without triggering the immune response
        iv. Sources include non-vascularized cancellous, cortical, or cortico-cancellous, bone, or vascularized bone (vascularized bone discussed in Chapter 13)
        v. There are limits to the amount of bone which can be transferred in addition to donor site morbidity considerations [20, 21]
        vi. Healing of Bone Grafts
            - Bone grafts can be used in healthy, non-radiated bony gaps up to 6 cm in length with survival dependent on immobilization to promote incorporation as well as good vascularity of the recipient bed
            - Primary Stage – 2 weeks; same for both cancellous and cortical bone
                - Characterized by a marked inflammatory response with recruitment of polynuclear cells, creation of a lattice of fibrous connective tissue and proliferation of capillary buds around the graft over the first week
                - In the second week, there is a shift to fibrous granulation tissue production and osteoclastic activity with osteocytic process within the bone graft itself and ingrowth of the capillaries and repopulation of the lacunae, haversian canals and trabeculae with primitive mesenchymal cells [24]
            - Secondary Stage - different between cancellous and cortical bone
                - *Cancellous bone graft*
                    - Revascularization completed within the primary repair timeframe owing to the large channels within the bone which facilitate both vascular penetration as well as influx of phagocytic cells and osteoclasts
                    - Highly osteogenic due to their inherently high concentrations of osteoblasts and osteocytes [25]
                    - Revascularization allows for the repopulation of the trabeculae of the bone graft with mesenchymal cells allowing for more rapid osteoconduction

    - Can integrate in 6-12 months, but due to low density, have less mechanical support [22, 25]
  - *Cortical bone grafts*
    - Revascularization process occurs in cortical bone through the small haversian canals with slow inward growth taking 1-2 months to complete
    - Via osteoclastic activity, the haversian canals are widened to facilitate ingrowth of the vascular supply and then influx of new lining mesenchymal cells which then differentiate into osteoblasts
    - It takes years for the cortical graft to be resorbed and replaced with new bone [21]

vii. Common Donor Sites

- *Iliac Bone*
  - Excellent source of both cortical and cancellous bone from which significant quantities can be harvested
  - Very dense allowing for excellent rigid fixation and high stress recipient areas
  - Unable to bend or shape the bone with ease
  - Large amounts of cancellous filler bone can be harvested for treatment of non-unions or alveolar defects
  - Major drawback is the morbidity of the surgery with risk of post-operative pain and in children risk to the cartilaginous apophysis which must remain undisrupted for normal growth
- *Rib Bone*
  - Provides cortical-cancellous bone grafts which are used for both cranial defects and for facial on-lay reconstruction for acquired or congenital facial deformities
  - Flexible nature allows for ease of shaping and molding but cannot withstand high stress forces
  - If periosteum is left in situ, the rib can regenerate, however if the periosteum is harvest with the graft, there is improved graft survival
  - Harvest of the graft does carry the risk of a pneumothorax but overall rib grafting can provide a large quantity of bone stock
- *Calvarial Bone*
  - Dense cortical bone which was first described by Tessier for use in facial reconstruction in 1982. [26]

- Limited risk of resorption due to the dense cortical nature, rapid revascularization, relatively easy harvest in close proximity to the surgical site and ability to obtain relatively large quantities of bone making it a commonly used source of bony grafting material. [27]
- Usually harvested as a split graft which preserved the inner table and thus the dura and brain.
- Inner and outer tables can be harvested with return of one of the tables to close the donor site defect

b. Bone Allografts
    i. Bone is transferred between genetically unmatched individuals
    ii. Higher failure rate than autologous bone due to immunogenic rejection factors
    iii. To prevent an immune reaction and prevent spread of disease, the cellular components are removed; however, these processes do affect the biologic properties of the graft
    iv. Increased risk of infection if graft is not properly sterilized
    v. Benefit of limitless quantity and lack of donor site morbidity
    vi. Usually reserved for patient for whom autografting is difficult or not possible [22]

c. Bone Xenografts - Rarely used due to reported complications such as infection, material displacement, immune reactions, chronic inflammation, foreign body reaction, and the risk of disease transmission

d. Synthetic Materials - May provide scaffolding and mimic bone, but may lack osteoinductive and osteoconductive properties; many different materials are being developed to enhance (i.e. demineralized bone matrix) or substitute (i.e. hydroxyapatite) bone grafts. (Described in Chapter 6)

Summary Points

1. There is no perfect grafting material.
2. Choice of grafting material must be made based on the defect characteristics, the patient characteristics, and expected morbidity with the goal of replacing "like with like" to restore form and function.
3. As medical science and technology continue to advance, tissue engineering and 3D printing offer new horizons for skin, cartilage and bone implants.

References

[1] Hazani, R., R. Whitney, and B.J. Wilhelmi, Article Commentary: Optimizing Aesthetic Results in Skin Grafting. *The American Surgeon*, 2012. 78(2): p. 151-154.

[2] Konior, R.J., Free composite grafts. *Otolaryngol Clin North Am*, 1994. 27(1): p. 81-90.

[3] Ruch, M.K., Utilization of composite free grafts. *J Int Coll Surg*, 1958. 30(2): p. 274-5.

[4] Caplan, A.I., Cartilage. *Scientific American*, 1984. 251(4): p. 84-97.

[5] Elves, M.W., A study of the transplantation antigens on chondrocytes from articular cartilage. *J Bone Joint Surg Br*, 1974. 56(1): p. 178-85.

[6] Kridel, R.W. and R.J. Konior, Irradiated cartilage grafts in the nose. A preliminary report. *Arch Otolaryngol Head Neck Surg*, 1993. 119(1): p. 24-30; discussion 30-1.

[7] Kridel, R.W., Ashoori, F., Liu, E.S. and Hart, C.G., Long-term use and follow-up of irradiated homologous costal cartilage grafts in the nose. *Arch Facial Plast Surg*, 2009. 11(6): p. 378-94.

[8] Saadi, R., Loloi, J., Schaefer, E. and Lighthall, J.G., Outcomes of Cadaveric Allograft versus Autologous Cartilage Graft in Functional Septorhinoplasty. *Otolaryngology–Head and Neck Surgery*, 2019. 161(5): p. 779-786.

[9] Ryu, Y.A., M. Jin, and N. Kang, Histological, Physical Studies after Xenograft of Porcine Ear Cartilage. *Arch Craniofac Surg*, 2017. 18(3): p. 155-161.

[10] Ortiz-Monasterio, F., A. Olmedo, and L.O. Oscoy, The use of cartilage grafts in primary aesthetic rhinoplasty. *Plast Reconstr Surg*, 1981. 67(5): p. 597-605.

[11] Murrell, G.L., Auricular cartilage grafts and nasal surgery. *Laryngoscope*, 2004. 114(12): p. 2092-102.

[12] Cobo, R., Correction of dorsal abnormalities in revision rhinoplasty. *Facial Plast Surg,* 2008. 24(3): p. 327-38.

[13] Mizuno, T., A New Technique for Augmentation Rhinoplasty Using Hybrid Autologous Grafts with Septal Extension Grafts in Asian Patients. *Facial Plast Surg*, 2019. 35(1): p. 58-64.

[14] Jang, Y.J., Song, H.M., Yoon, Y.J. and Sykes, J.M., Combined use of crushed cartilage and processed fascia lata for dorsal augmentation in rhinoplasty for Asians. *Laryngoscope*, 2009. 119(6): p. 1088-92.

[15] Pagan, A.D., D.A. Sterling, and B.T. Andrews, Cartilage Grafting Outcomes in Intermediate and Definitive Cleft Rhinoplasty. *Cleft Palate Craniofac J,* 2021. 58(8): p. 974-983.

[16] Brent, B., Auricular repair with autogenous rib cartilage grafts: two decades of experience with 600 cases. *Plast Reconstr Surg*, 1992. 90(3): p. 355-74; discussion 375-6.

[17] J, V.M., *Observation Medicochisurgicae.* 1670, Amsterdam: Henrici and T. Bloom.

[18] Smith, J.D. and M. Abramson, Membranous vs endochondrial bone autografts. *Arch Otolaryngol*, 1974. 99(3): p. 203-5.

[19] Zins, J.E. and L.A. Whitaker, Membranous versus endochondral bone: implications for craniofacial reconstruction. *Plast Reconstr Surg*, 1983. 72(6): p. 778-85.

[20] Elsalanty, M.E. and D.G. Genecov, Bone Grafts in Craniofacial Surgery. *Craniomaxillofacial Trauma & Reconstruction*, 2009. 2(3-4): p. 125-134.

[21] Khan, S.N., Cammisa, F.P. Jr, Sandhu, H.S., Diwan, A.D., Girardi, F.P. and Lane, J.M., The biology of bone grafting. *J Am Acad Orthop Surg*, 2005. 13(1): p. 77-86.

[22] Gillman, C.E. and A.C. Jayasuriya, FDA-approved bone grafts and bone graft substitute devices in bone regeneration. *Mater Sci Eng C Mater Biol Appl*, 2021. 130: p. 112466.

[23] Albrektsson, T. and C. Johansson, Osteoinduction, osteoconduction and osseointegration. *Eur Spine J*, 2001. 10 Suppl 2(Suppl 2): p. S96-101.

[24] Burchardt, H., Biology of bone transplantation. *Orthop Clin North Am*, 1987. 18(2): p. 187-96.

[25] Roberts, T.T. and A.J. Rosenbaum, Bone grafts, bone substitutes and orthobiologics: the bridge between basic science and clinical advancements in fracture healing. *Organogenesis*, 2012. 8(4): p. 114-24.

[26] Tessier, P., Autogenous bone grafts taken from the calvarium for facial and cranial applications. *Clin Plast Surg*, 1982. 9(4): p. 531-8.

[27] Zouhary, K.J., Bone graft harvesting from distant sites: concepts and techniques. *Oral Maxillofac Surg Clin North Am*, 2010. 22(3): p. 301-16, v.

Chapter 6

Implant Materials

Matthew B. Hirsch, MD

Introduction

1. Definitions
    a. *Alloplast*: a graft not taken from a human or animal source - may be synthetic (i.e., polymethylmethacrylate) or composed of a naturally occurring material (i.e., hydroxyapatite)
    b. *Allograft:* a graft taken from a genetically non-identical member of the same species
    c. *Biocompatible*: having little or no impact on the host tissue; not degraded by the host tissue and minimal immunologic response
2. Ideal implant material:
    a. Biocompatible
    b. Non-thermal conducting
    c. Radio-transparent
    d. Non-magnetic
    e. Lightweight
    f. Customizable
    g. Resistant to infection and trauma
3. Usage
    a. Aesthetic: tissue augmentation (i.e., chin implant) or camouflage (pre-jowl implant)
    b. Reconstructive: tissue defect (i.e., post-traumatic or post-ablative)
    c. Functional: structural support (i.e., batten grafts in rhinoplasty)
4. General advantages (vs. autologous materials)
    a. No donor site morbidity
    b. Large augmentation volume available
    c. Operative time savings (avoid additional time for graft or flap harvest)
    d. Technical simplicity (avoid expertise required for graft or flap harvest)
    e. Long shelf-life
    f. Customizable
    g. Low risk of graft resorption (with the exception of acellular dermal matrix which does show resorption) [1]
5. General disadvantages (vs. autologous materials)
    a. Infection risk

In: Essential Facial Plastic and Reconstructive Surgery. Volume 1 ISBN: 979-8-89113-306-8
Editors: Yan Ho Lee and Ira Papel © 2024 Nova Science Publishers, Inc.

   b. Extrusion risk
   c. Migration risk
   d. Lower resistance to trauma
   e. Resorption (acellular dermal matrix)
6. Basic principles
   a. Porosity
      i. *Smooth* (nonporous) implant surfaces: capsule forms around implant
         - May lead to higher risk of implant migration, late infection, skin or bone breakdown [2]
         - Easier to remove
      ii. *Porous* implant surfaces: more fibrous ingrowth "anchors" implant
         - Migration less likely
         - Larger pore size (100 μm) allows cells and immune components to reach implant and improve defense against infection [3]
         - More difficult to remove due to tissue ingrowth
         - Greater potential for biofilm formation
         - Potentially higher risk for early postoperative infection before fibrovascular ingrowth is achieved
   b. Fixation
      i. Rigid fixation reduces implant motion
      ii. Implant motion can lead to skin or bone breakdown, seroma formation, chronic inflammatory reaction
   c. Infection Risk
      i. All alloplasts are at risk of infection
      ii. Head and neck sites of implantation are often clean-contaminated, increasing infection risk compared to clean sites
      iii. Currently no evidence-based guidelines for implant infection prevention
      iv. Kullar et al in 2018 recommend peri- and post-operative antibiotics in rhinoplasties that utilize an alloplastic implant [4]
      v. Commonly employed measures to prevent implant infection:
         - Soak implants in antibiotic solution intraoperatively prior to implantation
         - Use perioperative and postoperative antibiotics [5]
         - Avoid over-augmentation or "pressure points" on overlying skin
         - Fixate implant when possible
         - Irrigate implant site with antibiotic solution prior to closure
         - Close meticulously (watertight closure)
      vi. No clear consensus exists on the relative risk of infection or extrusion of various alloplastic materials [5]

Implant Materials

1. Silicone
   a. Polysiloxane - polymer of silicon-oxygen backbone with methyl groups
   b. Soft, pliable, nonporous
   c. Easily carved intraoperatively
   d. Easily sterilized
   e. Easily removed
   f. Inexpensive and readily available
   g. Thick fibrous capsule forms around implant - no tissue integration or vascularization
   h. Commonly used for augmentation of chin, cheek, mandibular angle, nose
   i. May cause underlying bone resorption or thinning of overlying skin
   j. May have increased risk of late complications due to chronic peri-implant inflammation caused by implant micro-movements or bacterial seeding of capsule [6]
2. High Density Porous Polyethylene (HDPE) (i.e., MedPor)
   a. Porous 100 – 300 μm size interconnected pores
   b. Tissue ingrowth and vascularization occurs
   c. High tensile strength
   d. Readily accepts drilling and screw fixation without fracturing
   e. Available as preformed implants and solid carvable blocks
   f. Commonly used for orbital floor, cranioplasty, mandibular augmentation, microtia reconstruction
   g. May be combined with titanium mesh (i.e., orbital floor implants)
   h. Possible advantages: less migration, less bone erosion than smooth implants [7]
   i. More difficult to remove than smooth implants due to tissue integration
   j. Thought to be more resistant to infection and trauma than ePTFE, but this is still being elucidated
   k. Extrusion or infection can lead to breakup of the implant into small pieces which are difficult to extract.
3. Expanded polytetrafluoroethylene (ePTFE) (Gore-Tex)
   a. Woven carbon and fluorine-based synthetic polymer
   b. Porous (pore size 10 - 30 μm)
   c. Softer than silicone
   d. Available as preformed implants, solid tubes, and sheets
   e. Encourages fibrous ingrowth (although less than HDPE) leading to less risk of migration compared to smooth implants [8]
   f. Biocompatible, carvable
   g. Relatively easily removed
   h. Commonly used in malar, chin, mandibular angle, nasal and paranasal implants; also used in lip augmentation, nasolabial folds and marionette lines
   i. May lose pliability over time (contact with blood hardens implant edges)
   j. May be used in hybrid implant as a coating around a silicone implant core

4. Polyetheretherketone (PEEK)
    a. Thermoplastic polymer
    b. Smooth, rigid
    c. Commonly used for orbital, malar, and cranioplasty implants
    d. Easy to remove
    e. Craniofacial implants may be fully customizable and prefabricated with virtual surgical planning
    f. Elastic modulus similar to bone (limits resorption)
    g. Poor osseous integration and poor soft tissue adhesion
    h. Autoclavable, can be re-sterilized
5. Polyetherketoneketone (PEKK)
    a. Similar biomechanics properties to PEEK but 3D printed
    b. More porous than PEEK and may display greater osseointegration [9]
6. Polymethyl Methacrylate (PMMA)
    a. "Bone cement" commonly used in orthopedic surgery
    b. Formed by mixing liquid methyl methacrylate (MMA) monomer and a powdered MMA-styrene co-polymer
    c. Polymerization is a highly exothermic reaction (110 degrees C) which can cause tissue damage
    d. Active cooling via irrigation is required if curing is allowed to occur in-situ
    e. Implants may be preoperatively hand-fabricated by the surgeon or prefabricated with virtual surgical planning and then autoclaved
    f. Implants may be shaped (burred) intraoperatively to make small adjustments
    g. PMMA microspheres are an ingredient in Bellafill injectable filler
    h. May cause underlying bone resorption [2]
    i. Inexpensive, readily available
    j. Residual MMA monomer which does not undergo polymerization may be toxic
    k. No tissue ingrowth or vascularization
    l. Rigid
    m. Susceptible to fracture, infection
7. Hydroxyapatite
    a. Naturally occurring mineral form of calcium apatite
    b. One form of hydroxyapatite is a major component of human bone mineral
    c. Found naturally in enamel and dentin
    d. Originally used as a paste (mixed in-situ, then hardens in an exothermic reaction)
    e. Available as custom prefabricated implants alone or integrated with titanium mesh
    f. Hydroxyapatite is necessary for bone regeneration
    g. Main advantage in craniofacial implants is osseointegration
    h. Use in head and neck is mainly in cranioplasty, often combined with titanium mesh
    i. Found in dermal filler as calcium hydroxyapatite gel (i.e., Radiesse)
8. **Titanium mesh**
    a. Osseointegrates

   b. Available as custom prefabricated implant or fabricated intraoperatively
   c. May be combined/covered with hydroxyapatite in-situ or as a preformed hybrid implant to improve contour, simulate osseointegration, and reduce palpability through skin
   d. Used mainly in cranioplasty and reconstruction of larger facial bony defects due to rigidity and osseointegration capability
9. Cadaver Dermis (i.e., AlloDerm)
   a. Acellularized human dermal matrix (ADM)
   b. An *allograft,* not an *alloplast*
   c. Composed of collagen, elastin, vascular channels, and proteins that support tissue regeneration
   d. ADM allografts undergo incorporation into host tissue
   e. Vascularization demonstrated 1-2 weeks postoperatively
   f. Commonly used for nasal dorsum, tip camouflage, onlay grafts, middle lamellar eyelid reconstruction, face and neck reconstruction
   g. Formerly used in lip augmentation, facial slings, and oropharyngeal reconstruction, however many surgeons prefer autologous grafts for these indications
   h. ADM undergoes a variable amount of resorption after implantation making duration of effect unpredictable and most surgeons recommend overcorrection [1]
10. Infection Rates
   a. No clear consensus exists on the relative risk of infection or extrusion of various alloplastic materials; study results often yield conflicting data
   b. A systematic review and meta-analysis by Oliver et al in 2019 found a 1.58% infection rate for silicone, 1.17% for MedPor, 2.86% for Gore-Tex, and 2.43% for MMA [2]
   c. Infection data by site included 2.67% malar, 2.5% frontal, 1.75% nasal, and all others less than 1%.
   d. Peled et al found a 3.8% infection rate for silicone, 4% for ePTFE, and 6% for MedPor in a 2008 meta-analysis of alloplasts in rhinoplasty [6]
   e. Berghaus et al found Gore-Tex in rhinoplasty was more susceptible to infection than MedPor in 2006 [10]

Summary Points

1. Implants with higher porosity and greater tissue integration may lead to reduced risk of complications but are often more difficult to remove
2. Silicone, HDPE, and ePTFE are commonly used in cosmetic facial augmentation due to their ease of use, pliability, wide availability, carvability, and relatively low complication rates and high patient satisfaction rates.
3. Titanium, Hydroxyapatite, combination Titanium/Hydroxyapatite, PEEK, and PMMA are often used in craniomaxillofacial reconstruction due to their rigidity, osseointegrative potential (for Titanium and Hydroxyapatite), and their availability as custom prefabricated patient-specific implants.
4. Surgeons should consider each patient's needs individually and select accordingly from a wide range of safe alloplastic implant options
5. Rigid fixation of implants may promote stability and reduce the risk of complications
6. Avoiding over-augmentation and providing an adequate soft tissue covering may help reduce the risk of complications
7. Surgeons should consider preoperative and postoperative antibiotic prophylaxis when placing alloplastic implants and consider soaking implants in antibiotic solution
8. Further controlled studies are needed to understand each material's relative risk of infection and extrusion
9. Controlled studies or consensus guidelines are needed regarding measures to prevent implant infection

References

[1] Sclafani, A.P., Romo, T. 3rd, Jacono, A.A., McCormick, S.A., Cocker, R., Parker, A. "Evaluation of acellular dermal graft (AlloDerm) sheet for soft tissue augmentation: a 1-year follow-up of clinical observations and histological findings." *Archives of facial plastic surgery* 3.2 (2001): 101-103.

[2] Oliver, J.D., Eells, A.C., Saba, E.S., Boczar, D., Restrep,o D.J., Huayllani, M.T., Sisti, A., Hu, M.S., Gould, D.J., Forte, A.J. Alloplastic Facial Implants: A Systematic Review and Meta-Analysis on Outcomes and Uses in Aesthetic and Reconstructive Plastic Surgery. *Aesth Plast Surg* 43, 625–636 (2019). https://doi.org/10.1007/s00266-019-01370-0.

[3] Gui, L., Huang, L., & Zhang, Z. (2007). Genioplasty and Chin Augmentation with Medpore Implants: A Report of 650 Cases. *Aesthetic Plastic Surgery*, 32(2), 220–226. doi:10.1007/s00266-007-9106-6.

[4] Kullar R, Frisenda J, Nassif PS. The More the Merrier? Should Antibiotics be Used for Rhinoplasty and Septorhinoplasty?-A Review. *Plast Reconstr Surg Glob Open.* 2018 Oct 16;6(10):e1972. doi: 10.1097/GOX.0000000000001972. PMID: 30534507; PMCID: PMC6250483.

[5] Patel, Krishna, and Kathleyn Brandstetter. "Solid implants in facial plastic surgery: potential complications and how to prevent them." *Facial Plastic Surgery* 32.05 (2016): 520-531.

[6] Peled ZM, Warren AG, Johnston P, Yaremchuk MJ. The use of alloplastic materials in rhinoplasty surgery: a meta-analysis. *Plast Reconstr Surg* 2008;121(3):85e–92e.

[7] Hernandez, J. L., Woodrow, K. A., Medical Applications of Porous Biomaterials: Features of Porosity and Tissue-Specific Implications for Biocompatibility. *Adv. Healthcare Mater*. 2022, 2102087.

[8] Papel, Ira D. *Facial Plastic and Reconstructive Surgery*. 4th ed. New York, NY:Thieme, 2016. ISBN-13: 978-1604068481 CHAPTER: Synthetic and Biologic Implants.

[9] Yuan B, Cheng Q, Zhao R, Zhu X, Yang X, Yang X, Zhang K, Song Y, Zhang X. "Comparison of osteointegration property between PEKK and PEEK: Effects of surface structure and chemistry." *Biomaterials* 170 (2018): 116-126.

[10] Berghaus A, Stelter K. Alloplastic materials in rhinoplasty. *Curr Opin Otolaryngol Head Neck Surg* 2006;14(4):270–277.

Chapter 7

Imaging and Photography

Kaete Archer, MD
and Nancy Rothrock

Introduction

High-quality, standardized photographic documentation is essential for the practice of facial plastic and reconstructive surgery. So essential that learning about digital photography has become an expected learning objective of many fellowship programs in addition to the surgical and clinical management. The motivations behind medical photographic documentation extends beyond simply taking "pretty pictures". Medical images must be standardized in lighting, color, and position. This ensures a surgeon can accurately showcase outcomes in academic publications, advertising, medico-legal documentation, and as a pre-surgical communication tool.

Definitions

1. Photography
    a. Photograph – a recording of light using 4 variables: shutter speed, ISO, aperture, and white balance [1]
    b. Many makes and models of cameras can be used to produce high-quality medical photos utilizing these variables
        i. Shutter Speed - duration of exposure – how long light hits sensor of a digital single-lens reflex (DSLR) camera [1]
            - Slower shutter speed → longer exposure time required to get enough light onto sensor for a well-exposed image [1]
            - Expressed in seconds or fractions of a second [1]
            - Fast shutter speeds are used in bright daylight or to freeze motion (e.g., 1/500 of a second or faster) [1]
            - Slow shutter speeds are used in dimly lit conditions to achieve a motion blur or to increase depth-of-field [1]
        – If photographer is holding camera, speeds slower than 1/60 can create movement artifact
        – If photographer is shooting slower than 1/30, a tripod is likely needed
            - A "safe" *minimum* shutter speed is 1/focal length of the lens (e.g., 300mm lens = 1/300 of a second) [1]

In: Essential Facial Plastic and Reconstructive Surgery. Volume 1 ISBN: 979-8-89113-306-8
Editors: Yan Ho Lee and Ira Papel © 2024 Nova Science Publishers, Inc.

ii. ISO "International Standards Organization"
- Measures sensitivity of image sensor (lower ISO →less sensitive camera is to light; this results in finer noise, crisper picture [1]
- When there is plenty of light, as in medical photography, lowest possible ISO (i.e., 100, 200, 400, 800) should be used to retain most detail and have highest image quality [1]
- Higher ISO settings are generally used in darker situations to get faster shutter speeds (needed in action photography); higher ISO introduces more noise to images [1]

iii. Aperture
- Size opening of lens commonly referred to as f-stop which controls the amount of light that enters camera [1]
- Controls depth of field, which is the range within an image that is in sharp focus [1]
- Aperture Priority mode is when photographer sets aperture and ISO, and camera sets shutter speed [1]
- f2 aperture is a large opening with more light and f22 is a small opening with less light; bigger f-stop number → smaller aperture opening [1]
- Smaller f-stops create a shallow depth of field; larger f-stops create a deep depth of field [1]

iv. White Balance or Color Temperature - process of removing color casts, so that objects which appear white in person are rendered white in photo [1]

Camera Modes

1. Auto Mode
   a. Used when photographer wants to take photos without worrying about mechanics of photography [1]
   b. Sets all exposure levels automatically and usually prohibits minor adjustments manually [1]
   c. Although this is an "easy" setting, many medical photographers do not use Auto Mode
2. Manual Mode
   a. Gives photographer total control [1]
   b. Allows photographer to set shutter speed and aperture size [1]
   c. Adjustments to shutter speed and aperture can compensate for under- or over-exposure on patient photos which can be affected by an individual's skin tone
   d. Camera won't correct for under- or over-exposure [1]
3. Aperture (Priority) Mode
   a. Photographer sets size of aperture and camera automatically provides right shutter speed to deliver a correct exposure [1]

   b. Allows for blurring background or keeping entire image in sharp focus [1]
   c. Preferred by many medical photographers because it ensures that entire subject will be in focus using a high aperture setting such as f11-22
4. Shutter Mode
   a. Best option for taking action photography [1]
   b. Not commonly used in medical photography
   c. Shutter Mode allows photographer to freeze scene or blur photo [1]
5. Program Mode
   a. Like Auto Mode, this mode automatically sets aperture size and shutter speed for a perfect exposure [1]
   b. Permits photographer to tweak settings such as white balance, exposure, and shutter speed [1]

Focus Modes

1. Auto Focus
   a. Camera will only focus one time on one point [1]
   b. Can be used for portrait or medical photography
   c. Auto focus will fail in certain conditions:
      i. Plain, solid subjects without much detail or texture
      ii. Subjects in very low light
      iii. Extremely back-lit or reflective subjects
         - Motor in lens will zoom in and out trying to focus
         - When this happens, move the setting to "Manual Mode" and focus camera
      iv. Requiring focus on a specific point - camera may not focus on intended point (e.g., camera focuses on tip of nose when photographer intended focus to be on eyelashes)
2. Servo or Continuous
   a. Focus is constantly changing until picture is taken [1]
   b. Can be used for sports or when subject is moving [1]
3. Manual Focus
   a. Photographer controls focus [1]
   b. Best in low-light or low-contrast [1]
   c. Many professional medical photographers prefer to use Manual Focus as they are trained to see image snap into focus
   d. This also allows photographer to choose point of focus rather than allowing camera to choose

Lens

1. High quality lenses prevent distortion and provide a high depth of field so that entire face is in focus [2]

2. Lenses recommended for facial photography have a focal length between 90 to 105 mm (also known as 'portrait lenses') [2]
3. Gold standard facial lens is 105 mm macro fixed focus lens rather than zoom lens [3]
    a. Allows for focus at very close distances when documentation of a small area is needed [3]
    b. Macro lenses show details of small objects [1]
    c. Macro lenses also can manage focus when needing full face and neck photos
    d. Zoom lenses work IF you get a zoom that allows for close up work and wider shots although it is generally accepted that high quality fixed focus lenses will always allow for a sharper focus [3]
4. Shorter focal lengths such as 60mm can cause facial distortion (central bulging or "fishbowl effect") [2]

Setting Up a Medical Photography Room/Space

1. Dedicated photo room/space. (Figure 7.1)
    a. Photos should be taken in same space and under same conditions to create comparable, reproducible photos
    b. Good estimate for a photography room/space is 6 feet wide and 10 feet long at a minimum [3]
    c. Should be big enough to set up permanent lighting and a mounted wall background
2. Lighting
    a. Most important aspect to creating standardized, reproducible surgical photographs [2]
    b. In facial plastic surgery, surgeon needs to be able to utilize lighting to clearly and accurately demonstrate surface anatomy with contrast, textures and sharp lines by interpretation of highlights and shadows
    c. Harsher light source is sometimes used in rhinoplasty to bring out shadows, contours, and sharp lines of demarcation of external nasal anatomy [2]
    d. Diffusers such as umbrellas or soft boxes eliminate shadows and provide even lighting [2]
    e. Some surgeons use same lighting set up for rhinoplasty and facial rejuvenation
3. Light sources
    a. Can be a simple set up but flash lighting is needed to create well-illuminated and consistent pre- and post-operative photos [3]
    b. Ideal to have lighting above head of photographer and on either side of photographer [3]
    c. Two lights of equal power mounted to ceiling (or on stands) on either side of photographer work well to achieve even lighting [3]
    d. Harsh (rhinoplasty)
        i. On-camera flash, ring flash, or on-camera twin flash without diffuser
            - On-camera flashes can create uneven lighting [2]

- Ring flashes can create even, flat lighting but may wash out detail [2]
- On-camera twin flashes simulate a studio flash and are portable but may not be exactly reproducible since lighting is based on camera placement/position [2]

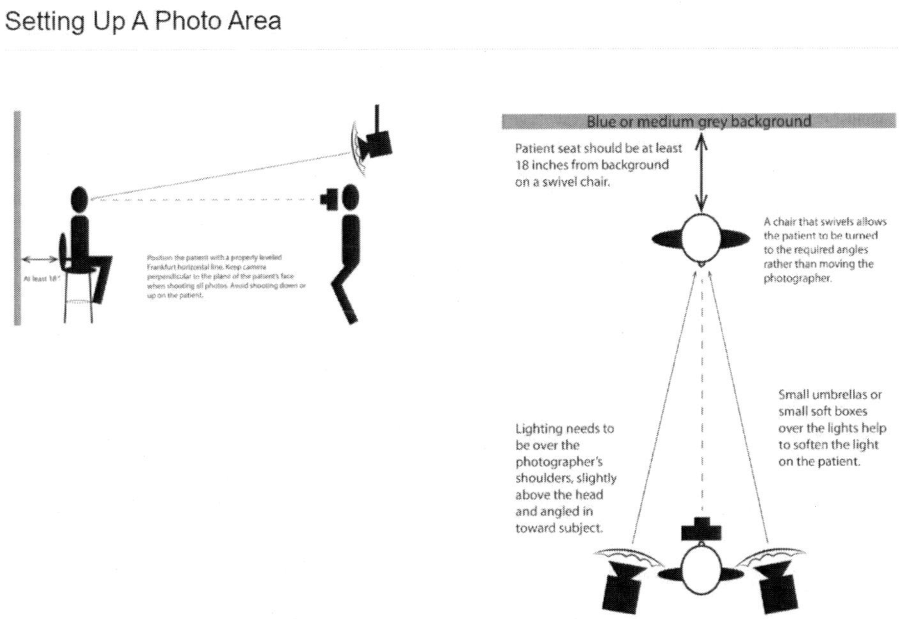

Figure 7.1. Photography setup.

   ii. In general, try to avoid using flash that is mounted to camera or a flash on a hot shoe (attachment to camera) because of harsh shadows appearing around subject [3]

e. Soft (facial rejuvenation)
   i. Multiple mounted/stationary flash units (e.g., 2 studio flashes)
   ii. Use soft boxes or umbrellas to diffuse [2]
f. Most common set up is with 2 studio flashes with or without diffusers [2]
g. A single backlight can be used to help separate patient from background or highlight facial anatomy [2]
h. At times, it may be advantageous to bounce light of a flash unit off a fairly low, white ceiling; can bring out facial detail that even lighting may not show such as lower eyelid bags

4. Lighting positions
   a. Even illumination is accomplished using 2 symmetrically-sized and symmetrically-powered lights located at 45-degree angles to patient [3]
   b. Single backlight (such as smaller flash unit) is mounted 1-3 feet in front of background centrally above and directed downward [2]
   c. Alternatively, backlight can be from 2 smaller flashes directed at 45-degrees towards background [2]

   d. Take care to keep background light soft enough to eliminate shadows but not strong enough for bright illumination
   e. Distance between 2 main lights can impact appearance of nasal tip anatomy
      i. The wider apart the lights are, the wider the spread of the shadows [2]
      ii. Keep lights no more than five to six feet apart
5. Backdrop
   a. Blue or cool colored background is preferred
      i. Cool colors such as blue, blue-green or grey give a warm cast to skin tone [3]
      ii. Warm-colored backgrounds such as red and orange give skin tones an unnatural greenish or blue cast [3]
   b. Black backdrops
      i. Sometimes used to avoid problems with shadows in background [3]
      ii. However, using black backdrops on patients who have darker skin or darker hair will cause subject to blend or fade into background and obscure true visualization of head, face, and neck [3]
   c. Even lighting minimizes shadows and decreases need to hide shadows with a dark background
6. Chair position
   a. Counter-height swivel chair should be positioned 18 inches away from background [3]
   b. Swivel chair is ideal for shooting from multiple angles

Patient Positioning

1. All views (except for base view and birds-eye view) should be taken with patient in Frankfort horizontal (a horizontal line, parallel with the floor, that runs across top of tragus to across top of infraorbital rim) [4]
2. Camera position should be perpendicular to plane of face [3]
3. Rhinoplasty-specific views [2]
   a. Frontal, side/profile
   b. Base view is included to visualize nostrils
   c. Right and left quarter views (in Frankfort horizontal, patient swivels 45 degrees to right and left; tip of nose should be flush with maxillary process of cheek
4. Hair
   a. Hair should be tucked behind ears and neck [4]
   b. In otoplasty, hair should be completely away from ears to accurately document ear position and angles [4]
   c. For forehead lifts, hair should be off forehead exposing hairline [4]
5. Framing
   a. Patient should be framed from top edge of head to clavicle [4]

   b. Patient should fill most of frame while minimizing empty space/distraction from backdrop
   c. Patient should be symmetric horizontally and vertically and centered in frame
   d. Earrings and other facial jewelry should be removed; if at all possible, makeup should be removed or minimized
   e. Photos should be taken with a relaxed, unsmiling (repose) expression; smiling photos may be added if appropriate

Trends in Photography and Videography

1. Growing use of 3D photography
   a. May help with documentation
   b. Can use morphing software to edit photos to help with patient counseling
2. Increased use of videography to help document dynamic movements and functional deficits [5]
3. Tools for photography and videography are increasingly available, portable, and have more functions, though cost can be a limiting factor [5]
4. Quality of photo-documentation via telemedicine platforms is not as high-quality or standardizable, but is feasible and likely to improve [5]

Summary Points

1. High-quality, standardized, reproducible photography is an essential part of a facial plastic and reconstructive surgery practice.
2. Lighting is perhaps the most important aspect to creating high-quality medical photographs. Two flash lights are ideal. Harsh lighting, such as an on-camera flash, will create unwanted shadows.
3. For all photographs, the patient should be in the Frankfort horizontal position, which is a horizontal line (parallel with the floor) that runs across the top of the tragus to across the top of the infraorbital rim.

References

[1] Kuhn, Walter. *Roberts Camera. Learn the Fundamentals course manual.* 4-Week Instructional Course. Indianapolis, Indiana. Unpublished.

[2] Galdino GM, DaSilva D, Gunter JP. Digital Photography for Rhinoplasty. *Plastic and Reconstructive Surgery*. April 1, 2002. 1421-1434.

[3] Perkins, Stephen. 02_*Photo Area Setup*. Unpublished.

[4] Perkins, Stephen. 01_*Photo Standardizatio*n. Unpublished.

[5] Tower JI, Lee JY, Lee YH. Screenshot Photography: Optimizing Photo-Documentation While Using Telehealth Video Platforms. *Facial Plast Surg Aesthet Med.* 2020 Jul/Aug;22(4):240-242. doi: 10.1089/fpsam.2020.0225. Epub 2020 May 27. PMID: 32460549.

Chapter 8

Anesthetics

Robert Deeb, MD

Introduction

The choice of anesthetic modality in facial plastic and reconstructive surgery and procedures is of the utmost importance.There are a variety of factors to consider in anesthetic choice including: type of procedure being performed, patient anatomy, comorbid conditions, airway considerations and patient/surgeon preferences. The surgeon must keep in mind that there are many procedures that can be performed under either general anesthesia or local anesthesia with or without sedation based on these factors. Proper anesthetic choice is a major factor in providing a safe, comfortable and efficient experience for the patient and contributes to achieving an optimal outcome. Accurate and effective use of local anesthesia can also help to decreased general anesthetic requirements.

This chapter will outline the pertinent anatomy of the head and neck as it relates to anesthesia in facial plastic and reconstructive surgery. It will also serve as an overview of the commonly used local anesthetics and how they can be implemented in a variety of surgeries and procedures. Lastly, some technical aspects to performing various local anesthetic injections will be reviewed.

Anatomy

1. Cutaneous head and neck innervation
    a. Cutaneous innervation to face provided by the ophthalmic (V1), maxillary (V2) and mandibular (V3) divisions of trigeminal nerve (Figure 8.1)
    b. Skin of anterior and lateral of neck supplied by sensory fibers derived from ventral rami of cervical spinal nerves via cutaneous branches of cervical plexus; primarily the anterior (transverse) cutaneous nerve of neck (C2, 3), great auricular nerve (C2, 3) and supraclavicular nerves (C3, 4)
    c. Skin on back of neck supplied by sensory fibers derived from dorsal rami of cervical spinal nerves; primarily greater occipital nerve (dorsal ramus of C2), third occipital nerve (dorsal ramus of C3) and dorsal ramus of (C4) [1]
2. Auricular Innervation
    a. External ear has complex pattern of innervation with contributions from C2, 3, cranial nerve V3, cranial nerve VII and cranial nerve X (Figure 8.2) [2]

In: Essential Facial Plastic and Reconstructive Surgery. Volume 1 ISBN: 979-8-89113-306-8
Editors: Yan Ho Lee and Ira Papel © 2024 Nova Science Publishers, Inc.

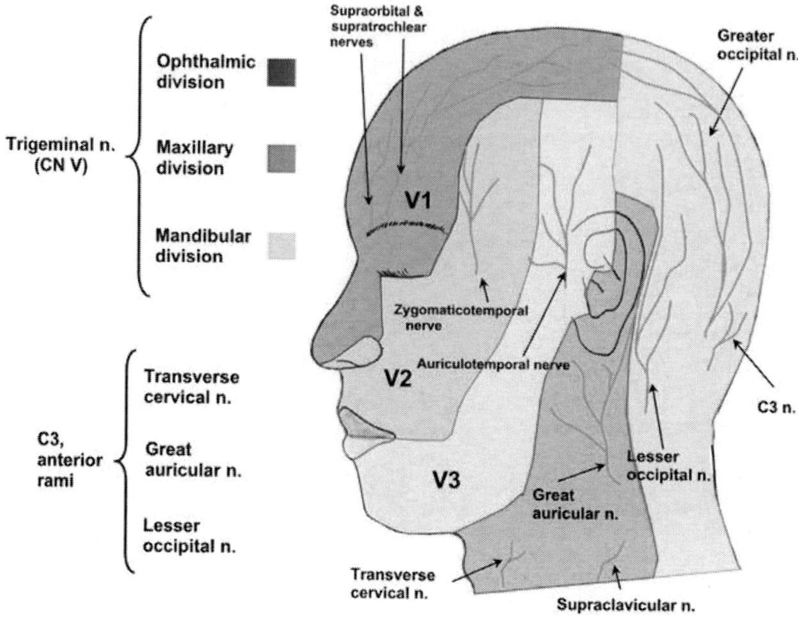

Figure 8.1. Cutaneous innervation of the head and neck [1].

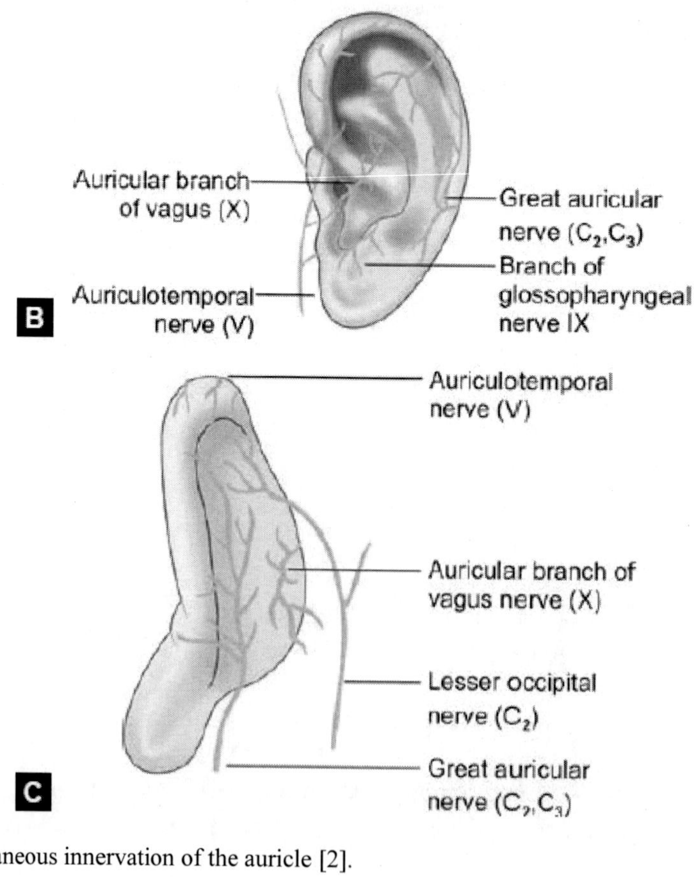

Figure 8.2. Cutaneous innervation of the auricle [2].

3. Nasal Innervation
   a. Internal and external innervation to nose is made up of branches of olfactory nerve (CNI), V1 and V2 (Figures 8.3a & 8.3b) [3]
   b. Nasal septum gets supply from the following nerves: [3]
      i. Olfactory nerves- supply upper part (one-third) just below cribriform plate
      ii. Internal nasal branch of anterior ethmoidal nerve, a branch from nasociliary- supplies anterosuperior part
      iii. Nasopalatine nerve, a branch of pterygopalatine ganglion- supplies posteroinferior part
      iv. Medial posterior superior nasal branches of pterygopalatine ganglion- supply posterosuperior part
      v. Nasal branch of greater palatine nerve- supplies posterior part
      vi. Anterior superior alveolar nerve, a branch of maxillary nerve-supplies anteroinferior part

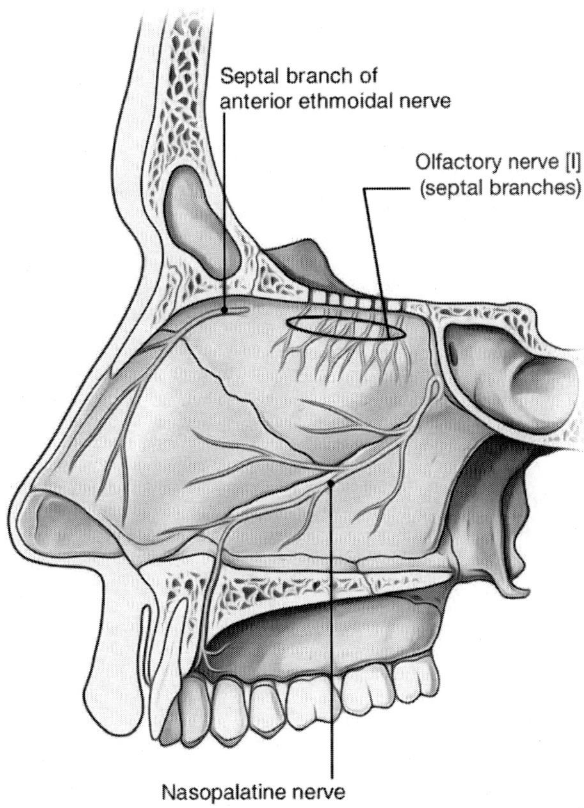

Figure 8.3a. Sensory innervation to the nasal septum. [3]

   c. The following nerves supply different parts of the lateral wall: [3]
      i. Olfactory nerves- supply upper part (one-third) just below cribriform plate of ethmoid up to superior concha

ii. Anterior ethmoidal nerve (from ophthalmic)-supplies anterosuperior quadrant
iii. Anterior superior alveolar nerve, a branch of infraorbital nerve (from maxillary)-supplies anteroinferior quadrant
iv. Posterior superior lateral branches, of pterygopalatine ganglion-supply posterosuperior quadrant
v. Nasal branches of greater palatine nerve, (from pterygopalatine ganglion)- supply posteroinferior quadrant

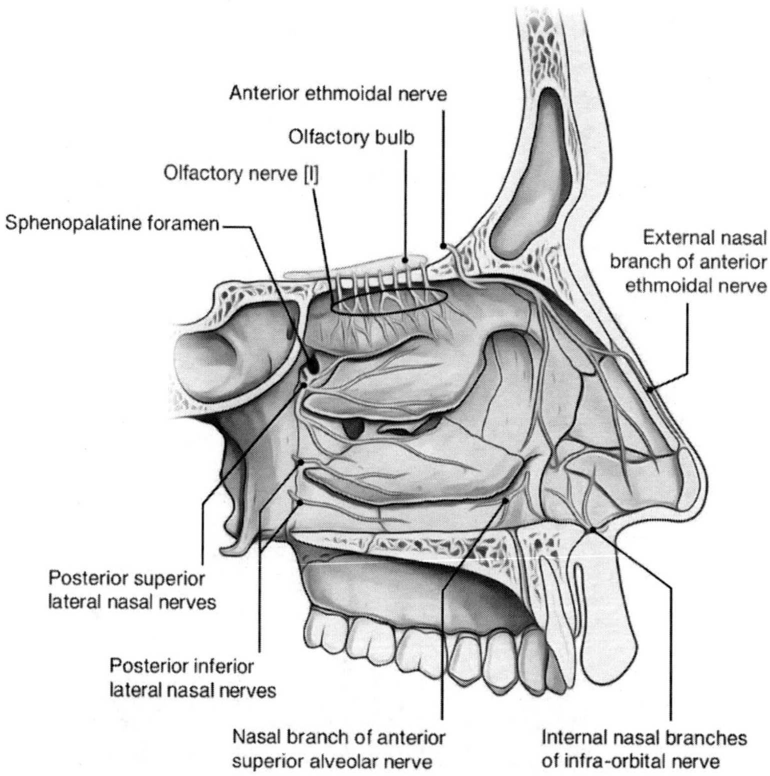

Figure 8.3b. Sensory Innervation to the lateral nasal sidewall. [3]

Local Anesthetics

1. Injectable local anesthetics divided into 2 broad categories:
   a. Amino amides
      i. Have an amide link between the intermediate chain and the aromatic end
      ii. Very stable in solution
   b. Amino esters
      i. Have an ester link between the intermediate chain and the aromatic end

ii. Unstable in solution
iii. Much more likely than amino amides to cause allergic hypersensitivity reactions [4]

2. Helpful guide for remembering which drug belongs to which class: all amino amides contain letter "i" twice, as does the term "amino amides" (Table 8.1)

Table 8.1. Injectable local anesthetics [4]

Drug	**Onset of action**	**Maximum dose (with epinephrine)**	**Duration (with epinephrine)**	**Class**
Lidocaine	Rapid	4.5 mg/kg (7 mg/kg)	120 min (240 min)	Amide
Mepivacaine	Rapid	5 mg/kg (7 mg/kg)	180 min (360 min)	Amide
Bupivacaine	Slow	2.5 mg/kg (3 mg/kg)	4 hours (8 hours)	Amide
Procaine	Slow	8 mg/kg (10 mg/kg)	45 min (90 mins)	Ester
Prilocaine	Medium	5 mg/kg (7.5 mg/kg)	90 min (360 min)	Amide
Tetracaine	Slow	1.5 mg/kg (2.5 mg/kg)	3 hours (10 hours)	Ester

Adverse Reactions and Their Management

1. Amino esters metabolized in plasma via pseudocholinesterases, whereas amino amides are metabolized in liver with renal excretion
2. Adverse reactions may result from injection of too much drug or from inadvertent intravascular injection
3. Signs and symptoms of toxicity include [4]:
   a. CNS affects: lightheadedness, tinnitus, circumoral numbness, metallic taste, double vision, tremors, seizures
   b. Cardiac affects: bradycardia, ventricular fibrillation or asystole
4. True allergic reactions occur in fewer than 1% of all reactions to local anesthetics
5. In suspected adverse reaction:
   a. Cease injection of local anesthetic
   b. Continuous monitoring of vital signs will help determine if more aggressive interventions are necessary
   c. Mild hypotension may require intravenous fluids, while more severe hypotension may necessitate use of vasoconstrictor drugs for circulatory support
   d. Seizure activity can be managed with anti-seizure medications such as diazepam
   e. Succinylcholine may be required to stop ongoing tremors, but its use requires intubation and mechanical ventilation
   f. Atropine and epinephrine may be indicated to treat bradycardia

Selection of Anesthesia Type

1. Dependent on patient, surgeon and circumstantial factors
2. Wide variety of procedures may be performed under general anesthesia or local anesthesia with or without intravenous sedation
3. Patient safety should guide decisions - a patient with multiple serious medical co-morbidities should undergo surgery in a hospital operating room setting under the care of an anesthesiologist
4. When deciding candidacy for local anesthesia, assess patient wishes and patient comfort with being partially or complete conscious - a significant history of anxiety or stress associated with other types of procedures, such as dental interventions, can be a red flag [5]
5. Duration of procedure is an important consideration as well - history of musculoskeletal disorders such as back pain, which may preclude a patient from lying still in the same position for an extended period of time, may also be a contraindication)
6. Airway disorders (i.e., obstructive sleep apnea or airway stenosis) can limit amount of sedation that can be safely administered. [6] The surgeon must tailor the anesthetic plan to the individual patient to minimize risk
7. Certain procedures amenable to local anesthesia: procedures in which the area of dissection can be easily anesthetized via a nerve block or tissue infiltration techniques E.g., eyelid reconstruction, blepharoplasty, auricular reconstruction, cosmetic otoplasty, nasal reconstruction, rhytidectomy, aesthetic and reconstructive lip procedures [7]

Safety Considerations

Procedures being performed under local anesthesia with IV sedation require additional safety considerations (compared to standard general anesthesia) procedures

1. Pay attention to use of oxygen in surgical field when electocautery is being employed
2. Tenting of oxygen must be avoided
3. Wide draping to allow for escape of oxygen is required
4. Flammable sterilizing products should be minimized [8]

Technical Aspects to Local Anesthetic Infiltration

Infraorbital Nerve Block

1. Useful technique when performing a variety of procedures including local flap reconstruction of cheek and associated structures, facial laceration repair, upper lip enhancement, energy or chemical treatments, or injectibles
2. Can be performed via intraoral (sublabial) approach or a transcutaneous approach

3. Infraorbital foramen located along a vertical line through the pupil just inferior to the inferior orbital rim. It should be palpated with either approach (Figure 8.4).

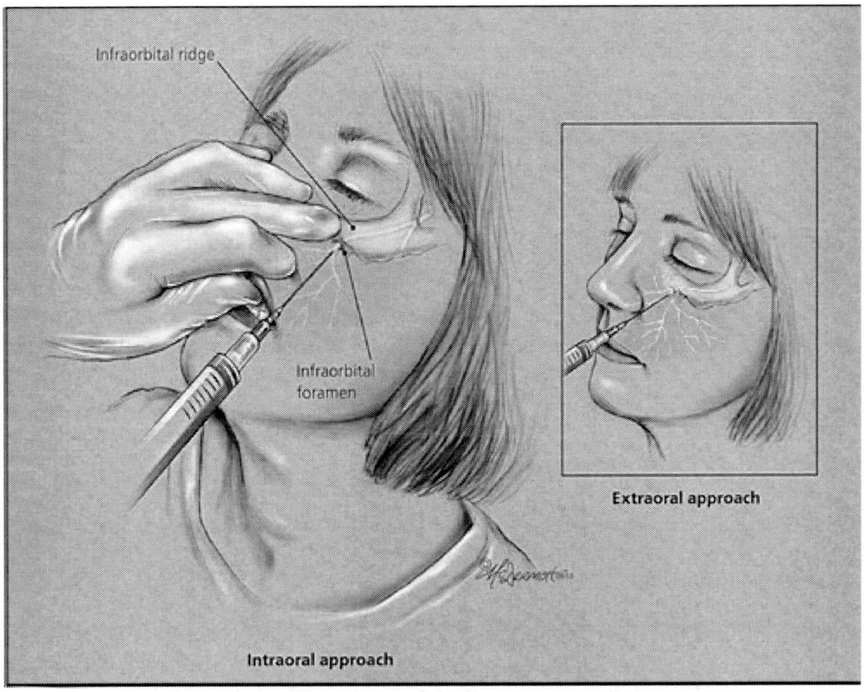

Figure 8.4. Infraorbital nerve block. [9]

Mental Nerve Block (Figure 8.5)

1. Inferior alveolar nerve is a branch of mandibular nerve, which is a branch of V3; enters mandibular foramen, runs within mandibular canal below teeth apices within ramus and body of mandible, exits mandible as mental nerve between the 1st and 2nd premolars
2. Mental nerve blockade useful to provide anesthesia to ipsilateral lower lip and can be useful in lower lip reconstructive surgeries as well as lower lip enhancement procedures along with chemical or energy treatments and injectibles. This is also very helpful for mentoplasty procedures.
3. To locate mental foramen, retract cheek and lip and locate space between 1st and 2nd mandibular premolars, look 1 cm inferior to gum line (just medial to the midline pupil). Note that this is in the same vertical line as the infraorbital foramen. [10]

Rhinoplasty Infiltration

1. Local anesthetic infiltration during rhinoplasty serves a dual purpose:
   a. Providing anesthesia to nose and surrounding structures
   b. Providing vasoconstriction to aid in dissection

2. Techniques may vary based on whether rhinoplasty approach is open or endonasal. Some examples are highlighted in the following figures (Figures 8.6a-c) [11].

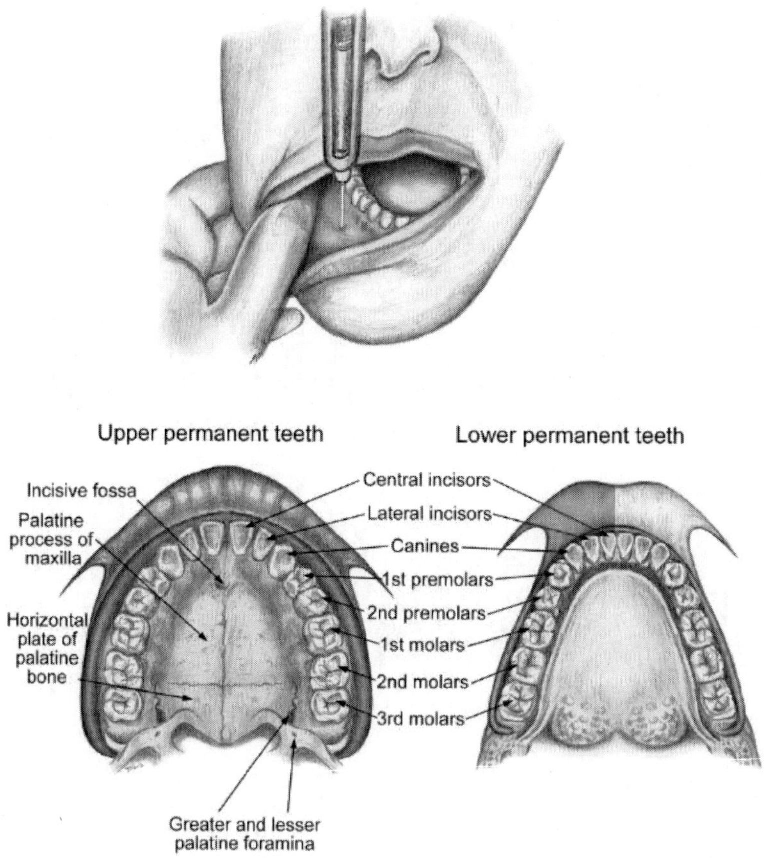

Figure 8.5. Mental nerve block. [10]

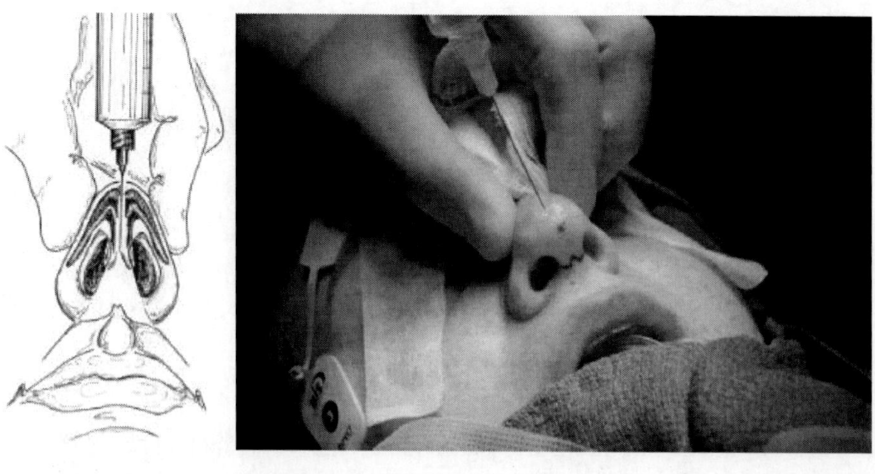

Figure 8.6a. Injection into subdermal plane in the midline of the columella from tip-defining points to the nasal spine in preparation for the external approach.

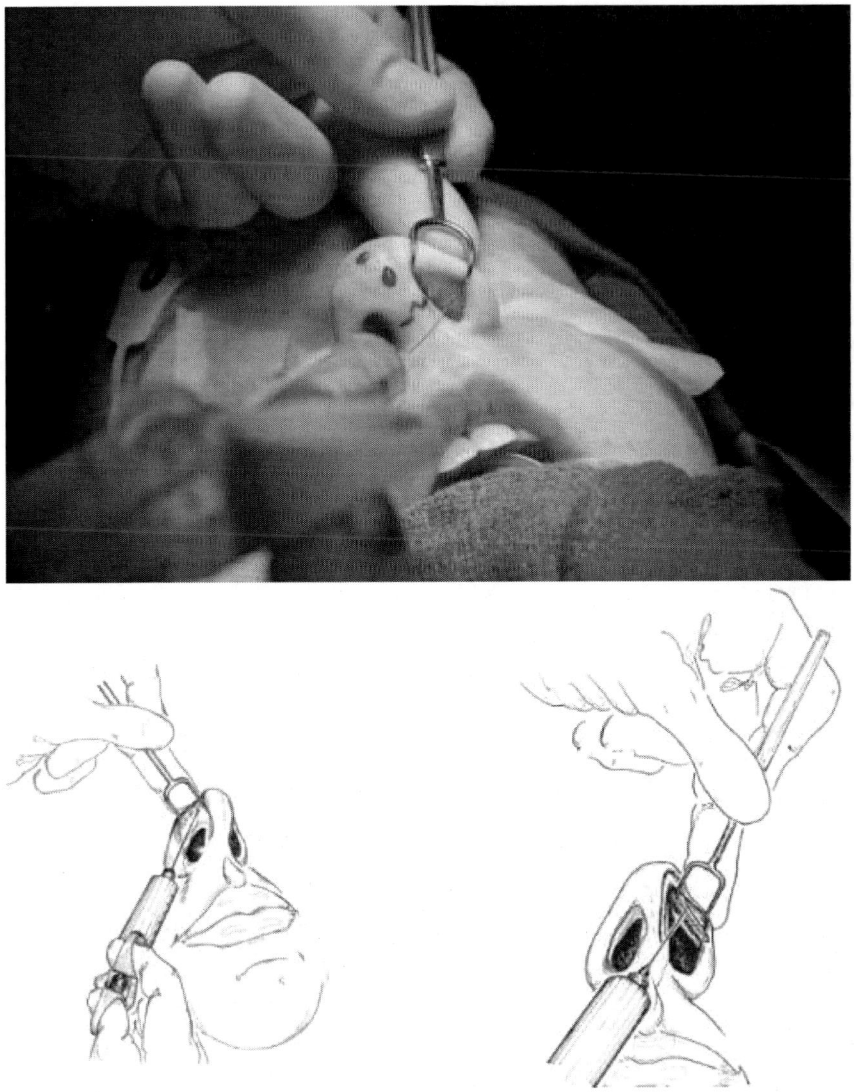

Figure 8.6b. Injection along the caudal margin of the lateral and intermediate crura of the lower lateral cartilage in preparation for marginal incision.

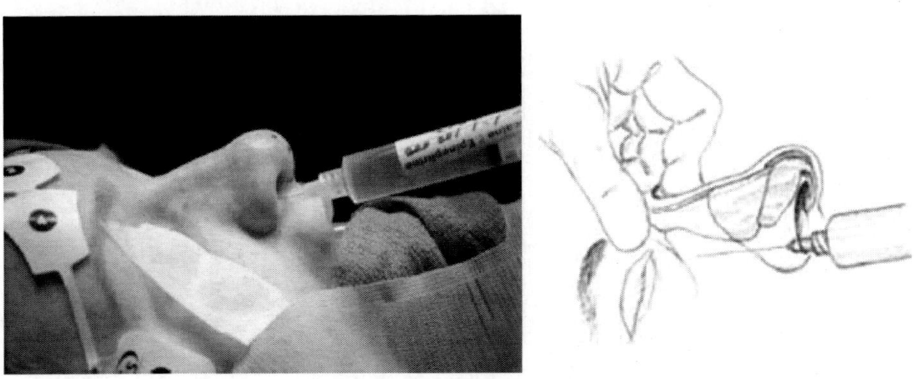

Figure 8.6c. Injection along the lateral nasal sidewall in preparation for lateral osteotomies.

Supraorbital Nerve Block

1. Useful technique when performing a variety of procedures including local flap reconstruction of forehead, glabella, eyebrows and associated structures, facial laceration repair, energy or chemical treatments, injection of filler or neuromuscular modulation as well as various brow lifting procedures (e.g. direct browlift, mid-forehead browlift)
2. Performed via transcutaneous approach
3. Supraorbital foramen/notch located along medial third of superior orbital rim. It should be palpated before injection.

Summary Points

1. Choice of anesthesia modality in facial plastic surgery procedures plays a critical role in successful patient outcomes
2. Knowledge of the various types of local anesthetics including dosing and adverse effects is essential in minimizing complications
3. Recognizing signs and symptoms of local anesthetic toxicity is critical so that emergency care in relation to the severity of the reaction can be administered
4. Appropriate pre-operative risk factor assessment as well as constant communication between the surgeon and anesthesiologist is necessary to ensure avoidance of complications
5. Proper techniques in performing various local anesthetic block procedures will aid in providing a comfortable experience for the patient as well as aiding the surgeon in a successful operation

References

[1] Themes, UFO. "Clinical Anatomy of the Head and Neck." *Anesthesia Key*, 22 Sept. 2016, https://aneskey.com/clinical-anatomy-of-the-head-and-neck/#.

[2] Kaur., Tuli BS, Tuli Isha Preet, Singh Amandeep, Tuli Navneet. "Chapter 1: Surgical Anatomy of the Ear." *Textbook of Ear, Nose and Throat*, 2nd ed., Jaypee Brothers Medical Publisher (P) Ltd., 2013, pp. 1–18.

[3] Volker, Dr. Joseph H. "Nasal Cavity." *Earth's Lab*, 4 Nov. 2021, https://www.earthslab.com/anatomy/nasal-cavity/.

[4] Ian K McLeod, MD. "Local Anesthetics: Introduction and History, Mechanism of Action, Chemical Structure." *Local Anesthetics: Introduction and History, Mechanism of Action, Chemical Structure*, Medscape, 23 Dec. 2021, https://emedicine.medscape.com/article/873879-overview#showall.

[5] DeJoseph L. Pou J. Local Anesthetic Facelift. *Facial Plast Surg Clin North Am.* Aug; 28(3): 409-418.

[6] Goldberg J, Silver M, Johnson M. Prevalence of Obstructive Sleep Apnea Risk According to the STOP-BANG Questionnaire in an Oral Surgery Office-Based Anesthesia Patient Population. *J Oral Maxillofac surg*. 2020 Dec; 78(12): 2156-2159.

[7] Prendiville S, Weiser S. Management of Anesthesia and facility in facelift surgery. *Facial Plast Surg Clin N Am* (2009) 531–538.

[8] Rinder C. Fire Safety in the operating room. *Curr Opin Anaesthesiol.* 2008. Dec (21) 6: 790-795.

[9] Latham, Joshua L., and Sean N. Martin. "Infiltrative Anesthesia in Office Practice." *American Family Physician*, 15 June 2014, https://www.aafp.org/afp/2014/0615/p956.html.

[10] "How Is the Mental Nerve Block Performed?" *Latest Medical News, Clinical Trials, Guidelines - Today on Medscape*, 3 May 2020, https://www.medscape.com/answers/82850-105904/how-is-the-mental-nerve-block-performed.

[11] Becker, Daniel G. "Infiltrative Anesthesia Technique." *Rhinoplasty Archive*, 16 Mar. 2020, https://www.rhinoplastyarchive.com/articles/rhinoplasty-fundamentals/infiltrative-anesthesia-technique.

Chapter 9

Patient Counseling and Ethics

Grant S. Gillman, MD
and Lauren A. Gardiner, MD

Introduction

The intent of facial plastic and reconstructive surgery is to improve appearance and function with the goal of enhancing patient quality of life. Self-confidence is critical to successful social interaction, and correction of a perceived defect can enhance self-esteem, reduce social anxiety, and enrich interpersonal relationships.

The ethical issues confronting facial plastic surgeons are not unlike those facing any other physician in regard to patient counsel as well as physician conduct. As compared to functional or medically necessary services, the cosmetic surgery arena has some unique considerations. These considerations include:

1. The distinctive interests, motivations and often heightened expectations of the cosmetic patient
2. The temptation of cosmetic surgeons to follow market trends
3. A different surgical payment and profit model.

These concerns present a different, additional set of ethical challenges to the facial plastic surgeon in the care of the cosmetic patient.

The Surgical Consultation - Patient Selection

The optimal physician – patient relationship is founded on open communication of expectations, risks, outcomes, and honest practices. A patient who is eager and willing to proceed surgically is not reason enough to commit oneself to being the surgical provider. The surgeon should feel comfortable with patient expectations and equally so with his / her ability to meet those goals. An ideal surgeon-patient match is more likely to result in a positive experience for both parties.

1. Appropriate patient selection should be as important to the surgeon as surgeon selection is to the patient.
2. The surgical consultation should prompt an honest and ethical self-assessment of the surgeon's ability to provide the service and the outcome requested.

In: Essential Facial Plastic and Reconstructive Surgery. Volume 1 ISBN: 979-8-89113-306-8
Editors: Yan Ho Lee and Ira Papel © 2024 Nova Science Publishers, Inc.

3. The ideal surgical patient would be one where:
    a. Surgical intervention can improve function or cosmesis
    b. Patient is likely to be reliable with follow up
    c. Expectations of surgical outcome are realistic, obtainable, confer no harm and the patient can be satisfied
4. "Red Flag" indicators may include: [1]
    a. Multiple revision surgeries
    b. Multiple surgical evaluations by different providers
    c. Motivation to please another individual
    d. Unrealistic expectations
    e. Pervasive unhappiness
    f. Concerns that are markedly disproportionate to objective physical findings
    g. Eagerness to proceed hastily to surgery but disinterest, inattentive, or dismissive of any discussion on risks or limitations of surgery
    h. Openly disparaging or angry comments regarding prior surgical providers
    i. Rude or demanding encounters with non-medical office staff coupled with overly flattering and complimentary behavior toward the surgeon
5. The surgeon must be aware that "do no harm" may also encompass post-operative psychological distress that could result from patient dissatisfaction or unhappiness.
6. Politely suggesting a second opinion with another provider is appropriate and potentially beneficial if for any reason the patient, their expectations, or the intended operation makes the surgeon feel uneasy at the time of the consultation.
7. Referral to a mental health provider may be a better option for some patients than a well performed surgical procedure.

The Pre-Operative Assessment

Sincere and frank patient counsel can only be meaningful if it follows a thoughtful, critical, and focused assessment of the patient and the area of concern.

1. The consulting surgeon should investigate motivations for surgery and remain cognizant of the social and racial contexts of beauty standards.
2. A thorough history and physical examination is the cornerstone of any pre-surgical evaluation.
3. Consideration of Medical Comorbidities
    a. General medical conditions which impede wound healing or might serve as relative contraindications to surgery should be noted, such as diabetes mellitus, tobacco use, vasculopathies, and nutritional status.
    b. The risk of a sub-optimal outcome in regard to a patient's pre-existing condition should be discussed and documented.
    c. Personality disorders and psychiatric conditions
        i. The consulting surgeon should appreciate the impact of psychiatric and personality disorders. These may influence patient reported outcomes as cosmetic interventions may play a role in bridging one's

perception of body image and self-esteem, irrespective of the technical success of a procedure.

ii. The incidence of psychiatric disorders in the plastic surgery patient population mirrors that of the general population with changing cultural and social norms over the last few decades. [2] The historical assertion that there is more psychological distress in the plastic surgery patient population is unfounded.

iii. Patients with psychiatric disorders may be poor surgical candidates as surgical interventions could worsen the underlying mental health condition. However, psychological factors should not serve as an absolute contraindication to surgery. Circumstances may vary from one patient to the next and should be considered on an individual basis.

iv. Younger age (<40), male sex, narcissistic personality disorder, and body dysmorphic disorder are negative predictive factors for patient satisfaction after a cosmetic intervention. [3]

v. It is not the surgeon's role to diagnose psychiatric conditions, but it is prudent to be aware of commonly encountered conditions:
  - Body Dysmorphic Disorder (BDD): defined as disproportionate obsession with a minimal or imagined defect of the body (see "Red Flag" indicators in Patient Selection). [4]
    - Cosmetic rhinoplasty is the most common requested surgical procedure in BDD patients. [4]
    - High potential for patient dissatisfaction. Avoid surgical interventions where surgical correction of a perceived flaw is near-impossible.
  - Borderline Personality Disorder (BPD): Defined as impulsivity, risk taking, self-destructive and self-harm behaviors. Surgical procedures can serve as an expression of self-harm [4]

vi. For some patients (psychiatric patients, BDD, gender dysphoria/transformation) surgical consultation should be performed as part of an interdisciplinary health team, specifically involving the patient's mental health professional, and when relevant, the hormone prescribing physician.

4. Photo-Documentation
   a. Photo-documentation serves as an effective and objective communication tool between patient and provider and, when needed, an accurate reference of the pre-operative state. Photographs serve as a vital component of the medicolegal record.
   b. Telemedicine or screenshots from patient encounters should not replace pre-operative photographs for elective surgery.
   c. Photographs are integral to surgical planning and as an intra- and post-operative reference.

   d. As an ethical consideration, in any pre/post photo gallery of patient outcomes for marketing materials, the photography should be standardized and consistent as not to misrepresent any particular post-surgical outcome.
   e. If a potential surgery patient will not allow preoperative photos to be taken this is a very concerning event and should disqualify this patient from surgery.

Patient Counseling and Informed Consent

Patients should be clearly counselled regarding the general procedural risks but also the limitations of surgery as it might relate to them specifically. Relevant specific observations from the physical examination that might guide the discussion include Fitzpatrick skin classification, skin thickness, skin tone, propensity to scarring, outcomes of prior surgery, and existing facial asymmetry. Informed consent should include:

1. Patient capacity (or ability) to make the decision
2. Surgeon disclosure of information on the diagnosis, indications, and treatment, including the expected risks and benefits (and the likelihood of such risks and benefits)
3. Patient ability to comprehend the relevant information
4. Patient voluntary agreement to proceed without coercion or duress
   a. The majority of medical malpractice claims come from inadequate informed consent and lack of communication of risks involved, followed by excessive scarring and disfigurement, functional complaints, and post-operative pain. [5, 6] The most litigated procedures are blepharoplasties and rhinoplasties. [7] Potential risks, limitations, or complications of surgery discussed should be thoroughly documented in the patient record.
   b. Patient counsel and informed consent should be carried out in a language that is comfortable and familiar to the patient. This might require the services of a translator.
   c. The ethically responsible surgeon should not limit pre-operative discussion solely to possible favorable outcomes. Any omission of limitations during the pre-operative discussion may be perceived by the patient as "an excuse" if it arises post-operatively following an unfavorable event.
   d. The surgeon should counsel patients on the potential need for revision surgery.
   e. Age considerations
      i. For patients <18 years of age, it is advisable to assess all functional issues, and/or longevity of patient dissatisfaction with a facial characteristic and to ensure the legal guardian is accepting of surgical intervention.
      ii. For elderly patients who are interested in elective surgery, pre-operative counseling should emphasize risk of poorer wound healing or a suboptimal cosmetic result given the skin's reduced tissue elasticity.

Ethics – General Considerations

1. Surgical experience
   a. Surgeons should limit their procedures and practice to areas in which they are properly trained and can reasonably be expected to perform to the standard of care. This is not the same as asking "am I the very best surgeon for the job?" but rather "am I reasonably comfortable and confident that I can achieve a certain outcome?"
   b. "Standard of care" refers to reasonably exercising the prudence, caution and quality of care that would be expected of a similarly qualified practitioner.
   c. When asked, surgeons should feel ethically bound to accurately disclose the extent of their experience to the patient, including any relevant limitations.
   d. The possible involvement of trainees in the surgery should be noted on any surgical consent form and the extent thereof further discussed openly if the patient expresses interest.
2. Continuing Medical Education (CME) / Scientific advancements
   a. All physicians have a duty to participate in CME activities throughout one's career
   b. The surgeon should have up-to-date knowledge of new medical advancements and therapies. These options should be discussed among the "alternatives to surgery" during the informed consent. If surgery is not recommended, alternative therapies should be communicated to the patient, including the possible limitations, and when relevant, lack of long-term data/outcomes.
3. Social Media/Marketing
   a. Competition with advertising, pricing, and the growing number of non-facial plastic surgeon providers has created a challenging marketplace. Despite the temptation to gain a competitive advantage, practitioners should ethically limit any claims made or implied through promotional materials to those that are honest, truthful and verifiable.
   b. Current trends support the notion that patients may select their provider based on social media and marketing presence over academic reputation and experience. [8]
   c. Aesthetic factors of a physician or group's media account may falsely instill trust and clinical acumen to patients.
   d. Unregulated media promotion of surgical and procedural outcomes threatens realistic expectations for patients who may seek surgery.
   e. When used thoughtfully - with the goal of education over garnering new business - social media channels afford an outlet to disseminate information, debunk false media medical claims, and promote clinical advancements within the field. [8]
   f. The role of academic societies and leadership within facial plastic surgery should be encouraged to disseminate accurate information on surgical procedures and for consumer protection. [9]
4. Economics and Ethical Billing practices

a. For cosmetic procedures, a complete accounting of costs (or accurate estimate) should be given to the patient beforehand and honored thereafter. There shouldn't be any "after-the-fact" supplemental billing.
b. Disclosure at the time of initial consultation for cosmetic surgery should include any out-of-pocket costs that may be incurred, should revision surgery be necessary.
c. It is unethical to over-represent the nature of any given condition in order to obtain preauthorization for surgery and to unbundle procedures to increase reimbursement and revenue.
d. Insurance companies should not be expected to cover costs implicit in cosmetic surgery. Cosmetic "add-ons" should not be misrepresented or bundled into functional surgery. The additional cosmetic work should be billed separately. Any documentation should explicitly state the combined functional and cosmetic nature of the surgery.

Summary Points

1. Ethical conduct and behavior affects every facet of patient care.
2. Facial plastic and reconstructive surgeons have unique considerations.
3. Implementation of ethical medical practice requires thoughtfulness, communication, thorough documentation, and recognition that medicine is a collaborative relationship between the patient and provider.

References

[1] Johnson, J. T, and Clark A Rosen. *Bailey's Head and Neck Surgery - Otolaryngology Volume 1.* Philadelphia: Wolters Kluwer Health, 2014.

[2] Ferraro, G.A., F. Rossano, and F. D'Andrea. "Self-Perception and Self-Esteem of Patients Seeking Cosmetic Surgery." *Aesthetic Plastic Surgery* 29, no. 3 (June 2005): 184–89. https://doi.org/10.1007/s00266-004-0124-3.

[3] Herruer, Jasmijn M., Judith B. Prins, Niels van Heerbeek, Godelieve W. J. A. Verhage-Damen, and Koen J. A. O. Ingels. "Negative Predictors for Satisfaction in Patients Seeking Facial Cosmetic Surgery: A Systematic Review." *Plastic and Reconstructive Surgery* 135, no. 6 (June 2015): 1596–1605. https://doi.org/10.1097/PRS.0000000000001264.

[4] Wever, Casper Candido (Capi), Ana Maria Elisabeth (Anita) Wever, and Mark Constantian. "Psychiatric Disorders in Facial Plastic Surgery." *Facial Plastic Surgery Clinics of North America* 28, no. 4 (November 2020): 451–60. https://doi.org/10.1016/j.fsc.2020.06.003.

[5] Atiyeh, Bishara S., Michel T. Rubeiz, and Shady N. Hayek. "Aesthetic/Cosmetic Surgery and Ethical Challenges." *Aesthetic Plastic Surgery* 44, no. 4 (August 2020): 1364–74. https://doi.org/10.1007/s00266-020-01821-z.

[6] Ong, Adrian A, Andrew Kelly, Geroline A Castillo, Michele M Carr, and David A Sherris. "Characterization of Medical Malpractice Litigation After Rhinoplasty in the United States." *Aesthetic Surgery Journal* 41, no. 10 (September 14, 2021): 1132–38. https://doi.org/10.1093/asj/sjaa380.

[7] Svider, Peter F., Brieze R. Keeley, Osvaldo Zumba, Andrew C. Mauro, Michael Setzen, and Jean Anderson Eloy. "From the Operating Room to the Courtroom: A Comprehensive Characterization of Litigation Related to Facial Plastic Surgery Procedures." *The Laryngoscope* 123, no. 8 (August 2013): 1849–53. https://doi.org/10.1002/lary.23905.

[8] "When Is Advertising a Plastic Surgeon's Individual 'Brand' Unethical?" *AMA Journal of Ethics* 20, no. 4 (April 1, 2018): 372–78. https://doi.org/10.1001/journalofethics.2018.20.4.msoc2-1804.

[9] Dayan, Steven. "Revision Plastic Surgery Reality Television: What's Good About *Botched*?" *JAMA* 319, no. 21 (June 5, 2018): 2156. https://doi.org/10.1001/jama.2018.5756.

Part 2. Reconstruction of Defects

Chapter 10

Local Flaps

Scott Stegemann, DO
and Jonathan Y. Lee, MD, MPH

Introduction

A flap is defined as a component of tissue that maintains its own blood supply while being transferred from donor to recipient site. Local flaps refer specifically to adjacent tissue transfer such that the vascularized donor tissue shares a border with the defect requiring closure. Local flaps are generally categorized by their movement: rotation, advancement, transposition. Within these movement categories, specific flaps are named by their design shape and/or epitomes. The use of local flaps is indicated in closing defects of a size that would incur unacceptably high tension in the setting of primary closure. The rearrangement of tissue is leveraging relative tissue laxity of adjacent areas to reduce tension of closure at both the donor and recipient sites. The varying movements and designs will have differing efficacy depending on the anatomic location, inherent tissue compliance, and defect size; however, it is common that multiple local flap options are viable.

Vascularity

1. Cutaneous Blood Supply Theory (Angiosomes and Fasciocutaneous Plexus)
    a. Knowledge of dermal blood supply anatomy is paramount when designing local flaps to ensure adequate perfusion postoperatively
    b. Angiosomes [1, 2]
        i. Angiosomes are macroscopic units that provide vascularity to skin and musculoskeletal systems
            - Defined as a three-dimensional segment of tissue perfused by a single arterial source, or perforator
            - Each perforator supplies a unique territory, which is called a perforasome [3]
        ii. Adjacent angiosomes are joined via arterio-arterial anastomoses and various arterial plexuses
        iii. This system provides sufficient arterial blood flow to cutaneous tissue, as a defective perforator can be overridden by the adjacent angiosomes

In: Essential Facial Plastic and Reconstructive Surgery. Volume 1 ISBN: 979-8-89113-306-8
Editors: Yan Ho Lee and Ira Papel
© 2024 Nova Science Publishers, Inc.

 iv. An increased number of arterio-arterial anastomoses exist in areas of overlapping vascular territories to provide smooth reliable blood flow
 c. Fasciocutaneous plexus [4, 5]
 i. Perfusion to cutaneous tissue is through a combination of various fascial vascular plexuses
 - Prefascial and subfascial plexuses are developed from various smaller musculocutaneous perforators, septocutaneous branches and direct cutaneous branches that anastomose at musculofascial junction
 - Prefascial plexus tends to be more thoroughly developed and mature
 ii. These plexuses and their multifaceted vascular supply provide arterial perfusion to cutaneous and subcutaneous tissue
2. Random pattern [6, 7, 8, 9]
 a. Defined as a flap perfusion pattern that derives vascular supply from interconnecting dermal and subdermal plexuses and not from a direct cutaneous arterial supply
 i. Plexuses exist at base of flap
 ii. Perfusion is random however reliable
 - Lacks significant bias in its vascular supply
 iii. Robust perfusion from this network preserves vascularity to flap following undermining
3. Axial pattern [6, 7, 8, 9]
 a. Defined as a flap vascular pattern based on an anatomically-recognized cutaneous arteriovenous system running along its axis
 b. Provides a large and robust option for wound closure
 c. Can incorporate a septocutaneous artery within flap-pedicle axis offering greater survival and length compared to random pattern flaps
 d. Design requires knowledge of vascular anatomy and various vascular territories associated with different facial arteriovenous bundles

Movement

1. General principles
 a. Local flap success is reliant on the degree of tissue laxity and resulting tissue tension at the inset site (i.e., primary defect site)
 i. Movement principles in local flap design is dependent on maximizing adjacent tissue laxity with minimizing tension at the repair
 ii. Other considerations include tissue color/texture, tissue thickness, presence of hair follicles, degree of undermining and size of the primary defect
2. Rotation Flaps
 a. General principle: flap is incised followed by adequate undermining to allow for adjacent tissue to pivot around an axis into a defect [8]

i. Flap is used to fill primary defect
ii. Secondary defect is cutaneous void created by flap movement
    - Secondary defect typically closed by primary closure, however larger defects may require an additional local flap depending on size and skin laxity

b. Movement [8]
    i. Curvilinear flaps which pivot into a defect
    ii. Rotation dependent on degree of undermining and skin elasticity
    iii. Typically there is minimal benefit to extending the arc of rotation beyond 180 degrees from the axis of primary defect

c. Common design options [8]
    i. Designed with a curvilinear orientation in direction of defect
        - Radius of arc of rotation should be 1-2 times height of defect; length of arc should be 4 times width of defect base
        - Height-width ratio of flap should be 2:1
        - Need wide undermining to allow for adequate, tension-free rotation of flap as it pivots to fill defect
    ii. O-Z flap [8]
        - Double rotation flap using two contralateral components to fill circular defect
        - Can be random or axial pattern depending on location
        - From defect, two lines are drawn extending laterally from opposite sides of defect along a common bisecting axis
            - Lines are mirror arcs of one another
            - Incision carried to subcutaneous tissue and flaps are undermined
            - Flaps are advanced and rotated to fill primary defect and sutured to one another
        - Minimizes tissue distortion of adjacent structures because tension vectors are parallel to two rotating flaps
    iii. L-plasty (A-L, O-L) [9]
        - Incision is extended along and beyond base of the defect, allowing for rotation around pivot point and inset of adjacent tissue into wound
    iv. T-plasty (A-T, O-T) [9]
        - Bilateral version of L-plasty
        - Allows for redistribution of tension between two advancing edges over a larger area
        - Linear incision carried along base of the defect in both directions
        - Opposing sides are then advanced and rotated to meet in middle at base of cutaneous defect
        - Burrow triangles can be used to excise redundant tissue
    v. Cervicofacial flap (Mustarde flap) [8, 9, 10]
        - Workhorse flap for large cheek defects

- Makes use of ample skin laxity in cheek and neck
- Random pattern
- Combination of advancement and rotation
- In traditional anterior advancement, incision runs superolaterally from defect along subciliary crease to lateral canthus then to preauricular crease, inferiorly around earlobe and along posterior hairline into inferior cervical crease
  - Incision and dissection are performed in a staged, as-needed manner with constant reassessment of arc of rotation to ensure excessive dissection is not performed
  - Allows for a lateral-to-medial advancement vector
  - Important consideration during design and dissection is possible blunting of nasolabial sulcus inferiorly and inferomedial tension on lower eyelid
    - Can minimize secondary movement and decrease tension flap by using tacking sutures (placed parallel to pedicle to stabilize flap and decrease tension)
    - Can use anchoring sutures to further secure flap to underlying periosteum of bony structures to further decrease tension
- Careful undermining in subcutaneous plane must to done to avoid damage to facial nerve
- Careless undermining can also disrupt blood supply and result in flap necrosis and failure

d. Pearls [8, 9]
  i. Rotational flaps have a great amount of flexibility
  ii. Due to broad design, these flaps tend to have robust vascular supply
  iii. Because of long, curved incision, need to be cognizant of skin incision as they will typically not lie cleanly within a relaxed skin tension line (RSTL)
  iv. Burrow triangles can be used to eliminate excess subcutaneous tissue

3. Advancement Flaps
  a. Advancement flaps are random pattern flap used in repair of cutaneous surgical defects [9]
  b. General principle: flap incised, undermined and advanced forward in a single linear vector to fill a defect
  c. Movement [8, 9, 11]
    i. Allows for reconstruction via unidirectional movement of flap into defect
    ii. Two types of movement
      - Primary movement: sliding or advancement of tissue into primary defect
      - Secondary movement: displacement of adjacent skin toward primary defect that results from tension after wound closure

(responsible for unfavorable cosmetic distortion of mobile facial structures, such as lips, lower eyes and nasal ala)

iii. Undermining done to provide adequate mobility of local tissue while preserving vascular supply

d. Common design options

i. Classic advancement flap (U-plasty) [9]
- Unilateral advancement flap
- Flap and pedicle move together in a single vector to fill defect
- Typical defect-to-flap length 1:3
- Can utilize Burrow triangles to excise redundant tissue and standing cones as needed to allow for incorporation of skin incisions into RSTLs

ii. Bilateral advancement flap (H-plasty) [8, 9]
- Two opposing unilateral advancing edges move to fill a common defect
- Allows tension to be redistributed over a greater area compared to classic unilateral advancement flap
- Resulting H-shaped scar can be masked in areas with natural parallel straight lines
- Opposing flap lengths do not need to be symmetrical
- Elasticity and redundancy of tissue from each site determine appropriate length
- Like unilateral flap, can use Burrow triangles to incorporate incisions into RSTLs

iii. V-Y advancement flap [8, 9]
- Flap design principles
  - Width of triangular flap is equal to the widest dimeter of primary defect
  - Length of flap is twice the height of primary defect
  - Apex angle of triangular flap should be 30 degrees
- Triangular flap incised and judiciously undermined taking care to avoid undermining pedicle
  - Movement mimics "pushing" motion into defect, allows for minimal tension at incision sites
- Can augment movement with rotation or transposition
  - At least one-fourth of flap area should be used as underlying pedicle when rotational or transposition component is used
  - If employed, there can be up to 180 degree of twisting of pedicle; should not exhibit more twisting motion as this can compromised blood flow
- V-Y advancement flaps typically provide excellent skin color and texture matching

iv. Cervicofacial advancement flap
- Combination of advancement and rotation

e. Pearls [8, 9, 11]
  i. Should consider facial RSTLs and cosmetic junctional units in preoperative planning
    - Scars with advancement flaps tend to be long and straight, so attention needs to be paid to appropriately hiding scar along these lines
  ii. Successful advancement flaps require appropriate adjacent tissue laxity
    - Any tension vector that does exist after repair should parallel axis of flap
  iii. Maximum tension is at distal border of flap

4. Transposition Flaps
  a. General principle: flap is incised, undermined and then pivoted toward defect over an incomplete skin bridge
  b. Movement [8, 10, 12]
    i. Linear flaps are undermined and then pivoted into a defect over an incomplete skin bridge, resulting in transposition of tissue from an area of laxity to an inelastic area
    ii. Specific flap movement is dependent on what flap is being used
  c. Common design options
    i. Z-plasty [13]
      - Random pattern transposition flap
      - Transposition of two triangular flaps results in partial closure of the defect
      - Can also be used to manipulate incision vector to better correspond with RSTLs or cosmetic junctions
    ii. Rhomboid flap (Limberg design) [8, 10, 12, 14]
      - Workhorse flap typically for small defects
      - Random pattern
      - Flap designed starts as creating a rhomboid over defect
        - Long axis between two 60 degree angles; short axis of flap between two 120 degree angles
      - o Lines of incision should try to be parallel to RSTL
      - o Short axis incision extension should be within lines of maximal extensibility, as this is where secondary defect will be
      - o Placement in line with maximal extensibility will decrease scar formation
        - First extension limb of flap should equal length of one side of defect toward the area of maximal laxity
        - Extension limb extends off short axis of rhombus, so cares need to be taken to orient flap properly
        - Second extension limb should be directed back toward defect at a 60 degree angle from first limb
        - Once area of maximal laxity is determined, incision of rhombus and extension limb is made and undermined

    - Rhomboid flap is then pivoted into defect
    - Secondary defect closed by primary repair
- Vascular supply is at base of the flap
- Modifications to Limberg rhomboid flap [8, 12]
    - Dufourmental (Figure 10.1)
        - Uses 90 degree to create shorter arc of rotation, decreasing pivotal restraint resulting in less tension at tip and wider pedicle
        - Used for more square defects
    - Webster
        - Uses 30 degree instead of 60 degree flap tip angle to transpose a more narrow flap into defect
        - Reduces tension and aids in closure of a smaller secondary defect
- Versatile flap with ability to match skin color and texture
- Has four possible orientations, allowing for proper orientation in accordance with RSTLs or at the junction of facial aesthetic subunit

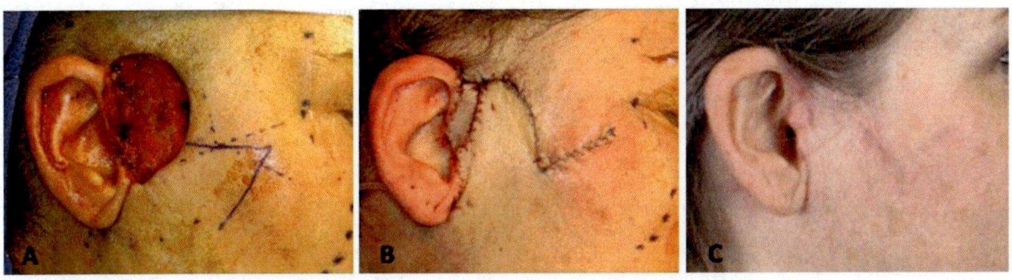

Figure 10.1. Rhomboid flap. A) Lateral cheek defect, 3x5cm. Markings of a rhomboid flap (dufourmental variant). B) Inset of the dufourmental flap. Full thickness skin graft for the ear component of the defect to maintain separate subunits. C) 12 months postoperative results.

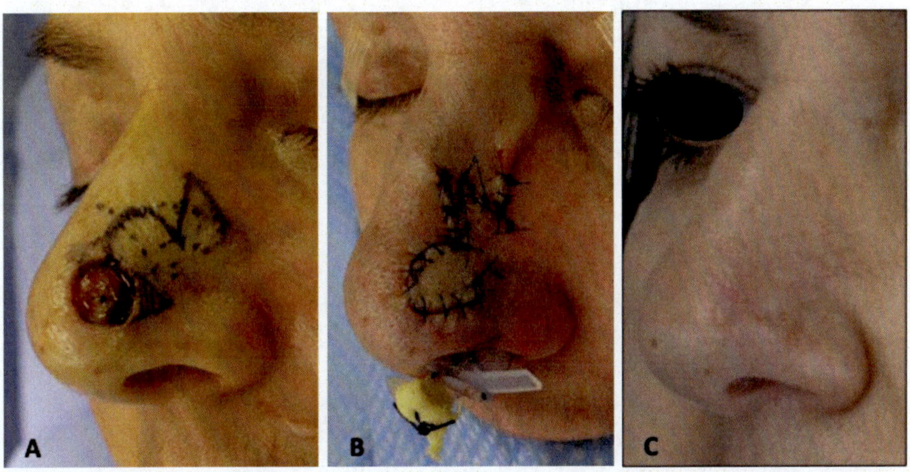

Figure 10.2. Bilobed flap. A) Nasal tip defect, 0.8mm. Markings of the bilobed flap with Zitelli modification. B) Inset of the bilobed flap. Nostril retainers sewn in place to help maintain alar shape. C) 12 months postoperative results.

iii. Bilobed flap [8, 10] (Figure 10.2)
- Workhorse flap for facial reconstruction
- Random pattern flap with rotational components
  - Two lobes based on single vascular pedicle
- Zitelli bilobed flap
  - Identify pivot point equal to radius of defect lateral to defect
  - Outer arc determined by rotating a length equal to 3 times radius around pivot point
  - Inner arc determined by rotating a length equal to 2 times radius around pivot point
  - Primary lobe is marked with a diameter equal to diameter of defect with axis measured 45 degrees from axis bisecting pivot point and defect (lobe extends from inner arc to outer arc)
  - Secondary lobe is marked with a diameter less than diameter of defect and centered 90 degrees from axis bisecting pivot point and defect (lobe extends from inner arc to outer arc with a triangular extension equal to length of radius of primary defect)
  - Flaps are raised, undermined and pivoted into position
    - Primary lobe pivots to cover primary defect
    - Secondary lobe pivots to cover defect of primary lobe
    - Defect of secondary lobe is closed primarily
  - Standing cone deformity excised
- Useful in areas where need to minimize tension directly adjacent to primary defect

d. Pearls [8, 10, 12]

i. Depth of incision should mirror depth of defect to maintain continuity

ii. Careful preoperative planning is needed to make sure there is tension-free closure

iii. Excellent color and texture matching with predictable flap viability

iv. Can cause dramatic distortion of distal nose if performed incorrectly

Anatomic Location of Defect

1. Scalp/Forehead

a. Considerations include general tissue inelasticity, preservation of function and aesthetic relationship to surrounding aesthetic units, location of hair follicles and proximity to neurovascular structures [15, 16]

b. Robust vascular supply

c. Key differences between scalp and forehead reconstruction [15, 16, 17]

i. Scalp is largely immobile compared to forehead

    ii. Forehead and temporal areas feature RSTLs and scars can be concealed in natural rhytides
    iii. Forehead is cosmetically noticeable so careful surgical planning and technique needed to avoid distortion of hairline or eyebrow (especially pertinent to large rotational flaps)
  d. Reconstructive options
    i. O-Z rotational flap
      - Useful in closure of larger scalp defects
      - Wide undermining increasing tissue movement to fill defect
      - Can utilize axial blood supply from STA laterally, occipital artery posteriorly or supratrochlear or supraorbital artery anteriorly
    ii. Orticochea flap [15, 18]
      - Useful in closure of large scalp defects
      - Local advancement and rotation flap comprised of three mobile segments; each segment receives axial pattern perfusion from superficial temporal, occipital and supratrochlear or supraorbital artery
      - Each flap is extensively undermined to allow for movement
      - Important to keep tips of individual flaps approximately 90 degrees to prevent vascular compromise
      - Useful reconstructive option for severely debilitated patients who cannot tolerated anesthesia
    iii. Unilateral or bilateral advancement flaps (U-plasty or H plasty)
      - Useful for small forehead lesions
      - Less efficacious for scalp lesions given inelastic nature of scalp tissue
      - Bilateral advancement flap reduces tension at defect site by redistribution over a greater area
      - Wide undermining allows for closure that can hide incisions in rhytides
    iv. Rhomboid flaps
      - Can be useful in temporal region
    v. A-T plasty
      - Can be useful in smaller scalp defects

2. Cheek
  a. Cheek is the largest facial aesthetic unit with a rich subdermal vascular plexus [19]
  b. Local flap reconstruction of the cheek must cover primary defect but also ensure adjacent aesthetic subunits are not distorted via secondary movement or excessive tension at repair site [19]
  c. Reconstructive options
    i. Cervicofacial advancement flap (Mustarde flap)
      - Workhorse flap of cheek reconstruction

- Random pattern flap that is elevated in sub-superficial muscular aponeurotic system (SMAS) plane
- Need to avoid distorting oral commissure, lower eyelid, nasal ala or tragus

ii. Unilateral advancement flap (U-plasty)
- Useful in reconstruction of medial cheek

iii. V-Y advancement flaps
- Useful in moderate-to-large medial cheek defects

iv. Rhomboid flap
- Transposition flaps useful for lateral cheek defects now amendable for V-Y advancement
- Useful reconstructive option for small medial cheek defects

3. Nose
   a. Reconstruction based on the various nasal aesthetic subunits [20]
      i. Subunits differ in skin texture, thickness, pilosebaceous structure and underlying subcutaneous framework
   b. Reconstruction options
      i. Z-plasty
         - Random pattern transposition flap
         - Useful in nasal dorsum and sidewall reconstruction
      ii. Dorsal nasal flap (Rieger flap) [21]
         - Axial pattern flap based on angular artery
         - Modified rotation flap that recruits excessive skin from glabella
            - Triangular-shaped flap incised over glabella
            - Curvilinear line drawn inferior passing along nasal sidewall-cheek junction to level of defect
            - Flap elevated and rotated to fill defect
            - Secondary defect then closed with a V-Y advancement flap
            - Useful in nasal dorsum and sidewall reconstruction
      iii. Bilobed flap
         - Workhorse flap for nasal tip reconstruction
         - Also useful in nasal dorsum and larger sidewall defects
      iv. V-Y advancement and cervicofacial flaps
         - Useful in nasolabial fold reconstruction
      v. Rhomboid flap
         - Useful in small lateral wall defects
4. Lip
   a. Lip can be a challenge for reconstruction [22]
      i. Distortion of vermillion border, Cupid bow, philtrum and oral commissure can lead to noticeable aesthetic deformities
      ii. Need to maintain normal facial animation and dental coverage as well
   b. Cutaneous tissue of lip is highly elastic however also adherent to underlying orbicularis oris muscle (OO) [22]

    i. Careful sharp dissection is necessary to advancement cutaneous tissue while preserving OO function
    ii. Disruption of muscle will impact function and need repair
c. Flap selection for vermillion border reconstruction depends on size and depth of defect
d. Reconstruction options [22]
    i. Perialar crescentic flap
        - Random pattern advancement flap
        - Used for lateral partial thickness defects affecting 1/3 of lip and full thickness defects affecting up to 2/3 of lip
    ii. Estlander flap
        - Axial pattern flap based on inferior labial artery
        - Utilizes tissue from opposing lip for reconstruction of lateral lip defects involving philtrum and commissure
        - Can lead to distortion of oral and facial animation
    iii. Gilles fan flap
        - Random pattern advancement rotation flap
        - Used for central full thickness defects up to 2/3 of lip that does not involve commissure
    iv. Karapandzic flap [23, 24, 25]
        - Axial pattern based on superior labial artery
        - Used in reconstruction of central defects up to 2/3 of upper lip
        - Bilateral advancement flap where full thickness adjacent labial tissue incised and inset to fill defect
            - Rectangular full thickness defect
            - Flaps are elevated from incisions running parallel to lip margin in nasolabial and mentolabial folds
            - Flaps then freed from underlying OO to increase mobility
            - Bilateral flaps advanced to fill defect and sutured to appropriate size to approximate height and width of lip
    v. V-Y advancement flap
        - Can be used to reconstruction vermillion border and commissure

Complications

1. Smoking - number one risk factor for local flap failure
    a. Increased risk of microvascular disease which can compromise postoperative perfusion and wound healing
2. Other risk factors: hypertension, diabetes, history of radiation and collagen disorders
3. Usually, complications with facial local flaps are mild
    a. Attributed to robust blood supply to face
4. Most common complication is venous congestion due to tension

5. Other complications
    a. Wound infection
    b. Seroma/hematoma
    c. Abnormal hair distribution
    d. Poor cosmetic outcomes
        i. Standing cone deformities
        ii. Trapdoor deformities
    e. Hypertrophic scarring
6. Major complications are extremely rare

Summary Points

1. The key to successful facial reconstruction with local flaps is vascularity. Random and axial pattern flaps are both useful reconstructive options
2. Flap viability is inversely proportional to tension. The more tension that exists at the site of local flap reconstruction, the less perfusion there will be
3. Reconstruction of skin defects of the face with local flaps requires analysis of skin anatomy, appropriate flap selection and design, analysis and matching of skin texture and color and delicate soft tissue manipulation. Normal anatomy and aesthetic landmarks should be preserved if possible
4. The commonly recognized workhorse flaps of facial reconstruction are the rhomboid, bilobed and cervicofacial advancement flaps, however there are numerous options available
5. Complications with local flap reconstruction tend to be mild. Patient history is an important predictive factor of flap success

Patient Case

A 65-year-old female is presenting with a biopsy positive melanoma of the central cheek. She has been indicated for wide local excision and a sentinel lymph node biopsy of the ipsilateral neck. An image of the cheek defect after excision of the lesion is shown (Figure 10.3).

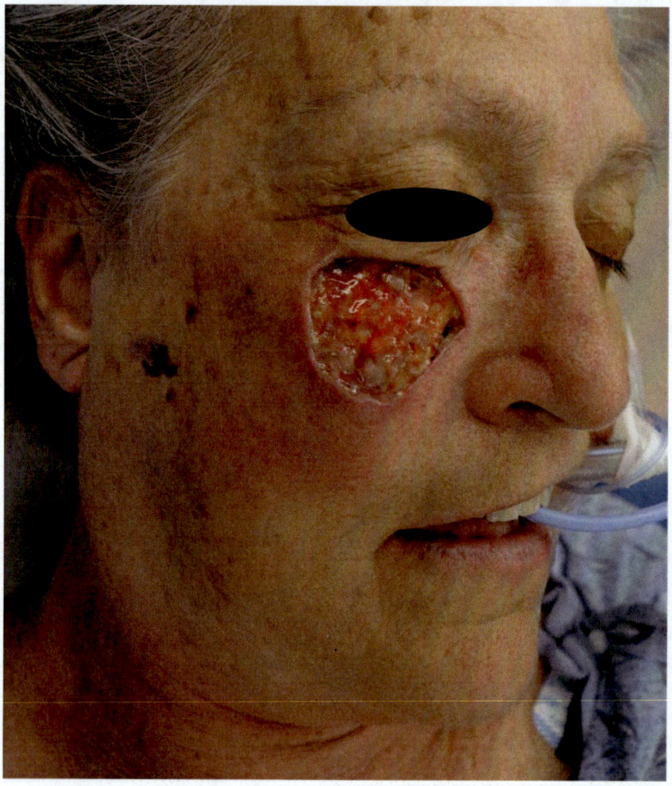

Figure 10.3. Patient case: cheek defect.

Q1. When choosing the reconstructive option in this patient, what are the advantages and disadvantages of local flap options?

A1. The main advantage of local flaps is the principle of replacing "like" with "like". A local flap, by definition, shares a border with defect. Therefore, the tissue of a local flap is most likely to match the lost tissue's characteristics including pigment, texture, and contour. In addition, a local flap maintains blood supply, which will result in relatively faster healing, compared to a graft. The disadvantages are in regard to design limitations, which are determined by the size and location of the defect. Since local flaps utilize rearrangement of tissue laxity to achieve closure, there can be significant distortion of the surrounding tissues which may preclude their use.

Q2 cervicofacial rotation advancement flap is determined to be the best option for reconstruction in this patient. How should the flap be designed to best maximize aesthetic outcome and minimize complications?

A2. When possible, the planned incisions should be placed in existing rhytids, Langer's lines, or borders between facial subunits to best camouflage subsequent scars. Although the defect does not extend to the junction of the cheek and nose, excising the tissue between the defect and the nasolabial fold as part of the burrows triangle of the flap should be considered. When designing the incision lateral to the lower eyelid, it should arc upward in the temple are to a level at or above the lateral canthus before transitioning downward in the preauricular area. This will help position the tension vector of the flap more superiorly to mitigate downward pull on the lower eyelid to avoid malposition postoperatively.

Q3. When elevating the cervicofacial flap, how can iatrogenic neurovascular injury be mitigated while optimizing flap survival?

A3. The cervicofacial flap can be elevated in either the sub-SMAS plane or in the subcutaneous plane. Similar to a skin-only rhytidectomy, elevation in the subcutaneous plane can be done quickly and safely with a tunneling technique using curved scissors. Albeit, the blood supply to the flap is not as robust compared to a deeper plane dissection and partial flap loss is more common with larger defects that require more extensive flap elevation. A deeper sub-SMAS plane elevation requires a relatively slower dissection under direct vision to avoid nerve injury; however, the vascularity is more robust and should be considered when needing to elevate a larger flap.

References

[1] Taylor, G.I., Palmer, J.H. The vascular territories (angiosomes) of the body: experimental study and clinical applications. Mar 1987. *Br J Plast Surg*, *40*(2): pp 113-141.

[2] Fujii, M., Terashi, H. Angiosomes and Tissue Healing. Jun 2019. *Ann Vasc Disease,* 12(2): 147-150.

[3] Saint-Cyr, M., Wong, C., Schaverien, M., Mojallal, A., Rohrich, R. The Perforasome Theory: Vascular Anatomy and Clinical Implications. Nov 2009. *J Plast Recon Surg,* 124(5): pp 1529-1544.

[4] Cormack, G.C., Lamberty, B.G. Fasciocutaneous Vessels: Their Distribution on the Trunk and Limbs and Their Clinical Application in Tissue Transfer. 1984. *J Clin Anat,* 6(2): pp 121-131.

[5] Boretto, J.G., De Cicco, F.L. *Fasciocutaneous Flaps*. Jul 2022. NCBI StatPearls Pub [Internet]. Treasure Island (FL). StatPearls Publishing.

[6] McGregor, A., Morgan, G. Axial and Random Pattern Flaps. Jul 1973. *Br J Plast Surg*, 26(3): pp 202-213.

[7] Hashimoto, I., Soshi Ishida, Y.A., Kashkiwagi, K., Yutaro Yamashita, K.M., Yamato, R., Toda, A., Fukunaga, Y., Yoshimoto, S., Tsuda, T., Nagasaka, S., Keyama, T. Development of Skin Flaps for Reconstructive Surgery: Random Pattern Flap to Perforator Flap. 2016. *J Med Invest*, 63(3-4): pp 159-162.

[8] Starkman, S.J., Williams, C.T., Sherris, D.A. Flap Basics I. Aug 2017. *J Facial Plast Surg Clin Nor Am*, 25(3): pp 313-321.

[9] Shew, M., Kriet, J.D., Humphrey, C.D. Flap Basics II. Aug 2017. J *Facial Plast Surg Clin Nor Am*, 25(3): pp 323-335.

[10] Chu, E.A., Byrne, P.J. Local Flaps I: Bilobed, Rhombic and Cervicofacial. Aug 2009. *Facial Plast Surg Clin Nor Am*, 17(3): pp 349-360.

[11] Kruter, L., Rohrer, T. Advancement Flaps. Oct 2015. *J Derm Surg*, 41: pp 239-246.

[12] Hon, H.H., Chandra, S.R. Rhomboid Flap. Mar 2020. A*tlas Oral Max Facial Surg Clin Nor Am*, 28(1): pp 17-22.

[13] Larrabee, W.F. Design of local skin flaps. 1990. *Otolaryngol Clin North Am*, 23: pp 899-923.

[14] Larrabee W.F., Trachy R., Sutton D., Cox K.: Rhomboid flap dynamics. *Arch Otolaryngol* 1981; 107: pp. 755-757.

[15] Desai, S.C., Sand, J.P., Sharon, J.D., Branham, G., Nussenbaum, B. Scalp Reconstruction: An Algorithmic Approach and Systematic Review. Jan 2015. *JAMA Facial Plast Surg*, 17(1): pp 56-66.

[16] Bradford, B.D., Lee, J.W., Reconstruction of the Forehead and Scalp. Feb 2019. *Facial Plast Surg Clin Nor Am*, 27(1): pp 85-94.

[17] Fowler, N.M. Futran, N.D. Achievements in Scalp Reconstruction. Apr 2014. *Orolaryngol Head Neck Surg*, 22(2): pp 127-130.

[18] Badhey, A., Kadakia, S., Abraham, M.T., Rasamny, J.K., Moscatello, A. Multiflap Closure of Scalp Defects: Revisiting the Orticochea Flap for Scalp Reconstruction. Sept 2016. *Am J Otolaryngol*, 37(5): pp 466-469.

[19] Pepper, J.P., Baker, S.R. Local Flaps: Cheek and Lip Reconstruction. Sept 2013. *JAMA Facial Plast Surg*, 15(5): pp 374-382.

[20] Joseph, A.W., Truesdale, C., Baker, S.R. Reconstruction of the Nose. Feb 2019. *Facial Plast Surg Clin Nor Am*, 27(1): pp 43-54.

[21] Johnson, T.M., Swanson, N.A., Baker, S.R., Brown, M.D., Nelson, B.R. The Reiger Flap for Nasal Reconstruction. Jun 1995. *Arch Otolaryngeal Head Neck Surg*, 121(6): pp 634-637.

[22] Boson, A.L., Boukovalas, S., Hays, J.P., Hammel, J.A., Cole, E.L., Wagner, R.F. Upper Lip Anatomy, Mechanics of Local Flaps and Considerations for Reconstruction. Mar 2021. *Cutis*, 107(3): pp 144-148.

[23] Teemul, T.A., Telfer, A., Singh, R.P., Telfer, M.R. The Versatility of the Karapandzic Flap: A Review of 65 Cases with Patient-Reported Outcomes. Feb 2017. *J Cran Max Facial Surg*, 45(2): pp 325-329.

[24] Ethunandan, M., Macpherson, D.W., Santhanam, V. Karapandzic Flap for Reconstruction of Lip Defects. Dec 2007. *J Oral Max Facial Surg*, 65(12): pp 2512-2517.

[25] Wo, L.M., Singh, D., Thaller, S.R. Local Flaps for Reconstruction in the Head and Neck. May 2021. *J Craniofacial Surg*, 32(3): pp 832-835.

Chapter 11

Regional Flaps

Mingyang Gray, MD
and Shaun C. Desai, MD

Introduction

The evolution of head and neck reconstruction accelerated as the use of free tissue transfer became more readily available. However, regional flaps must be considered due to:

1. Ease of dissection
2. Decreased donor site morbidity
3. Faster recovery

Situations that call for regional flaps include [1, 2]:

1. Patient considerations
    a. High risk co-morbidities
    b. Post-radiated tissue
2. Surgical considerations
    a. Failed free flap
    b. Vessel-depleted neck

General advantages [3, 4]:

1. Shorter operating time
2. Less donor site morbidity
3. Shorter length of stay
4. Increased vasculature
5. No need for microvascular training

General disadvantages

1. Limited arc of rotation
2. Unpredictable distal tip vasculature
3. Inadequate for large/complex reconstruction
4. Increase in certain donor site morbidity

In: Essential Facial Plastic and Reconstructive Surgery. Volume 1 ISBN: 979-8-89113-306-8
Editors: Yan Ho Lee and Ira Papel © 2024 Nova Science Publishers, Inc.

In this chapter, we will discuss the following regional flaps in a defect-oriented approach:

1. Pericranial
2. Temporoparietal fascia
3. Paramedian
4. Temporalis
5. Temporalis tendon transfer
6. Facial artery musculomucosal (FAMM)
7. Pectoralis
8. Submental island
9. Supraclavicular
10. Latissimus dorsi
11. Trapezius island

1. Scalp and Skullbase
    a. Patient Evaluation
        i. Examine extent and depth of defect
            - Scalp
            - Bone
            - Dura
        ii. Goals of reconstruction
            - Skin thickness and color
            - Hair bearing skin
            - Dural coverage without calvarial exposure
        iii. Challenges
            - Previous scars
            - Need for postop radiation
    b. Regional flap options
        i. Pericranial flap
            - Design and Dissection [5]
                - Blood supply: supraorbital and supratrochlear arteries
                - Elevate flap in subgaleal plane to the supraorbital rim
                - Size: up to 15x20cm
            - Donor site
                - Cover with remainder of scalp or adjacent tissue transfer
                - Can use skin graft over pericranial flap or heal by secondary intention
            - Benefits
                - Thin, pliable tissue
                - Well vascularized
            - Complications and Considerations
                - Incorporating galea in the flap design can risk skin necrosis
                - Back cuts to increase arc of rotation can compromise flap vascularity

ii. Temporoparietal fascia flap [6]
- Design and dissection
  - Blood supply: superficial temporal artery
  - Dissect superior to inferior off the deep layer of temporalis fascia
- Donor site
  - Contour defect
  - Potential alopecia
- Benefits
  - Very thin (2-4mm) and pliable
- Complications and considerations
  - Use a Doppler to mark the pedicle
  - Avoid temporal branch of facial nerve by limiting anterior flap dissection
  - Avoid excessive cautery of skin flap as can lead to alopecia

2. Nasal

a. Patient Evaluation

i. Nasal subunits
- 9 nasal subunits
- >50% of subunit involved: redesign defect to incorporate entire subunit

ii. Depth of defect
- Skin/soft tissue
- Cartilage
- Mucosa

b. Regional flap options

i. Paramedian flap
- Design and Dissection [7]
  - Blood supply: supratrochlear artery located 1.7 to 2.2 cm lateral to midsagittal plane
  - Pedicle width should be between 1.2 - 1.5cm width
  - Size: dependent on defect, can increase with tissue expanders
  - Consider laminating or prelaminating flap for full thickness defects [8]
  - Delayed flap transfer can improve distal vasculature
- Donor site
  - Undermine widely to close primarily (temporal line to temporal line)
  - Distal aspect can heal by secondary intention
- Benefits
  - Low failure rate
  - Color match
- Complications and Considerations

- Require multiple stages depending on defect and patient expectations
- Pedicle width or flap thinning can compromise distal vascularity
- Use doppler to confirm blood supply
- Active smoking can compromise blood supply (important to delay takedown of flap for extra few weeks)
- Wound infection can be caused by poor sterile technique or necrosis of nasal lining or cartilage
- Excessive tension can lead to poor flap perfusion

3. Facial paralysis
   a. Patient Evaluation
      i. Etiology of paralysis predicts likelihood of recovery and reconstructive options
         - Trauma
         - Neoplasm
         - Viral
         - Idiopathic
         - Congenital
      ii. Assess movement of upper, middle, and lower thirds of the face
      iii. Assess function of facial nerve and donor nerves
   b. Regional flap options
      i. Temporalis muscle flap [9]
         - Design and Dissection
            - Blood supply: deep temporal artery
            - Transfer temporalis muscle sling over zygoma
            - Neurovascular bundle on the undersurface of muscle must be kept intact
         - Donor site
            - Raise the temporoparietal fascia to fill the defect after the temporalis muscle is harvested
            - Minimize donor site deformity with TPF flap
         - Benefits
            - Most reliable for midface and lower face paralysis
            - Initiate semi-volitional movement with jaw clenching
            - Can be divided into multiple strips to distribute equal tension
         - Complications and Considerations
            - Bulky flap
            - Single vector
            - Expose second molar intraoperatively as the muscle will extend with time
            - Include pericranium with flap to enforce distal suture line

- Passing temporalis under zygoma limits motion

ii. Temporalis tendon transfer [10]
- Design and Dissection
  - Temporalis tendon freed from the medial aspect of the mandibular ramus
  - Intraoral dissection
  - Minimally invasive incision through nasolabial fold
- Donor site
  - Minimal comorbidity
  - Pterygoid muscles compensate for temporalis
- Benefits
  - Single stage surgery
  - Immediate symmetry
- Complications and Considerations
  - Coronoidectomy can extend the reach and prevent potential trismus [11]
  - Soft diet for 6 weeks will prevent dehiscence
  - Use of temporalis tendon transfer does not preclude future reanimation procedures
  - There is a fixed single vector for oral commissure excursion
  - No spontaneity of excursion
  - Additional length can be achieved with tensor fascia lata extension
  - Degree of excursion is inconsistent

4. Oral cavity

a. Patient Evaluation

i. Goals of reconstruction [12]
- Preserve movement of remaining native tongue
- Provide bulk for speech and swallowing and prevent trismus
- Consider dynamic closure of velopharyngeal sphincter

b. Regional flap options

ii. Facial artery musculomucosal (FAMM) flap [13] (Figure 11.1)
- Design and Dissection
  - Blood supply: facial artery
  - Size: 1.5-2.0cm width
  - Identify superior labial artery at oral commissure
  - Establish depth of dissection
  - Inferiorly based or superiorly based depending on defect

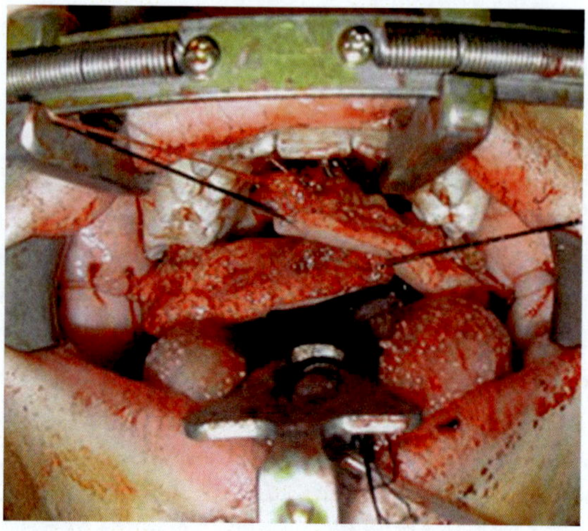

Figure 11.1. Bilateral sFAMM raised.

- Donor site
  - Close primarily
  - Buccal fat advancement
- Benefits
  - Low morbidity
  - No additional donor site
  - Replace like with like tissue in the oral cavity
- Complications and Considerations
  - Typically performed as two-stage procedure with pedicle release after 2-3 weeks
  - Patients need to use bite block in interim
  - Facial artery damaged during neck dissection would compromise flap viability
  - Potential for trismus at donor site may be exacerbated by postoperative radiation [12, 14]

iii. Pectoralis flap [15]

- Design and Dissection
  - Blood supply: pectoral branch of the thoracoacromial artery with internal mammary perforators and lateral thoracic artery perforators
- Donor site
  - Skin paddle generally medial to nipple
  - Skin paddle design inferior to breast tissue in women
  - Close primarily or with adjacent tissue transfer
- Benefits
  - Robust blood supply
  - Large skin paddle
  - Easy harvest
  - Can reach temporal line with modifications

- Complications and Considerations
  - Assess for Poland syndrome, previous chest wall trauma or surgery
  - Skeletonize pedicle and release humoral head attachments to increase arc of rotation
  - Including lateral thoracic artery improves vascularity but limits arc of rotation
  - Carefully ligate intercostal perforators to avoid bleeding, try to preserve 2nd and 3rd perforators if need deltopectoral flap in future

5. Face/Neck
   a. Patient evaluation
      i. Depth of defect affects form and function
         - Facial muscles affect speech and swallow
         - Oral competency should be restored or maintained
         - Extension to buccal space can cause trismus
      ii. Consider aesthetic effects of reconstructive options
         - Color and texture match is difficult
         - Facial paralysis can further complicate reconstruction
         - Flap design can affect eyelid and oral commissure position
   b. Regional flap options
      iii. Supraclavicular artery island flap
         - Design and Dissection [16]
           - Blood supply: superficial transverse cervical artery, suprascapular artery
           - Size: up to 10x22cm [17]
           - Vascular pedicle located in triangle formed by
             - o Posterior edge of SCM
             - o External jugular vein
             - o Clavicle
         - Donor site
           - Close primarily or with adjacent tissue transfer
           - Wound tension can cause hypertrophic scarring
         - Benefits [18]
           - Good color match
           - Long pedicle
           - Wide arc of rotation
           - Thin and versatile flap
         - Complications and Considerations
           - Sporadic use and high learning curve
           - Wound dehiscence
           - Seroma at donor site
           - Distal vasculature commonly compromised
      iv. Submental artery island flap
         - Design and Dissection [19]

- Blood supply: submental artery and vein
- Size: up to 7x18cm
- Submental artery is a branch of the facial artery
  - Medial aspect of submandibular gland
  - Between mandible and mylohyoid muscle
- Can be raised as osteocutaneous flap with a rim of mandible
- Raise with anterior belly of digastric or mylohyoid to capture more perforators [20, 21]

- Donor Site
  - Close primarily
- Benefits
  - Long pedicle (up to 8cm)
  - Extend pedicle length with microvascular transfer of vein to recipient site
  - Wide arc of rotation
  - Thin and versatile flap
  - Faster recovery and lower overall cost
- Complications and Considerations
  - Close proximity to level one neck dissection, although no compromise to oncologic outcome [22, 23]
  - Risk to marginal mandibular nerve
  - Arc of rotation may be limited by submental vein
  - Excess adipose tissue limits flap design

v. Latissimus dorsi transfer [24]

- Design and Dissection
  - Blood supply: thoracodorsal artery
- Donor site
  - Potential compromise in activity
  - Seroma
- Benefits
  - Large thin muscular flap
- Complications and Considerations
  - Can be harvested with rib
  - Tunnel between pectoralis major and minor to improve reach
  - Can be innervated with thoracodorsal nerve
  - Pedicle may kink when used as a pedicled flap

vi. Trapezius island flap [25]

- Design and Dissection
  - Blood supply: transverse cervical artery, dorsal scapular artery
  - Skin flap between medial border of scapula and spine
  - Raise flap superficial to rhomboid muscles
  - Ligate dorsal scapular artery for greater arc of rotation

- Donor site
- Benefits
- Complications and Considerations
  - Require decubitus positioning
  - May need skin grafting

Summary Points

1. The main goal of head and neck reconstruction is to restore form and function.
2. Regional flaps are viable options that can be harvested with less operative time and patients recover with shorter postoperative hospitalizations.
3. These flaps are comparable to free tissue transfer and play a complementary role in the reconstructive ladder.

Patient Cases

Case 1.

Q1. A 60 year-old male presents with a 2cm infiltrative lesion on the right lateral tongue. He underwent hemi-glossectomy and right selective neck dissection for squamous cell carcinoma. The intraoral defect measured 1/3 of the right tongue with resection of the adjacent floor of mouth. What are the options for reconstruction of this defect?

A1.

- Secondary intention - allow it to granulate
- Primary closure
- Skin graft or mucosal graft
- Regional: FAMM flap, submental island flap
- Free tissue transfer: radial forearm

Q2. A FAMM flap was chosen for reconstruction. What are the benefits and disadvantages of this flap?

A2.

- Advantages
  - Low morbidity
  - No distal donor site
  - Replace like-with-like tissue in the oral cavity

- Disadvantages
  - Requires two-stages with pedicle release after 2-3 weeks
  - Patients need to use bite block in interim
  - Facial artery damage during neck dissection may compromise flap viability
  - Potential for trismus at donor site may be exacerbated by postoperative radiation

Q3. What are the steps of performing this flap?

A3.

- Blood supply: facial artery (optional: doppler this artery intraorally and follow course)
- Width of the pedicle should be 1.5-2.0cm
- Inferiorly based or superiorly based depending on defect
- Measure out defect and mark the flap
- Identify superior labial artery at oral commissure
- Establish depth of dissection (dissect just deep to the buccinator muscle)
- Rotate flap and inset onto defect making sure there is enough laxity to preserve pedicle
- Place bite block and secure (may wire to adjacent teeth) or may use a custom dental device (designed and made pre-operatively)
- May avoid bite block if tunneled inferiorly around the mandibular body
- May close donor site primarily or may use buccal fat advancement to close defect

Q4. Four hours after surgery, the flap looks edematous and slightly dark, but doppler signals are present. What can cause this?

A4.

- The venous drainage of this flap is less predictable. Keeping the pedicle slightly wider may facilitate venous drainage.

Case 2.

Q5. A patient elects a submental island flap for buccal reconstruction. What artery is this flap based on?

A5.

- Submental artery - branch of the facial artery; it is found:
  - On medial aspect of submandibular gland
  - Between mandible and mylohyoid muscle

Q6. What are the advantages and disadvantages of this flap?

A6.

- Advantages:
  - Can cover defects up to 7x18cm
  - Can be raised as osteocutaneous flap with a rim of mandible
  - Long pedicle (up to 8cm)
  - Wide arc of rotation
  - Thin and versatile flap
  - Fast recovery and low overall cost

- Disadvantages:
  - Close proximity to level one neck dissection so must be careful to protect vasculature (although no compromise to oncologic outcome)
  - Risk to marginal mandibular nerve
  - Arc of rotation may be limited by submental vein
  - Excess adipose tissue limits flap design

Q7. What are the operative steps for this flap?

A7.

- Doppler the artery in the submental region (behind the mandible, next to anterior belly of digastric muscle)
- Design flap (after measuring defect) so that the anterior edge is just posterior to the mandible.
- Dissect this flap prior to the neck dissection to preserve vasculature
- Dissect in subplatysmal plane until identification of ipsilateral submandibular gland and bilateral anterior belly of the digastric muscles
- Identify facial and submental vessels adjacent to submandibular gland, preserve subplatysmal skin island up to the lateral border of the mylohyoid.
- Protect the marginal mandibular nerve.

- Once the submental vessels are visualized as they pass under the anterior belly of the digastric, raise flap distal to proximal.
- Raise with anterior belly of digastric or mylohyoid to capture more perforators
- The underlying mylohyoid muscle is either cut or a strip is included with the pedicle if the flap needs to be tunneled medial to the mandible for intraoral reconstruction.
- Mylohyoid is detached from the mandible and hyoid and is bluntly dissected off ipsilateral geniohyoid muscle to mobilize flap
- Extend pedicle length with microvascular transfer of vein to recipient site
- Close donor site primarily

Q8. Unfortunately, after raising the appropriately sized flap, it does not reach to the distal aspect of the defect. What is the best next step?

A8.

- Ligate the submental vein and anastomose it to the contralateral facial vein

References

[1] Desai SC, Seth R. Shifting Paradigms in Head and Neck Reconstructive Surgery During the COVID-19 Crisis. *Facial Plast Surg Aesthet Med.* 2020;22(3):152-154.

[2] Ranasinghe V, Mady LJ, Kim S, Ferris RL, Duvvuri U, Johnson JT, Solari MG, Sridharan S, Kubik M. Major head and neck reconstruction during the COVID-19 pandemic: The University of Pittsburgh approach. *Head Neck.* 2020;42(6):1243-1247.

[3] Zhang J, Wang Y, Han X, Chen H. Comparison of Clinical Results and Quality-of-Life in Tongue Cancer Patients Undergoing Submental Island Flap and Radial Forearm Free Flap Reconstruction. *J Oral Maxillofac Surg.* 2020;78(9):1639-1644.

[4] Jorgensen MG, Tabatabaeifar S, Toyserkani NM, Sorensen JA. Submental Island Flap versus Free Flap Reconstruction for Complex Head and Neck Defects. *Otolaryngol Head Neck Surg.* 2019;161(6):946-953.

[5] Gishen K, Yoo J, Plotsker E, Thaller SR. Revisiting the Pericranial Flap for Scalp Reconstruction. *J Craniofac Surg.* 2021;32(Suppl 3):1275-1280.

[6] Jaquet Y, Higgins KM, Enepekides DJ. The temporoparietal fascia flap: a versatile tool in head and neck reconstruction. *Curr Opin Otolaryngol Head Neck Surg.* 2011;19(4):235-241.

[7] Shokri T, Kadakia S, Saman M, Habal MB, Kohlert S, Sokoya M, Ducic Y, Wood-Smith D. The Paramedian Forehead Flap for Nasal Reconstruction: From Antiquity to Present. *J Craniofac Surg.* 2019;30(2):330-333.

[8] Ziegler JP, Oyer SL. Prelaminated paramedian forehead flap for subtotal nasal reconstruction using three-dimensional printing. *BMJ Case Rep.* 2021;14(1).

[9] Cheney ML, McKenna MJ, Megerian CA, Ojemann RG. Early temporalis muscle transposition for the management of facial paralysis. *Laryngoscope.* 1995;105(9 Pt 1):993-1000.

[10] Lu GN, Byrne PJ. Temporalis Tendon Transfer Versus Gracilis Free Muscle Transfer: When and Why? *Facial Plast Surg Clin North Am.* 2021;29(3):383-388.

[11] Owusu Boahene KD. Temporalis Muscle Tendon Unit Transfer for Smile Restoration After Facial Paralysis. *Facial Plast Surg Clin North Am.* 2016;24(1):37-45.

[12] Comini LV, Spinelli G, Mannelli G. Algorithm for the treatment of oral and peri-oral defects through local flaps. *J Craniomaxillofac Surg.* 2018;46(12):2127-2137.

[13] Pribaz J, Stephens W, Crespo L, Gifford G. A new intraoral flap: facial artery musculomucosal (FAMM) flap. *Plast Reconstr Surg.* 1992;90(3):421-429.

[14] Ayad T, Xie L. Facial artery musculomucosal flap in head and neck reconstruction: A systematic review. *Head Neck.* 2015;37(9):1375-1386.

[15] Patel K, Lyu DJ, Kademani D. Pectoralis major myocutaneous flap. *Oral Maxillofac Surg Clin North Am.* 2014;26(3):421-426.

[16] Lamberty BG. The supra-clavicular axial patterned flap. *Br J Plast Surg.* 1979;32(3):207-212.

[17] Sandu K, Monnier P, Pasche P. Supraclavicular flap in head and neck reconstruction: experience in 50 consecutive patients. *Eur Arch Otorhinolaryngol.* 2012;269(4):1261-1267.

[18] Kokot N, Kim JH, West JD, Zhang P. Supraclavicular Artery Island Flap: Critical Appraisal and Comparison to Alternate Reconstruction. *Laryngoscope.* 2020.

[19] Martin D, Pascal JF, Baudet J, Mondie JM, Farhat JB, Athoum A, Le Gaillard P, Peri G. The submental island flap: a new donor site. Anatomy and clinical applications as a free or pedicled flap. *Plast Reconstr Surg.* 1993;92(5):867-873.

[20] Faltaous AA, Yetman RJ. The submental artery flap: an anatomic study. *Plast Reconstr Surg.* 1996;97(1):56-60; discussion 61-52.

[21] Zenga J, Emerick KS, Deschler DG. Submental Island Flap: A Technical Update. *Ann Otol Rhinol Laryngol.* 2019;128(12):1177-1181.

[22] Patel UA. The submental flap for head and neck reconstruction: Comparison of outcomes to the radial forearm free flap. *Laryngoscope.* 2020;130 Suppl 2:S1-S10.

[23] Wang J, Tan Y, Shen Y, Lv M, Li J, Sun J. Oncological safety of submental island flap for reconstruction of pathologically node-negative and node-positive T1-2 oral squamous cell carcinoma-related defects: A retrospective study and comparison of outcomes. *Oral Oncol.* 2020;102:104507.

[24] Ong HS, Ji T, Zhang CP. The pedicled latissimus dorsi myocutaneous flap in head and neck reconstruction. *Oral Maxillofac Surg Clin North Am.* 2014;26(3):427-434.

[25] Ramirez CA, Fernandes RP. The supraclavicular artery island and trapezius myocutaneous flaps in head and neck reconstruction. *Oral Maxillofac Surg Clin North Am.* 2014;26(3):411-420.

Chapter 12

Free Flaps and Microvascular Reconstruction

Melina J. Windon, MD
and Chaz L. Stucken, MD

Introduction

1. Free tissue transfer, which came into use in the 1970s for head and neck reconstruction, is the harvest of a tissue bed supplied by a named vascular pedicle, with division and microvascular anastomosis of this donor artery and vein to recipient vessels in or near the resection bed [1]
2. Indications
    a. Large and complex defects in head and neck for which form and function would be superiorly restored with free tissue compared to locoregional tissue (or has failed prior locoregional reconstruction)
    b. Osseous defects to restore occlusion
    c. History of prior radiation therapy conferring higher risk of fistula and wound dehiscence
    d. Anticipated post-operative radiation therapy where vascularized tissue is prudent to protect structures i.e. carotid system, facial nerve, pericranium, hardware
    e. Functional loss that can be addressed with vascularized, innervated tissue (i.e. defects of pharynx or tongue, parotid with facial nerve sacrifice)

Patient Evaluation

1. A careful history includes:
    a. Prior head/neck surgery
    b. Deep vein Thrombosis (DVT)
    c. Handedness
    d. Lifestyle and occupation
    e. Risk factors for flap failure (scleroderma, peripheral vascular disease, radiation therapy, tobacco use, frailty, diabetes mellitus, renal failure) [2]
2. Exam (and intra-operative evaluation) includes attention to primary tumor and reconstructive needs. This includes:
    a. Extent of planned neck dissection

In: Essential Facial Plastic and Reconstructive Surgery. Volume 1 ISBN: 979-8-89113-306-8
Editors: Yan Ho Lee and Ira Papel © 2024 Nova Science Publishers, Inc.

b. Composition (skin, soft tissue, bone, muscle, mucosa, floor of mouth, nerve), and function (speech/swallow, role of motor and sensory innervation) of resected tissue
c. Dental restoration plans
d. Pedicle length requirements, vessel availability and quality/size
e. Need for post-operative radiation; may require coverage of vital structures and hardware, and overcorrection for flap volume loss (42% at 1 year [3])

Management [4]

1. Perioperative Considerations
    a. Smoking cessation
    b. Optimize nutritional status
    c. Anesthesia considerations:
        i. Minimize fluids, correct underlying causes of hemodynamic instability prior to vasopressor use
        ii. Consider arterial line to ensure perfusion is maintained and hypertension is not overtreated.
        iii. Goal hemotocrit >25 and hemoglobin> 7.0.
        iv. Post-operative extubation/weaning from ventilatory support as early as safely possible
    d. Airway management [5].
        i. Nasotracheal intubation for oral cavity resections
        ii. Consider tracheostomy if:
            - Resection includes substantial floor of mouth
            - Bulky flap
            - Greater than hemiglossectomy
            - Microstomia
            - Micrognathia/retrognathia and/or trismus
            - Segmental mandibulectomy
            - Lip-split and/or lingual release (transcervical delivery of tongue)
            - Double free flap reconstruction
            - Longer operative time, to allow for weaning during resolution of edema
            - Anticipated depressed mental status post operatively rendering inability to communicate airway distress
        iii. Where performed, efforts should be taken to keep tracheostomy site separate from surgical bed containing flap pedicle
2. Radial Forearm Free Flap
    a. Uses:
        i. Thin, pliable skin and fascia with long pedicle

    ii. For intraoral mucosal or any cutaneous defect, dural repair and pharyngeal repair including radical tonsillectomy defects for coverage of vessels
  b. Donor site morbidity:
    i. Arm contracture (should incision cross antebrachial fossa)
    ii. Paresthesia
    iii. Poor cosmesis
    iv. Fracture of the radius if osseous flap harvested
  c. Technical considerations:
    i. Preoperative Allen's test confirms ulnar-based vascularization of thumb and index finger after radial artery is harvested
      - In 12% of cases, two anomalies exist that preclude this flap:
        - Incomplete superficial palmar arch
        - Lack of communication between deep and superficial palmar arches)
      - Perform by compression of radial and ulnar arteries and pumping hand open and closed
      - Then, with hand open in a relaxed position, release ulnar artery
      - A "negative" result is blushing of thumb/index finger within 10 seconds, an indication of adequate perfusion by ulnar artery.
    ii. Split thickness skin graft is harvested to close donor site; improve take by preservation of paratenon and/or coverage with muscular turnover flaps using extensor compartment muscles
    iii. Often harvested with tourniquet to 250 mm Hg
  d. Anatomy/Harvest:
    i. Fasciocutaneous flap with or without radius bone
    ii. Based off of radial artery and venae comitantes in lateral intermuscular septum between brachioradialis and flexor carpi radialis muscles giving 7-9 fascial branches
    iii. Cephalic vein can be harvested
    iv. May include 10 cm and 40% cross-section of radius bone, antebrachial cutaneous nerve for sensation, palmaris longus when present for suspension, and brachioradialis muscle

3. Anterolateral Thigh Free Flap
  a. Uses:
    i. Bulky or thin (perforator dissection) soft tissue
    ii. For large glossectomy, cutaneous, scalp, total laryngopharyngectomy, salvage laryngectomy, open maxillectomy defects
  b. Donor site morbidity:
    i. Minimal, although seromas are common
    ii. Leg weakness associated with harvest of tensor fascia lata (TFL)
  c. Technical considerations:

i. Thickness of thigh varies widely among individuals; for this reason body habitus must be considered when planning reconstruction
ii. A perforator dissection (harvest of a cutaneous or fasciocutaneous flap without muscle bulk) requires identification of perforators and, if musculocutaneous, tracing them through muscle to their origin from the pedicle
iii. A skin defect less than 9 cm can be closed primarily

d. Anatomy/Harvest:
i. Fasciocutaneous flap with or without skin, fat, and vastus lateralis
ii. Supplied by 1-3 septocutaneous branches of lateral femoral circumflex artery (LCFA) and its accompanying venae comitantes
iii. Septum between vastus lateralis and rectus femoris located along line from lateral patella to anterior superior iliac spine
iv. Most perforators take a musculocutaneous course, otherwise septocutaneous
v. Perforators [6]:
- Type I: (90%) originate from descending branch of LCFA
- Type II: (4%) arise from transverse branch and have a long course;
- Type III (4%) from profundal femoris; too small for microvascular anastomosis

vi. TFL and/or anterior branch of the lateral cutaneous nerve of the thigh may be included
vii. Rectus femoris muscle and its pedicle may be harvested together with vastus lateralis as a chimeric flap

4. Fibula Free Flap

a. Uses:
i. Mandibulectomy, maxillectomy defects
ii. Limited accompanying soft tissue with fickle vascular supply to skin and poor relative mobility of osseous and soft tissue components

b. Donor site morbidity:
i. Slight reduction in ankle motion, strength
ii. Cold intolerance, foot edema
iii. Post-operative pain while driving (may be consideration to avoid right leg)

c. Technical considerations:
i. Virtual surgical planning allows for bone cutting guides saving intra-operative time
ii. Preoperative consultation with dentistry for discussion of endosteal dental implants versus obturator
iii. Closure may require skin grafting
iv. Preoperative arterial-phase CTA or MRA to evaluate three-vessel runoff of peroneal, posterior tibial and anterior tibial vessels and presence of atherosclerosis; if either tibial vessel is diminutive,

vascular supply to foot may depend on communication from peroneal, and this vessel should not be harvested
   v. Low height of fibular bone compared to native mandible can be addressed using a double-barreled design
   vi. Choice of leg for composite defects is guided by desired position of skin paddle relative to neomandible
   vii. Typically harvested with tourniquet
  d. Anatomy/Harvest:
   i. Osseous, osteocutaneous, osteomuscular flap
   ii. Can include up to 25 cm of fibula
   iii. Supplied by 4-5 septocutaneous perforators within posterior crural septum dividing posterior (soleus and gastrocnemius) and lateral anterior (peroneus longus and brevis) muscular compartments
   iv. Septum estimated on surface anatomy along a line from fibular head to lateral malleolus
   v. Additional cutaneous vascular supply from musculocutaneous perforators
   vi. 6 cm of bone distally and proximally must be preserved
   vii. Lateral sural cutaneous nerve may be harvested in addition for sensate flap
5. Scapula/Parascapular Free Flap
  a. Uses:
   i. Multiple variations used for wide applications including any large soft tissue and/or osseous defect
   ii. Especially useful where independent orientations of osseous and soft tissue components are required
  b. Donor site morbidity:
   i. Minimal to moderate shoulder dysfunction
   ii. Advantage of early mobilization after surgery compared with fibular free flap
  c. Technical considerations:
   i. Presence of peripheral vascular disease makes scapula preferable to fibula
   ii. Endosteal implantation is possible [7] although bone stock less than fibula
   iii. Harvest can be done in tandem in semidecubitus position with a bean bag and upper extremity limb positioner [8]
  d. Anatomy/Harvest:
   i. Fasciocutaneous and osteocutaneous flaps
   ii. Supplied by branches of the subscapular artery
   iii. Flap may include up to 14 cm of lateral border of scapula, and/or a 10 x 13 cm horizontally oriented fasciocutaneous paddle based off circumflex scapular branch
   iv. Scapular tip free flap, based off angular branch of thoracodorsal artery, is a favorable alternative as it is curved allowing favorable

reconstruction of mandibular or midface defects of up to 9 cm [9] and has a longer vascular pedicle

v. Latissimus and/or serratus anterior muscle may be included, based off thoracodorsal artery

vi. Vertically oriented fasciocutaneous skin paddle based off descending branch of circumflex scapular artery may also be included

6. Rectus Abdominis Free Flap
   a. Uses:
      i. Complex wounds, radiated beds, salivary fistulas requiring large volume of muscle and/or skin
      ii. Skull base reconstruction for separation of cranial and nasal cavities
   b. Donor site morbidity:
      i. Abdominal hernia or asymmetry
      ii. Closure may include mesh to minimize risk of this
   c. Technical considerations:
      i. Prior abdominal surgery may have compromised vascular supply of rectus muscle
      ii. Surgical history must be carefully elicited
   d. Anatomy/Harvest:
      i. Muscular, musculofasciocutaneous, or fasciocutaneous flap
      ii. Based on deep inferior epigastric artery (DIEA) and vein
      iii. Most commonly two dominant DIEA branches; larger caliber DIEA branches arborize with smaller deep superior epigastric artery on lateral and inferior muscular surface
      iv. Rectus abdominis muscle arises from pubis and inserts into thorax
      v. Periumbilical perforators arise from 2 cm cephalad to 3 cm caudad to umbilicus
      vi. Dissection, commonly through a transverse suprapubic incision, should stay above arcuate line at level of anterosuperior iliac spine to minimize risk of herniation
      vii. Above this line, posterior rectus sheath is comprised of aponeuroses of transversus abdominis and internal oblique muscles and anterior rectus sheath includes contributions from internal and external obliques muscles
      viii. May include 6th rib, or 6-10th rib costal cartilage [10, 11]

Complications

1. Flap failure
   a. Due to arterial ischemia or vascular congestion occurs around 5%, mostly within first 48 hours.
   b. Most often due to poor geometry causing kinking of or extrinsic compression of vein (i.e. hematoma)

c. Leech therapy or intradermal bivalirudin can be employed for venous congestion, or operative revision
d. Arterial size mismatch can cause turbulent flow and arterial thrombosis detected on loss of doppler signal on post-operative monitoring or by clinical exam (pallor, cool to touch, lack of bright red bleeding to needle stick/scratch)
e. Although arterial spasm can be reversed by warming flap or head position, arterial occlusion refractory to these maneuvers is reason for operative exploration with thrombectomy with or without thrombolytic agents
f. Microcirculatory compromise with thrombus can be treated with thrombolytic injection [12]
g. Flap failure is associated with pedicle revision at time of surgery and intraoperative prolonged ischemia time [13]
h. Ischemic tolerance [14]:
    i. Dermis and subcutaneous tissues 4-6 hours
    ii. Muscle 2 hours
    iii. Bone 3 hours

2. Fistula
    a. Persistent communication between upper aerodigestive tract and neck through a dehiscence along inset suture line causing leakage of saliva and infection
    b. Heralded by erythema, neck fullness and leukocytosis 3-7 days post operatively
    c. Often managed by nil per os (NPO), wound exploration/washout and serial packing
3. Lingual tethering
    a. Common sequela of oral tongue and floor of mouth reconstruction
    b. Minimize risk via flap design with adequate soft tissue to reconstruct floor of mouth and oral tongue with tissue paddles that are partially mobile relative to each other, in a bilobed flap design
4. Malunion and nonunion
    a. Typically forms at junction of neomandible or neomaxilla and native bone when segments are plated greater than 1 mm apart
    b. Associated with wound healing issues such as plate extrusion, infection, and osteonecrosis [15]

Summary Points

The advent and generalization of free tissue transfer with microvascular anastomotic techniques has revolutionized the field of reconstructive head and neck surgery and brought markedly improved functional and cosmetic outcomes to patients requiring large extirpative defects.

Patient Case

59 year-old female with past medical history of diabetes mellitus and extensive sun exposure due to her occupation is found to have a 6 cm ulcerated, invasive mass of the preauricular area that was biopsied and returned squamous cell carcinoma. She has paralysis of the frontal branch of the facial nerve. Imaging demonstrates direct invasion into the parotid gland and external auditory canal. She undergoes wide local excision, auriculectomy, lateral temporal bone resection, total parotidectomy with sacrifice of the facial nerve extending from the mastoid segment to the peripheral nerve branches due to direct invasion, and neck dissection. Post operative radiation therapy is planned.

Question 1: What are your reconstructive needs?

Answer: Large volume of fat for coverage of the facial nerve during radiation therapy, skin, nerve, and fascia. A large skin paddle is necessary for coverage of the cutaneous defect. In anticipation of facial nerve or facial nerve branches sacrifice, may need facial nerve reconstruction (static and/or dynamic).

Question 2: What are your reconstructive options?

Answer: The best option in this case is an anterolateral thigh free flap, harvest of the nerve to vastus for use in cable grafting the proximal end of the main trunk of the facial nerve to any remaining distal branches, and tensor fascia lata grafting to suspend the midface. Alternatives include a fat-fasciocutaneous scapular free flap or pedicled submental island flap should the patient have substantial submental tissue, with nerve harvest at a separate site.

Question 3: What is the vascular supply of an ALT free flap?

Answer: supplied by 1-3 septocutaneous branches of lateral femoral circumflex artery (LCFA) and its accompanying venae comitantes. Most perforators take a musculocutaneous course, otherwise septocutaneous. 90% of perforators are Type I that originate from descending branch of the LCFA. Type II (4%) arise from the transverse branch and have a long course, and Type III (4%) from the profundal femoris. Type III are too small for microvascular anastomosis (Yu 2004). TFL as well as anterior branch of the lateral cutaneous nerve of the thigh may be included.

Question 4: What are possible complications of free flap reconstruction?

Answer: flap failure, hematoma/hemorrhage, infection, non-healing wounds, dehiscence, donor site morbiditiy, scar, need for revision or another type of reconstruction.

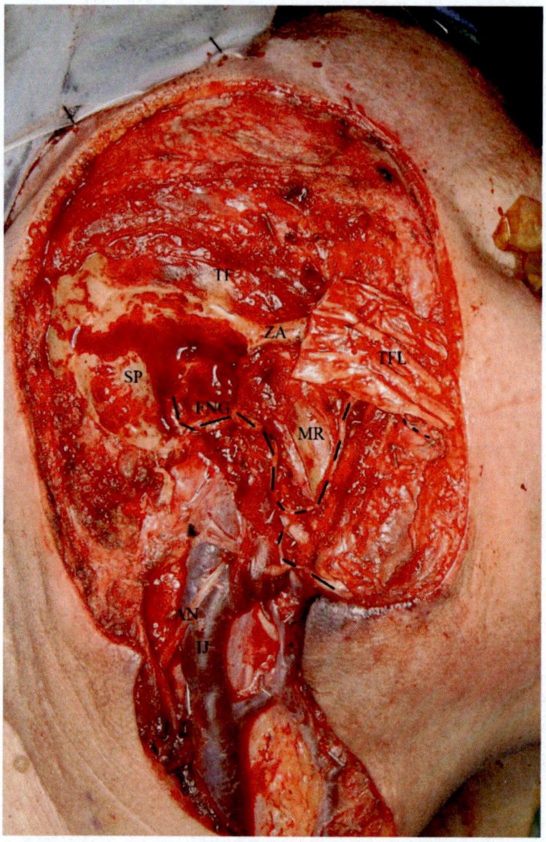

Figure 12.1. Defect shown, AN- accessory nerve, IJ- internal jugular vein, TF- temporalis fossa, TFL- tensor fascia lata graft, FNG- facial nerve graft (hash marks from mastoid segment to multiple facial branches), MR- mandibular ramus, SP- sigmoid plate in mastoid defect, ZA- zygomatic arch.

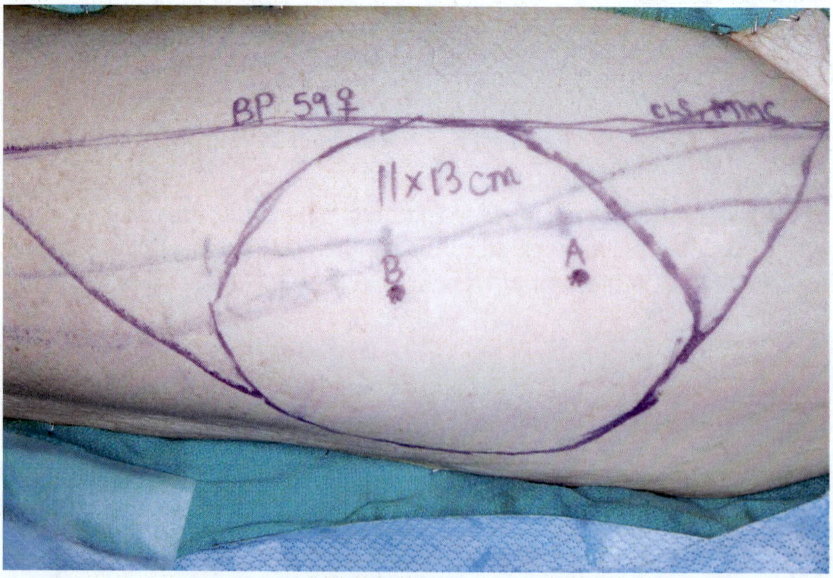

Figure 12.2. Left anterolateral thigh free flap donor site. A and B perforators marked.

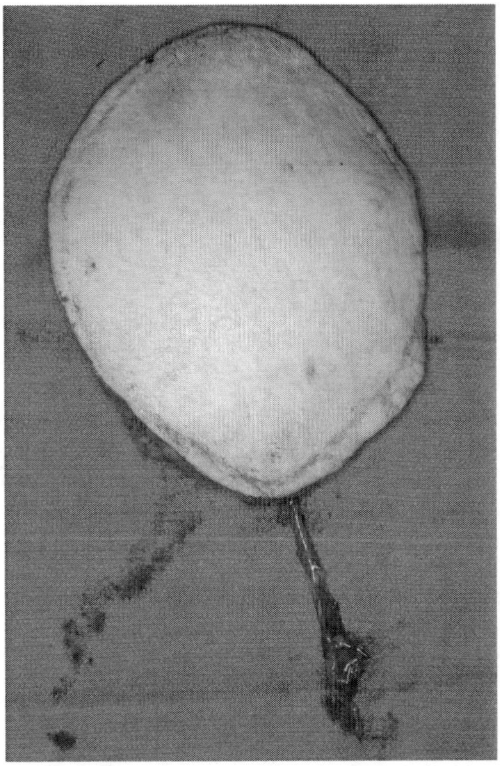

Figure 12.3. Perforator based fasciocutaneous anterolateral thigh free flap without muscle.

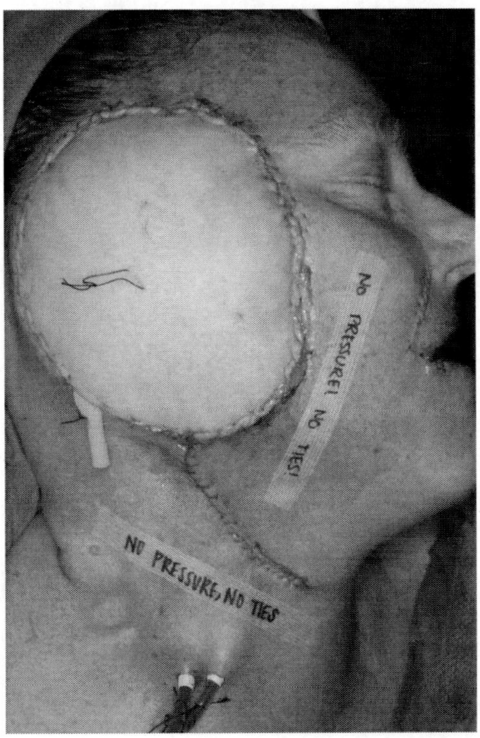

Figure 12.4. After flap inset.

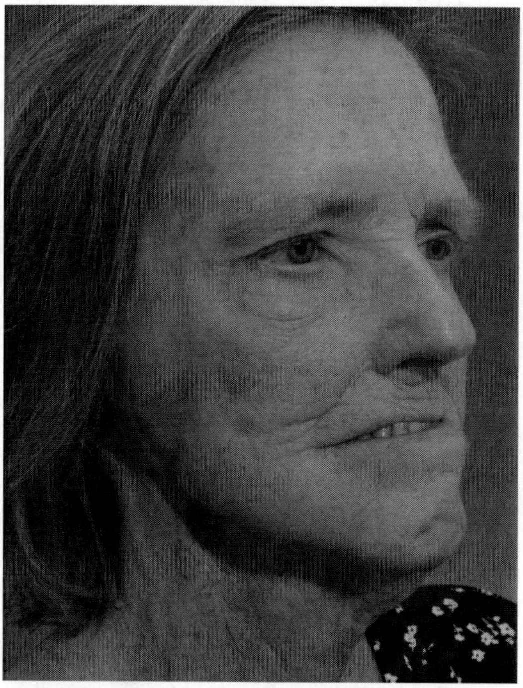

Figure 12.5. After completion of radiation.

References

[1] Pellini, Raul, and Gabriele Molteni. 2020. *Free Flaps in Head and Neck Reconstruction A Step-By-Step Color Atlas: A Step-By-Step Color Atlas*. https://doi.org/10.1007/978-3-030-29582-0.

[2] Ishimaru, Miho, Sachiko Ono, Sayaka Suzuki, Hiroki Matsui, Kiyohide Fushimi, and Hideo Yasunaga. 2016. "Risk Factors for Free Flap Failure in 2,846 Patients With Head and Neck Cancer: A National Database Study in Japan." *Journal of Oral and Maxillofacial Surgery : Official Journal of the American Association of Oral and Maxillofacial Surgeons* 74 (6): 1265–70. https://doi.org/10.1016/j.joms.2016.01.009.

[3] Razavi, Christopher R., Jason Hostetter, Aishwarya Shukla, Zhi Cheng, Nafi Aygun, Kofi Boahene, Patrick J. Byrne, Jeremy Richmon, Harry Quon, and Shaun C. Desai. 2022. "Predictors of Free Flap Volume Loss in Nonosseous Reconstruction of Head and Neck Oncologic Defects." *Ear, Nose & Throat Journal* 101 (1): 48–53. https://doi.org/10.1177/0145561320938903.

[4] Healy DW, Cloyd BH, Straker T, Brenner MJ, Damrose EJ, Spector ME, Saxena A, Atkins JH, Ramamurthi RJ, Mehta A, Aziz MF, Cattano D, Levine AI, Schechtman SA, Cavallone LF, Abdelmalak BB. Expert Consensus Statement on the Perioperative Management of Adult Patients Undergoing Head and Neck Surgery and Free Tissue Reconstruction From the Society for Head and Neck Anesthesia. *Anesth Analg.* 2021 Jul 1;133(1):274-283.

[5] Dawson, Rebecca, Daniel Phung, James Every, Dulan Gunawardena, Tsu-Hui Low, Sydney Ch'ng, Jonathan Clark, James Wykes, and Carsten E. Palme. 2021. "Tracheostomy in Free-Flap Reconstruction of the Oral Cavity: Can It Be Avoided? A Cohort Study of 187 Patients." *ANZ Journal of Surgery* 91 (6): 1246–50. https://doi.org/10.1111/ans.16762.

[6] Yu, Peirong. 2004. "Characteristics of the Anterolateral Thigh Flap in a Western Population and Its Application in Head and Neck Reconstruction." *Head & Neck* 26 (9): 759–69. https://doi.org/10.1002/hed.20050.

[7] Lanzer, Martin, Thomas Gander, Klaus Grätz, Claudio Rostetter, Daniel Zweifel, and Marius Bredell. 2015. "Scapular Free Vascularised Bone Flaps for Mandibular Reconstruction: Are Dental Implants Possible?" *Journal of Oral & Maxillofacial Research* 6 (3): e4–e4. https://doi.org/10.5037/jomr.2015.6304.

[8] Stevens JR, Rosko AJ, Marchiano E, Haring C, Chinn SB, Malloy KM, Prince ME, Casper K, Moyer J, Chepeha D, Stucken CL, Spector ME. 2018. "The Spider Limb Positioner in Subscapular System Free Flaps." *Oral Oncology* 85 (October): 24–28. https://doi.org/10.1016/j.oraloncology.2018.08.004.

[9] Marchiano, Emily, Jayne R. Stevens, Eric Liao, Andrew J. Rosko, Allison R. Powell, Steven B. Chinn, Chaz L. Stucken, and Matthew E. Spector. 2020. "Three-Dimensional Modeling of the Scapular Tip for Anterolateral and Lateral Mandibular Defects." *Oral Oncology* 107 (August): 104718. https://doi.org/10.1016/j.oraloncology.2020.104718.

[10] Urken, Mark L., Cheney, Mack L., Blackwell, Keith E., Harris, Jeffrey R., Hadlock, Tessa A., and Futran, Neal. 2012. *Regional and Free Flaps for Head and Neck Reconstruction*. Second. Baltimore, MD: Wolters Kluwer and Lippincott Williams & Wilkins.

[11] Myers, Eugene N. and Snyderman, Carl H. 2018. *Operative Otolaryngology: Head and Neck Surgery*. Third. 2 vols. China: Elsevier.

[12] Olinde, Lindsay M., Nicole I. Farber, and Joshua J. Kain. 2021. "Head and Neck Free-Flap Salvage." *Current Opinion in Otolaryngology & Head and Neck Surgery* 29 (5): 429–36. https://doi.org/10.1097/MOO.0000000000000739.

[13] Crawley, Meghan B., Larissa Sweeny, Prasanti Ravipati, Ryan Heffelfinger, Howard Krein, Adam Luginbuhl, Richard Goldman, and Joseph Curry. 2019. "Factors Associated with Free Flap Failures in Head and Neck Reconstruction." *Otolaryngology–Head and Neck Surgery* 161 (4): 598–604. https://doi.org/10.1177/0194599819860809.

[14] Griffin, John R. 2005. "Microsurgery: Free Tissue Transfer and Replantation." *Selected Readings in Plastic Surgery* 10 (5).

[15] Swendseid, Brian, Ayan Kumar, Larissa Sweeny, Tingting Zhan, Richard A. Goldman, Howard Krein, Ryan N. Heffelfinger, Adam J. Luginbuhl, and Joseph M. Curry. 2020. "Natural History and

Consequences of Nonunion in Mandibular and Maxillary Free Flaps." *Otolaryngology–Head and Neck Surgery* 163 (5): 956–62. https://doi.org/10.1177/0194599820931069.

Chapter 13

Cranioplasty

Gabriel F. Santiago, MD, FNPS
and Chad R. Gordon DO, FNPS

Introduction

Cranioplasty is the term used to describe reconstruction and/or restoration of a skull defect which can result from both trauma, congenital malformation, and/or surgical intervention of the cranium. [1] While cranioplasty has typically been a procedure performed by neurosurgeons, plastic & reconstructive surgeons are increasingly being consulted to assist in the evaluation and treatment of patients undergoing cranioplasty given the improved outcomes that can be achieved with multi-disciplinary care. [2] Historically, cranioplasty techniques date back to 3000 BC where the Inca civilization was found to have performed cranioplasty using precious metals, and other natural materials such as shells and gourds, while xenografts using canine craniums were found to be used in 16th century Europe to as late as 1917 in the United States. [3] Currently, the primary categories of reconstruction materials consist of autologous bone and alloplastic materials, each having their own distinct advantages and disadvantages. [4]

Regardless of the method used, the goal of cranioplasty is to provide protection for the brain, normalize shape of the cranium, and restore the native fluid dynamics (CSF and Blood Flow) of the brain which can be affected by lack of cranial support of the overlying scalp producing *Syndrome of the Trephined* or, *Sinking Scalp Syndrome.* [5] Importantly, one should recognize that cranioplasty is not just a cosmetic procedure, but can improve both physical form, and brain function.

Patient Evaluation

When evaluating a patient for cranioplasty, there are many factors which need to be considered, as these will ultimately guide your choice of timing, material and technique.

1. Consider the etiology of craniectomy and suitability for surgery.
2. Assess the level of neurologic deficit
3. Given risks of cranioplasty, patients with devastating brain injury may not ultimately realize the benefits of cranioplasty and therefore may not be suitable candidates for surgery

In: Essential Facial Plastic and Reconstructive Surgery. Volume 1 ISBN: 979-8-89113-306-8
Editors: Yan Ho Lee and Ira Papel © 2024 Nova Science Publishers, Inc.

4. Given that decompressive craniectomy is often performed to accommodate edematous brain tissue, excessive brain edema may necessitate surgical delay in order to fit within the reconstructed cranium
    a. It is important to distinguish parenchymal edema vs. pseudomeningocele
    b. Patients in the latter category may often be managed with a combination of CSF drainage (either at the time of surgery or with shunting) and cranioplasty
5. Thorough evaluation of the scalp:
    a. Identify all pre-existing incisions which may affect scalp perfusion
    b. Assess for insults to the scalp such from prior surgeries, history of radiation, or presence/absence of existing soft tissue infection
    c. Presence or absence of these factors may necessitate adjunctive measures to prevent extrusion of cranioplasty construct. For example:
        i. In patients with very thin scalps, can employ augmentation techniques using rectus fascia or other biologic materials sutured to deep aspect of scalp to improve integrity [6, 7]
        ii. In patients with signs of soft tissue infection, consult infectious disease for targeted antibiotic therapy (critical to avoid infection of cranioplasty construct)
        iii. For patients with multiple incisions in the scalp, anticipate whether post-operative perfusion will be sufficient to maintain wound integrity over cranioplasty construct (if a soft-tissue defect is likely, scalp rotation over primary defect with full-thickness skin grafting to secondary defect (typically from lower abdomen in order to hide the scar) is a good option, and avoids need for free-tissue transfer in many cases (Figure 13.1)

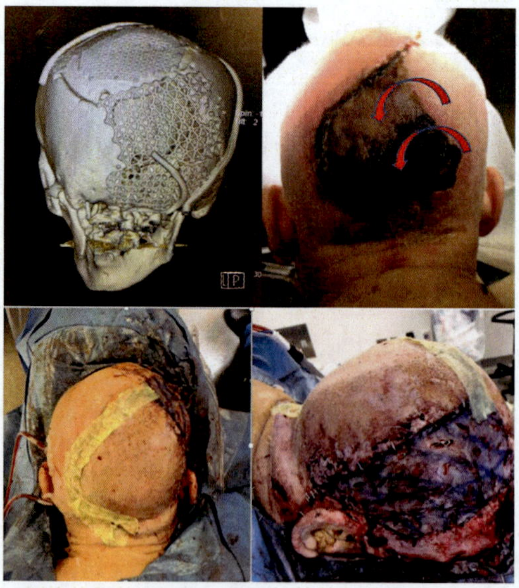

Figure 13.1. Patient with posterior scalp necrosis following a tumor resection. Patient underwent rotational scalp flap from the left parietal scalp and reconstruction of the donor site with full thickness skin graft from the abdomen allowing for closure of the primary defect without need for free-tissue transfer.

iv. In authors' experience, patients with significant sinking of the scalp do not require use of tissue expanders, as loss of elasticity can almost uniformly be overcome with wide-undermining of scalp [2]

Management

Choice of Materials

In cases of large-size cranial defects, use of alloplastic cranial implants has the following advantages over autologous bone:

1. No risk of resorption (especially high risk in younger patients with large cranial defects) [8]
2. Ability to use computer assisted design and manufacture (CAD/CAM) to match both bony and soft-tissue contours of non-injured side of head resulting in improved cosmesis
3. Improved sterility given lack of need for cold storage and handling
4. Ability to modify intra-operatively to fit the contours of cranial defect

Design

1. Planning for cranioplasty involves a multi-disciplinary team of biomedical engineers and surgeons working together to create ideal design
2. To avoid post-cranioplasty temporal hollowing, implant should be designed in a manner which adds bulk over temporal region (Figures 13.2 and 13.3) to account for absence of temporalis muscle rather than just following the skull contour of normal side [9]

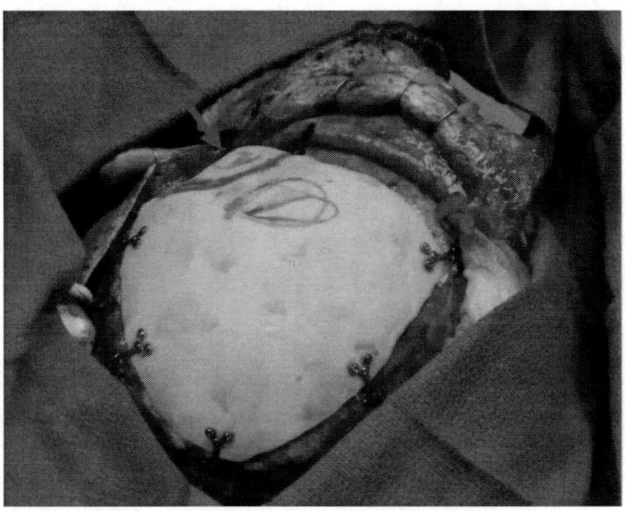

Figure 13.2. Cranioplasty Construct with augmented temporal region.

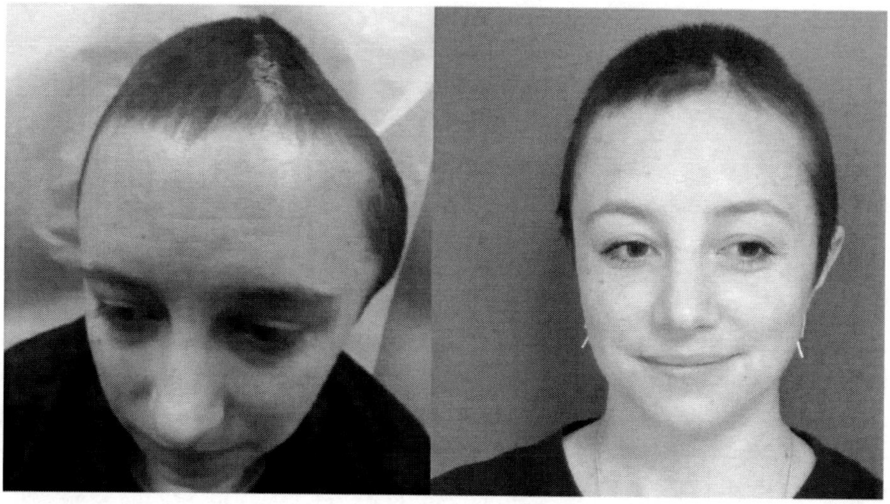

Figure 13.3a. and 13.3b. 13.3a. Patient with history of craniectomy following trauma presenting with skull defect and pseudomeningocele. 13.3b. Patient 3 months following cranioplasty using temporally bulked custom cranial implant to avoid temporal hollowing complication.

Surgical Procedure

1. Shave head whenever possible with use of surgical clippers (razors should be avoided)
2. Horse-shoe headrest preferred as it will allow for access to a greater percentage of scalp during surgery
3. Scrub scalp with a scrub-brush prior to formal sterile prep in order to remove any loose debris from scalp
4. Prep with betadine
5. Drap patient's head to allow for maximal exposure of majority of patient's head (not just area of defect); wide under-mining of the scalp often required to achieve tension free closure
6. Perform a second alcohol-based prep over surgical site
7. Mark cranial defect and planned incision with surgical skin-marker
8. To minimize bleeding, inject tumescent solution consisting of 1:1 1% Xylocaine with 1:100,000 Epinephrine and Normal Saline in sub-galeal space (30-40 ml in total); use extreme caution to avoid intra-parenchymal injection of tumescent solution
9. Minimize blood-loss and maximize preservation of hair follicles:
    a. Avoid use of Rainey clips
    b. Incision scored with a 15 blade to dermis, then completed with needle-tip cautery in segmented fashion on low settings
    c. Any arteries encountered coagulated using bipolar cautery
10. Once the skull defect is encountered, dissection continues with use of needle-tip cautery focusing on dissection in the loose areolar plane
    a. Use the pericranial-onlay technique: leave existing peri-cranium down on top of dura to serve as an additional protective barrier for brain (Figure 13.4)
    b. Correct dissection plane identified by white vertically oriented fibrous tissue

    c. Cautery tip should preferentially be angled slightly towards galeal layer of scalp as opposed to dura in order to avoid accidental durotomy [10]
11. Once flap has been completely elevated, bring cranial implant into field and assess fit
    a. Often, some minor contouring of implant is required
    b. A high-speed drill with pineapple burr often used to smooth sharp edges of cranial implant or improve fit within existing craniectomy.
12. Secure implant well to avoid delayed implant mobility
    a. Titanium neuro-plates often used around circumference of implant to achieve this (Figure 13.2)
    b. Perform final stability test by gently pressing on edges of implant to ensure rigid fixation
13. Bluntly undermine scalp 360 degrees around skull to improve scalp laxity, as tension-free closure is paramount for success
14. Two round 15 french drains used to avoid excess fluid/blood collection over cranioplasty construct
15. Close scalp in 3 layers using 3-0 PDS, followed by 3-0 Vicryl, followed by 3-0 nylon for skin layer
16.

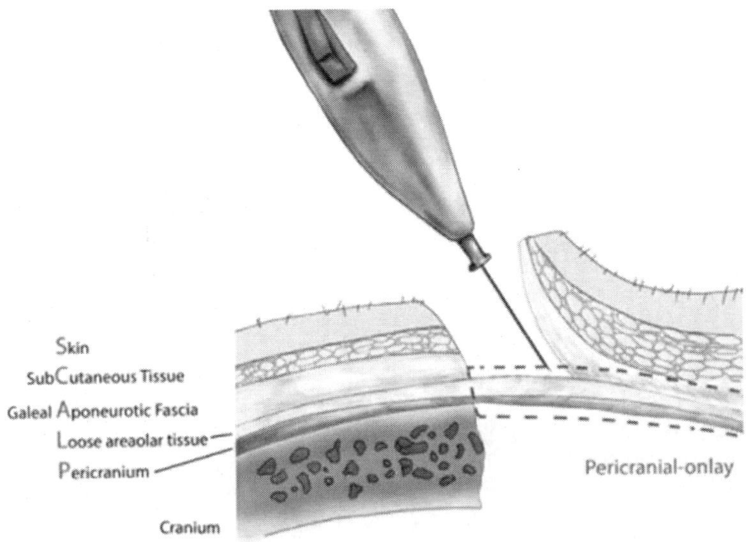

Figure 13.4. Diagram of the dissection plane for pericranial-onlay technique for scalp elevation during cranioplasty.

Postoperative Management

1. Typically remove drains on post-operative day 2 and 3 with discharge on post-operative day 3
2. Sutures left in for 2 weeks at a minimum and removed once adequate healing is noted at post-operative visit

Complications

1. In a series of 500 cranioplasty patients published by the authors (GS, CG), the most common complications include [2]:
    a. Infection (7.8%)
    b. Epidural hematoma (2.2%)
    c. Wound dehiscence (1.8%)
2. Minor complications:
    a. Superficial surgical site infections and transient alterations in mentation (3.6%)
    b. New onset seizures (1.2%)
3. Risk factors for complications: low BMI, long-term anti-coagulation therapy, liver disease, trauma as etiology for craniectomy (vs. vascular event or tumor resection), history of > 2 surgeries, presence of shunting
4. Use of autologous bone was found to be associated with a significantly increased risk of major complications when compared to synthetic material used
5. No difference was found between individual synthetic materials with regards to risk of major complication [2]

Summary Points

1. Cranioplasty is a procedure which improves both form and function in patients with a history of craniectomy.
2. Reconstructive surgeons have a unique perspective with regard to scalp flap design and complex wound closure that can improve outcomes of neurosurgical patients undergoing the cranioplasty procedure.
3. A multi-disciplinary approach involving neurosurgery, reconstructive surgeons and other medical specialists is key to mitigating risk-factors in patients prior to cranioplasty.
4. The use of the pericranial-onlay technique along with special considerations of skin flap design and cranial implant design has been found to minimize post-surgical complications, and maximize success in patients undergoing cranioplasty.[2]

Patient Case

Q1. You are called to evaluate a patient with history of decompressive craniectomy interested in reconstruction. What history would you obtain? (Figure 13.3a.)

A1. The patient appears to have a left sided cranial defect with persistent brain edema vs. pseudomeningocele causing expansion of the left sided scalp. One should obtain a full history regarding the craniectomy with care to note timing of injury and prior treatment history. Additionally, inquiry regarding risk factors for cranioplasty complications should be performed such as medical co-morbidities, prior surgical history, presence of current or prior infection, presence or absence of shunt and neurologic symptoms.

Q2. What should you include in your physical exam?

A2. Head and neck exam especially evaluating the number and locations of prior scalp incisions, integrity of the scalp, signs of soft tissue infection of the scalp, as well as a full neurologic exam to document any pre-existing neurologic deficits. All deficits should be documented to serve as a baseline for post-surgical changes.

Q3. What type of studies should you obtain prior to taking to surgery? What information are you looking to obtain with these studies?

A3. A fine-cut CT Maxillofacial series along with MRI of the brain should be obtained to evaluate the etiology of the left-sided swelling noted on physical exam. In patients with persistent brain parenchymal edema, delay of the cranioplasty should be considered. In patients with meningocele or pseudomeningocele, consultation with neurosurgery should be obtained to determine whether CSF drainage, or shunting can be performed at the same time or prior to cranioplasty. The CT scan can be used for pre-operative design of the patient's cranial implant. It is important to note both the contour of the of the cranium, as well as thickness of the temporalis muscle on the normal side of the head to avoid 'temporal hollowing' appearance following cranioplasty.

Q4. What are the risks of cranioplasty surgery, and what are risk factors for complications?

A4. In a single-surgeon series of 500 patients undergoing cranioplasty, major risks include infection (7.8%), followed by epidural hematoma (2.2%) and wound dehiscence (1.8%). Minor complications include superficial surgical site infections and transient alterations in mentation (3.6%), and new onset seizures (1.2%). Risk factors for complications identified in this cohort included low BMI, long-term anti-coagulation therapy, and liver disease, as well as trauma as the etiology for craniectomy (vs. vascular event or tumor resection), history of > 2 surgeries, and presence of shunting. Notably as well, use of autologous bone was found to be associated with a significantly increased risk of major complications when compared to synthetic material. No difference was found between individual synthetic materials with regards to risk of major complication. [2]

Q5. What is Syndrome of the Trephined, and how can cranioplasty improve brain function?

A5. Syndrome of the Trephined is a complication of craniectomy resulting from atmospheric pressure exerting itself on the brain via the unsupported scalp. Its symptoms include motor, cognitive and language deficits. It has been shown that absence of scalp support by the cranium or cranial construct can result in a reversible alteration in cerebral blood flow and cerebrospinal fluid. Improvement in these factors and the resulting symptoms can be achieved by relieving this atmospheric pressure on the brain. [5]

References

[1] Pasick CM, Margetis K, Santiago GF, Gordon C, Taub PJ. Adult Cranioplasty. *J Craniofac Surg.* 2019 Oct;30(7):2138-2143. doi: 10.1097/SCS.0000000000005659. PMID: 31478955.

[2] Belzberg M, Mitchell KA, Ben-Shalom N, Asemota AO, Wolff AY, Santiago GF, Shay T, Huang J, Manson PN, Brem H, Gordon CR. Cranioplasty Outcomes From 500 Consecutive Neuroplastic Surgery Patients. *J Craniofac Surg.* 2022 Mar 4. doi: 10.1097/SCS.0000000000008546. Epub ahead of print. PMID: 35245275.

[3] Sanan A, Haines SJ. Repairing holes in the head: a history of cranioplasty. *Neurosurgery.* 1997 Mar;40(3):588-603. doi: 10.1097/00006123-199703000-00033. PMID: 9055300.

[4] Wolff A, Santiago GF, Belzberg M, Huggins C, Lim M, Weingart J, Anderson W, Coon A, Huang J, Brem H, Gordon C. Adult Cranioplasty Reconstruction With Customized Cranial Implants: Preferred Technique, Timing, and Biomaterials. *J Craniofac Surg.* 2018 Jun;29(4):887-894. doi: 10.1097/SCS.0000000000004385. PMID: 29489570.

[5] Ashayeri K, M Jackson E, Huang J, Brem H, Gordon CR. Syndrome of the Trephined: A Systematic Review. *Neurosurgery.* 2016 Oct;79(4):525-34. doi: 10.1227/NEU.0000000000001366. PMID: 27489166.

[6] Wolff A, Santiago G, Weingart J, Huang J, Gordon CR. Introducing the Rectus Fascia Scalp Augmentation Technique: A New Method for Improving Scalp Durability in Cranioplasty Reconstruction. *J Craniofac Surg.* 2018 Oct;29(7):1733-1736. doi: 10.1097/SCS.0000000000004686. PMID: 29944559.

[7] Kinsella CR Jr, Grunwaldt LJ, Cooper GM, Mills MC, Losee JE. Scalp reconstruction: regeneration with acellular dermal matrix. *J Craniofac Surg.* 2010 Mar;21(2):605-7. doi: 10.1097/SCS.0b013e3181d08cee. PMID: 20489465.

[8] van de Vijfeijken SECM, Groot C, Ubbink DT, Vandertop WP, Depauw PRAM, Nout E, Becking AG; CranioSafe Group. Factors related to failure of autologous cranial reconstructions after decompressive craniectomy. *J Craniomaxillofac Surg.* 2019 Sep;47(9):1420-1425. doi: 10.1016/j.jcms.2019.02.007. Epub 2019 Feb 16. PMID: 31353299.

[9] Zhong S, Huang GJ, Susarla SM, Swanson EW, Huang J, Gordon CR. Quantitative analysis of dual-purpose, patient-specific craniofacial implants for correction of temporal deformity. *Neurosurgery.* 2015 Jun;11 Suppl 2:220-9; discussion 229. doi: 10.1227/NEU.0000000000000679. PMID: 25710104.

[10] Gordon CR, Fisher M, Liauw J, Lina I, Puvanesarajah V, Susarla S, Coon A, Lim M, Quinones-Hinojosa A, Weingart J, Colby G, Olivi A, Huang J. Multidisciplinary approach for improved outcomes in secondary cranial reconstruction: introducing the pericranial-onlay cranioplasty technique. *Neurosurgery.* 2014 Jun;10 Suppl 2(0 2):179-89; discussion 189-90. doi: 10.1227/NEU.0000000000000296. PMID: 24448187; PMCID: PMC4703091.

Practice Guidelines – Reconstruction of Defects

When a particular set of basic criteria is met, then the Qualified Options for treatment, testing, or management below are reasonable and justifiable recommendations.

- When the patient presents with defects of the scalp, face, or neck, then healing by secondary intension with or without local wound care, primary closure, local flap, regional flap, microvascular reconstruction, allographs, xenographs, tissue expansion, neuromuscular modulation, and filler are qualified options.
- When the patient presents with defects of the scalp, or face involving soft tissue, bone/cartilage, then in addition to the above options, grafts, implants, hair restoration, and prosthetics are qualified options.
- When the patient presents with defects of the neck involving soft tissue, then in addition to the above options, grafts, are qualified options.

Patient Characteristics	Qualified Option(s)
Defects of the Scalp, Face, Neck (Any)	Healing by secondary intention with or without local wound care Primary closure Local flap Regional flap Microvascular reconstruction/free flap Allografts/xenografts Tissue expansion Neuromuscular modulation, filler*
Defects of the Scalp, Face (Soft tissue or bone/cartilage)	Graft(s): skin/mucosal/dermal/fat/composite/ cartilage/bone/nerve Implants Hair restoration Prosthetics (e.g., ear, nose, hair)
Defects of the Neck (Soft tissue)	Graft(s): skin/mucosal/dermal/fat/nerve

*Note: while some autologous filler material (e.g., fat, dermis) may be covered by payors, certain materials may not be covered

Part 3. Congenital Anomalies

Chapter 14

Microtia

Magdalena Soldanska, MD
and Alexis Tashima, MD

Introduction

1. Microtia translates to mean "small ear", however, the term is used to refer to a wide spectrum of congenital auricular anomalies where any portion of the ear is deficient or missing
2. Presentation can range from complete absence of an ear, to mild anomalies in shape, and is frequently associated with aural atresia (absence of external auditory canal) and conductive hearing loss
3. Microtia is the second most common congenital deformity of the head and neck, after cleft lip and palate
4. Incidence of microtia is 1 in 6,000-10,000 live births (slightly higher in Asian and Hispanic populations
5. More common in males than females, and right side more common than left [1]
6. Most often unilateral (90%), however can be bilateral. 60%-70% isolated.
7. Can be associated with hemifacial microsomia/Goldenhar syndrome, or Treacher Collins syndrome [2]
8. Can be classified by area of affected anatomy
    a. Nagata classification:
        i. Lobular microtia (also called Grade 3)
        ii. Small conchal microtia
        iii. Large conchal microtia
        iv. Anotia (also called Grade 4)
    b. Grades:
        i. Grade 1: ear is smaller than normal; key features are present; may have minor alterations in shape or form
        ii. Grade 2: some features of ear are missing, though usually much of the lower two-thirds of the ear is still present; sometimes called "conchal type microtia"; ear canal may be present, but may have canal stenosis
        iii. Grade 3: most common type of microtia, featuring small peanut-shaped remnant ear lobe; sometimes called "lobular type microtia"; aural atresia (Figure 14.1)

In: Essential Facial Plastic and Reconstructive Surgery. Volume 1 ISBN: 979-8-89113-306-8
Editors: Yan Ho Lee and Ira Papel © 2024 Nova Science Publishers, Inc.

iv. Grade 4: Complete absence of external ear without any remnant; "anotia"; rarely seen [3]

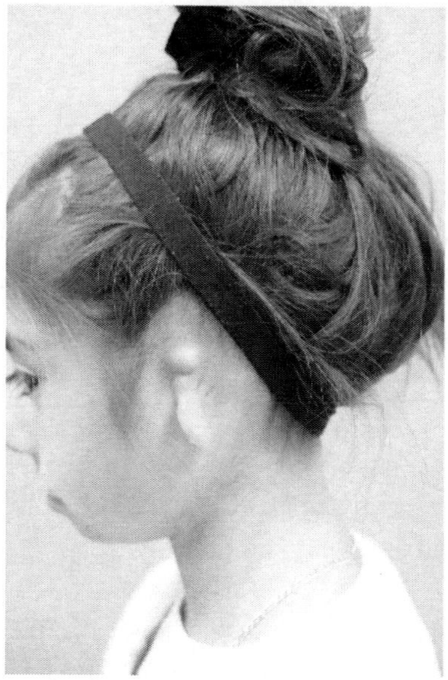

Figure 14.1. Pt is a 9 year old female with craniofacial microsomia and bilateral lobular type microtia.

Patient Evaluation

1. Look for:
    a. Associated first and second brachial arch anomalies or hemifacial microsomia
    b. Facial symmetry including occlusal cant, malocclusion, facial nerve weakness
    c. Type of microtia (Nagata classification)
    d. Presence or absence of external auditory canal (If present, assess if it is normal)
    e. Hairline (may be inferiorly positioned, especially in syndromic patients, such as in hemifacial microsomia or Treacher Collins)
    f. Previous hearing evaluation
2. Inquire about previous surgeries:
    a. Previous ear reconstruction
    b. Cochlear implants
    c. Tympanoplasties
    d. Bone-anchored hearing aid (BAHA) placement
        i. Implant to improve conductive hearing loss (i.e., in patient with aural atresia)
        ii. If bilateral conductive hearing loss, may need hearing augmentation earlier to improve speech development
    e. Any surgery requiring coronal incision (due to potential disruption of the superficial temporal artery)
3. Consider imaging:

   a. Preop CT scan not necessary
   b. Can be performed to assess anatomy of thorax
   c. Can allow for 3D modeling of cartilage harvest and cartilage construct
4. Collaborate with multiple teams: craniofacial, ENT, audiology
   a. Audiology may already be involved if newborn screening revealed hearing loss
   b. If BAHA placed before ear reconstruction, coordinate with ENT surgeon placing BAHA to ideally place implant and processor away from normal postauricular skin and away from the temporoparietal fascia (TPF) [4]

Management

1. Options for reconstruction
   a. Autologous reconstruction (costal cartilage)
      i. most widely used technique for total ear reconstruction [5, 6]
      ii. Benefits: patient's native tissue = better incorporation, less risk of infection or extrusion [7-9]
      iii. Risks: donor site morbidity, multiple surgeries, possible resorption
   b. Synthetic based reconstruction (High-density Porous Polyethylene, e.g., Medpor/Supor)
      i. Benefits: ability to perform surgery at younger age (3-7), no donor site, possible improved definition and shape, fewer surgical procedures, may be 3D printed [10-14]
      ii. Risks: higher risk of infection and extrusion, need to utilize a large TPF flap, thus less soft tissue available for salvage [15, 16]
   c. Auricular prosthesis
      i. Benefits: best appearance and likeness to normal ear, less involved surgery, only option if poor surrounding skin quality (burns), failed reconstruction with no usable superficial temporal artery or other fascia
      ii. Risks: does not change color with patient's natural skin, may dislodge, requires daily maintenance (poor compliance in children), high cost (usually not covered by insurance), need to replace every few years.
2. Timing:
   a. 8-10 years of age for autologous reconstruction
   b. Allow for growth of the normal ear to make framework for reconstruction (ear growth complete around age 7) [17]
   c. Sufficient cartilage needed to create a construct for the ear (chest circumference around 60cm for sufficient costal cartilage to create a complete ear construct) [18]
   d. Child is mature enough to express their own desire to have a reconstructed ear
   e. Compliance with post-operative care
3. Surgical technique of autologous reconstruction

a. Stage 1: Creation of pocket, harvesting rib and carving construct:
   i. Fabricating template:
      - Trace contours of normal ear (contralateral or parent's if bilateral microtia) on transparent plastic film
      - Account for skin thickness (1.5-2mm) by making framework slightly shorter/smaller than the target auricle
   ii. Markings for ear placement:
      - General landmarks: lateral canthus and oral commissure
      - Position may vary in patients with hemifacial microsomia and ear must be placed in aesthetically pleasing position, especially with concern for any possible future jaw reconstruction
      - Most important aspects of symmetry include the craniocaudal position of the ear and the angle from vertical meridian (most commonly 15 degrees)
      - Doppler trajectory of superficial temporal artery (often aberrant, especially in setting of syndromic microtia), and protect throughout dissection of pocket
   iii. Skin Incision:
      - Auricular skin is best for reconstructing an ear (fascial flaps used only when auricular skin not available) [19]
      - "W" incision designed to allow for rotation of lobule and allow for adequate dissection of pocket to place the framework (Nagata technique) [20]
      - May use transverse incision to preserve normal earlobe (Firmin technique)
      - Carefully dissect pocket 1cm outside of proposed placement to decrease skin tension
      - Remove any abnormal cartilage remnant, preserve normal cartilage where present
      - Keep skin over pocket thin to allow for natural contours (subcutaneous dissection with scissors and minimal use of electrocautery)
   iv. Graft harvest and carving:
      - Costal cartilage is the only cartilage with sufficient quantity and ability to hold its shape in the setting of deforming forces of the skin
      - Make oblique skin incision over 6th and 7th rib. Dissect down to perichondrium preserving as much muscle integrity as possible
      - Graft harvest from the ipsilateral or contralateral side (Figure 14.2)
        - Base piece to be carved from the synchondrosis of two ribs (6 and 7)

  - Eighth costal cartilage rib used for helix (at least 7 cm in length to recreate curvature)
  - Additional cartilage harvested for tragus, antitragus, and antihelix
  - Ideally, preserve as much perichondrium (especially posterior) in the chest to minimize deformity (except on rib 8 or 9, which are floating ribs)
- Carve all anatomic pieces on side table with specialized microtia carving gauges based on previously-made template, and combine pieces with double armed 5-0 wire suture, burying the twisted wire ends into the construct to prevent palpability or extrusion
- Maintain enough cartilage thickness to minimize collapse under skin tension; requires cartilage thicker than conchal cartilage to maintain stability
- Close muscle and skin of donor site over the catheter of a local anesthetic releasing pump (e.g., On-Q pump) for post-operative pain management, or perform intercostal nerve block [21]
  - Donor site often source of highest pain post operatively
  - Any left-over cartilage can be banked in chest soft tissues and saved for second stage if possible

v. Cartilage graft placement in ear pocket:
- Set the angle from vertical meridian, anchor construct to underlying fascia
- Place 2 small suction drains (e.g. 4mm TLS drains)
- If revision ear reconstruction is being done in area with scarred skin, or if low hairline, use TPF flap to cover construct where there is lack of normal quality or hairless skin, and then place skin graft over fascia

vi. Post-operative care
- Chest X-ray should be considered to rule out pneumothorax from rib harvest
- Admit patient until pain adequately controlled (usually 1-2 days)
- Remove drains prior to discharge
- Keep ear covered for at least 1 week
- Consider prophylactic antibiotics

b. Stage 2: Elevation of construct and creation of retroauricular sulcus (Figure 14.3)

i. Elevation of construct
- Performed 6 months after 1st stage, 1 year if TPF used in 1st stage

- Goal is to provide projection of the reconstructed ear that is symmetric, and to create a retroauricular sulcus with normal depth
- Graft is elevated up to the level of the concha keeping a thin layer of soft tissue over cartilage construct

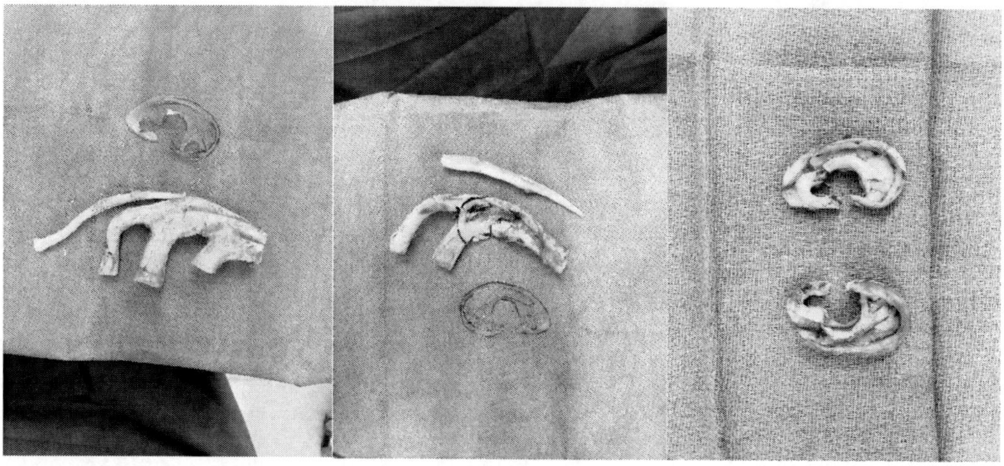

Figure 14.2. After cartilage harvest, the ear template is traced onto the harvested rib cartilage to create individual anatomic components, which are then carved and connected with wire suture.

ii. Creation of retroauricular sulcus
   - Support/projection of the construct can be achieved with banked cartilage or polyethylene implant placed medial to the antihelix to mimic the concha
   - Coverage of projection cartilage or implant often involves vascularized fascia with overlying full thickness or split thickness skin graft
   - Options for fascial flaps: superficial or deep TPF (must have an intact superficial temporal artery), random-pattern mastoid fascia, occipital fascia
   - Skin graft harvest may be from scalp (STSG), contralateral post-auricular sulcus, or trunk
   - Bolster the graft to prevent hematoma and promote full adherence

iii. Post-operative care
   - Patient may be discharged same day or observed overnight
   - Headwrap dressing for at least 1 week
   - Consider prophylactic antibiotics

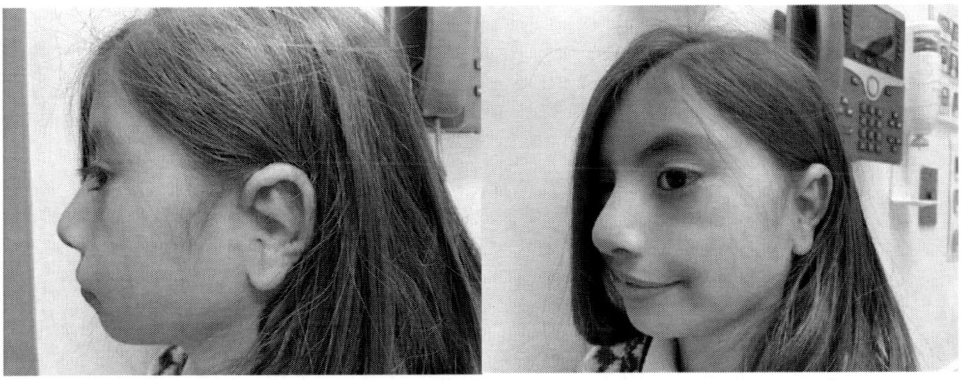

Figure 14.3. 9 year old patient underwent Nagata two stage autologous ear reconstruction with elevation of construct 6 months after first stage reconstruction.

Complications

1. Most common: skin necrosis and resulting exposure or infection of the underlying framework [22]
2. Any amount of skin necrosis must be addressed and cartilage construct must be completely covered as soon as possible with return to operating room (within 1 week) to prevent resorption of cartilage [23]
3. Soft tissue coverage from post-auricular skin or fascial flap and skin graft [24]
4. Less common: exposed wire, hypertrophic scar or keloid, chest wall deformity
5. Challenging cases include bilateral microtia, hemifacial microsomia, revision surgery, thick skin, ectopic meatus, low hairline
6. Well-vascularized temporoparietal fascia flap (superficial or deep), mastoid fascia and occipital fascia are all "lifeboats" to salvage reconstruction in instances of exposure or in revision surgery

Summary Points

1. Autologous ear reconstruction using a costal cartilage framework is the most commonly used technique for total ear reconstruction
2. Reconstruction of the ear is one of the most challenging surgical procedures with inconsistent results (even by experienced auricular reconstructive surgeons) and should be only performed by those with adequate training and experience
3. Newer techniques and future directions of total ear reconstruction include 3D modeling of the normal ear, tissue expansion of fascial flaps, and tissue engineering [25]
4. Challenges include creating a natural scaffold that withstands the tension of contracting deficient skin in microtia patients

Patient Case

Q1. A 7 year-old male patient sees you in the office with an external ear below. (Figure 14.4) What would you ask about the patient's history?

A1.

1. Medical and surgical history
2. Family history of congenital malformations
3. Hearing history

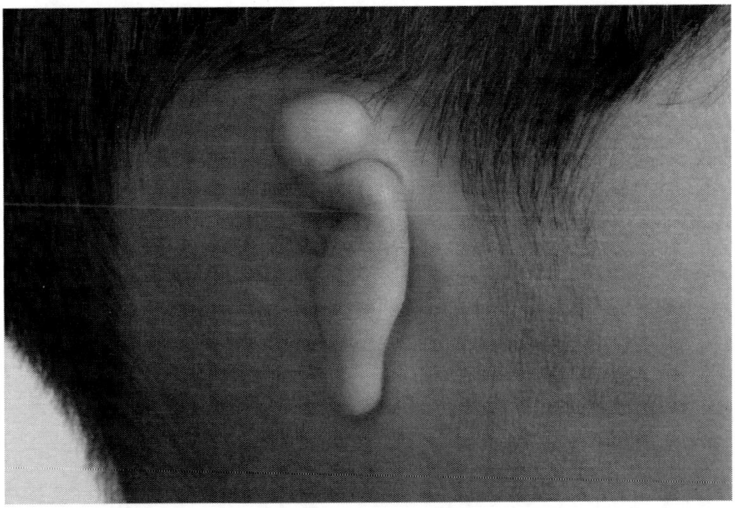

Figure 14.4. Case Figure.

Q2. What would you look for on physical exam?

A2.

1. Associated first and second brachial arch anomalies or hemifacial microsomia
2. Facial symmetry including occlusal cant, malocclusion, facial nerve weakness
3. Type of microtia (in this case: Grade 3 or Nagata classification small conchal type)
4. Presence or absence of external auditory canal (If present, assess if it is normal)
5. Hairline (may be inferiorly positioned, especially in syndromic patients, such as in hemifacial microsomia or Treacher Collins)
6. Signs of previous surgeries:
    a. Previous ear reconstruction
    b. Cochlear implants
    c. Tympanoplasties
    d. Bone-anchored hearing aid (BAHA) placement
        i. Implant to improve conductive hearing loss (i.e., in patient with aural atresia)
        ii. If bilateral conductive hearing loss, may need hearing augmentation earlier to improve speech development
    e. Any surgery requiring coronal incision (due to potential disruption of the superficial temporal artery)

Q3. What other diagnostic tests would you consider?

A3.

1. Hearing tests/evaluations
2. Imaging:
    a. Preop CT
    b. Chest Xray: an be performed to assess anatomy of thorax
    c. CT imaging can allow for 3D modeling of cartilage harvest and cartilage construct

Q4. What other specialties/teams would you consider involving?

A4.

1. Craniofacial
2. ENT
3. Audiology

Q5. How would you counsel the patient and his family regarding timing of repair?

A5.

1. Timing of surgery depends on a variety of factors:
    a. Usually 8-10 years of age for autologous reconstruction
    b. Should allow for growth of the normal ear to make framework for reconstruction (ear growth complete around age 7)
    c. Sufficient cartilage needed to create a construct for the ear (chest circumference around 60cm for sufficient costal cartilage to create a complete ear construct)
    d. Child should be mature enough to express their own desire to have a reconstructed ear
    e. Consider compliance with post-operative care

Q6. What is the 2-stage technique for microtia repair? (Nagata)

A6.

1. Stage 1 - harvesting costal cartilages; fabricate 3D costal cartilage framework; place graft in anatomic position underneath soft tissue flap
2. Stage 2 - elevate reconstructed auricle to achieve desired projection

Q7. What is the 4-stage technique for microtia repair? (Brent)

A7.

1. Stage 1 - harvest the rib cartilage to create basic size and shape of the ear; place graft in anatomic position underneath soft tissue
2. Stage 2 - create the earlobe; at least 2 months after stage 1
3. Stage 3 - elevate the cartilage framework; at least three months after stage 2
4. Stage 4 - create the tragus; at least three months after stage 3 is completed

References

[1] Wilkes GH, Wong J, Guilfoyle R. Microtia reconstruction. *Plast Reconstr Surg*. 2014 Sep;134(3):464e-479e.

[2] Hartzell LD, Chinnadurai S. Microtia and Related Facial Anomalies. *Clin Perinatol*. 2018 Dec;45(4):679-697.

[3] Kim A, Lee H, Oh KS. Review of 602 Microtia Reconstructions: Revisions and Specific Recommendations for Each Subtype. *Plast Reconstr Surg*. 2020 Jul;146(1):133-142.

[4] Zhang TY, Bulstrode N, Chang KW, Cho YS, Frenzel H, Jiang D, Kesser BW, Siegert R, Triglia JM. International Consensus Recommendations on Microtia, Aural Atresia and Functional Ear Reconstruction. *J Int Adv Otol*. 2019 Aug;15(2):204-208.

[5] Joukhadar N, McKee D, Caouette-Laberge L, Bezuhly M. Management of Congenital Auricular Anomalies. *Plast Reconstr Surg*. 2020 Aug;146(2):205e-216e.

[6] Bonilla A. Pediatric Microtia Reconstruction with Autologous Rib: Personal Experience and Technique with 1000 Pediatric Patients with Microtia. *Facial Plast Surg Clin North Am*. 2018 Feb;26(1):57-68.

[7] Im DD, Paskhover B, Staffenberg DA, Jarrahy R. Current management of microtia: a national survey. *Aesthetic Plast Surg*. 2013 Apr;37(2):402-8.

[8] Ikeda AK, Bhrany AD, Sie KCY, Bly RA. Management of patients with unilateral microtia and aural atresia: recent advances and updates. *Curr Opin Otolaryngol Head Neck Surg*. 2021 Dec 1;29(6):526-533.

[9] Siegert R, Magritz R. Otoplasty and Auricular Reconstruction. *Facial Plast Surg*. 2019 Aug;35(4):377-386.

[10] Wang Y, Zhang J, Liang W, Xiao X, Zhang J, Zhang J, Su Z, Liu M, Chen Y, Ji C. Ear Reconstruction with the Combination of Expanded Skin Flap and Medpor Framework: 20 Years of Experience in a Single Center. *Plast Reconstr Surg*. 2021 Oct 1;148(4):850-860.

[11] Jiang C, Zhao C, Chen B, Lu L, Sun Y, Yan X, Yi B, Wu H, Shi R. Auricular reconstruction using Medpor combined with different hearing rehabilitation approaches for microtia. *Acta Otolaryngol*. 2021 Jun;141(6):572-578.

[12] Li Y, Li D, Xu Z, Zhang R, Zhang Q, Xu F, Chen X. New strategies for base frame fabrication in microtia reconstruction. *Sci Rep*. 2021 Aug 5;11(1):15947.

[13] Mao X, Li X, Jia J, Kang D, Miao Y, Lu Z, Hu Z. Validity and reliability of three-dimensional costal cartilage imaging for donor-site assessment and clinical application in microtia reconstruction patients: A prospective study of 22 cases. *Clin Otolaryngol*. 2020 Mar;45(2):204-210.

[14] Leto Barone AA, Redett RJ. Pursuing Mirror Image Reconstruction in Unilateral Microtia: Customizing Auricular Framework by Application of Three-Dimensional Imaging and Three-Dimensional Printing. *Plast Reconstr Surg*. 2018 Jun;141(6):973e-974e.

[15] Constantine KK, Gilmore J, Lee K, Leach J Jr. Comparison of microtia reconstruction outcomes using rib cartilage vs porous polyethylene implant. *JAMA Facial Plast Surg*. 2014 Jul-Aug;16(4):240-4.

[16] Tahiri Y, Reinisch J. Porous Polyethylene Ear Reconstruction. *Clin Plast Surg*. 2019 Apr;46(2):223-230.

[17] Sun Z, Yu X, Chen W, Yang Q, Song Y, Zhou J, Jiang H. Costal Cartilage Assessment in Surgical Timing of Microtia Reconstruction. *J Craniofac Surg*. 2017 Sep;28(6):1521-1525.

[18] Kim A, Moon J, Lim SY, Oh KS. The Interchondral Joints of Thorax in Microtia Surgery: Classification and Fabrication Strategies. *Ann Plast Surg*. 2021 Jul 1;87(1):98-104.

[19] Hwang E, Kim YS, Chung S. A new skin flap method for total auricular reconstruction in microtia patients with a reconstructed ear canal: extended scalp and extended mastoid postauricular skin flaps. *J Plast Reconstr Aesthet Surg*. 2014 Jun;67(6):770-4.

[20] Yamada A. Autologous Rib Microtia Construction: Nagata Technique. *Facial Plast Surg Clin North Am*. 2018 Feb;26(1):41-55.

[21] Woo KJ, Kang BY, Min JJ, Park JW, Kim A, Oh KS. Postoperative pain control by preventive intercostal nerve block under direct vision followed by catheter-based infusion of local analgesics in rib cartilage harvest for auricular reconstruction in children with microtia: A randomized controlled trial. *J Plast Reconstr Aesthet Surg*. 2016 Sep;69(9):1203-10.

[22] Saadi RA, Snyder D, Shokri T, Lighthall JG. Postoperative outcomes of autologous rib graft for microtia repair in children: A NSQIP study. *Int J Pediatr Otorhinolaryngol.* 2021 Jul;146:110733.

[23] Cugno S, Bulstrode NW. Cartilage exposure following autologous microtia reconstruction: An algorithmic treatment approach. *J Plast Reconstr Aesthet Surg*. 2019 Mar;72(3):498-504.

[24] Kim YS, Yun IS, Chung S. Salvage of Ear Framework Exposure in Total Auricular Reconstruction. *Ann Plast Surg.* 2017 Feb;78(2):178-183.

[25] Fu YY, Li CL, Xie YZ, Zhu YY, Zhang TY. Functional ear reconstruction strategies for microtia with congenital aural stenosis in seventy-six patients. *Clin Otolaryngol.* 2020 Jul;45(4):611-615.

Chapter 15

Cleft Lip and Nose

Miles J. Pfaff, MD
and Joseph E. Losee, MD

Introduction

Embryology

1. Nasolabial complex development
    a. Timing: fourth to sixth weeks gestation
    b. Columella, nasal tip, philtrum, frenulum, labial tubercle, and primary palate
        i. Arise from intermaxillary segment, which forms from fusion of bilateral medial nasal prominences
    c. Ala formation
        i. Fusion of medial and lateral nasal processes
2. Cleft lip and nose deformity
    a. Failure of fusion of medial nasal and maxillary prominences [1, 2]

Anatomy of the Unilateral Cleft Lip and Nose Deformity

1. Lip [3] (Figure 15.1A and 15.1B)
    a. Separated into medial (noncleft) and lateral lip (cleft) elements
    b. Medial lip element
        i. Orbicularis oris inserts into anterior nasal spine and columella
        ii. Median tubercle deficiency (more than lateral lip element)
    c. Lateral lip element
        i. Orbicularis oris inserts into alar base
        ii. Median tubercle deficiency
2. Nose [4, 5, 6]
    a. Caudal septal deviation towards noncleft side
    b. Nasal tip deviation towards cleft side
    c. Septal bowing towards cleft side
    d. Cleft side lower lateral cartilage is diminutive and flat relatively to non-cleft side
    e. Increased alar base width on cleft side (displaced laterally); alar base is also displaced posteriorly and inferiorly

In: Essential Facial Plastic and Reconstructive Surgery. Volume 1 ISBN: 979-8-89113-306-8
Editors: Yan Ho Lee and Ira Papel © 2024 Nova Science Publishers, Inc.

f. Vertical height deficiency of columella

3. Alveolus

a. Incomplete or complete cleft of alveolus

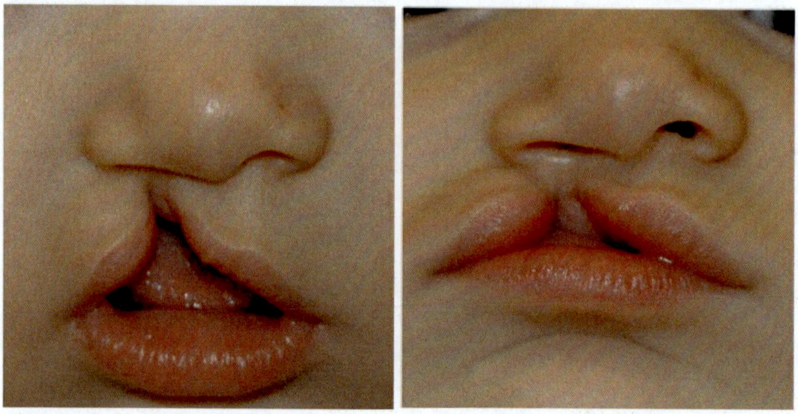

Figure 15.1. Pre-operative 6-week-old male with a right unilateral incomplete cleft lip. A) Frontal and B) basal views.

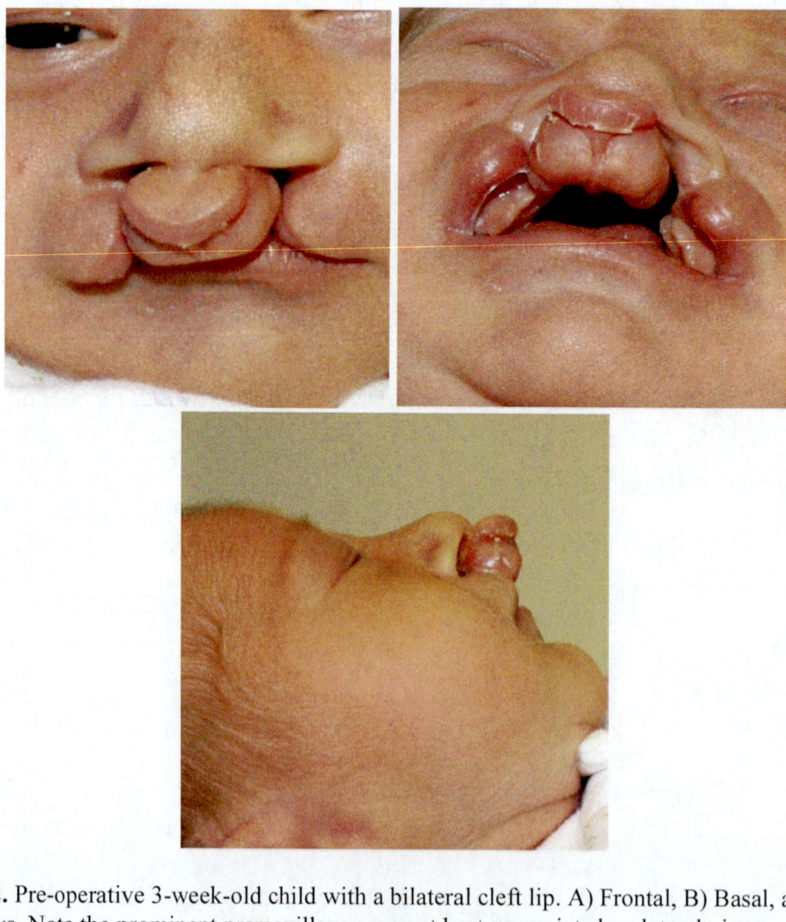

Figure 15.2. Pre-operative 3-week-old child with a bilateral cleft lip. A) Frontal, B) Basal, and C) Lateral views. Note the prominent premaxillary segment best appreciated on lateral view.

Anatomy of the Bilateral Cleft Lip and Nose Deformity (Figure 15.2A-C)

1. Lip [7]
    a. Premaxilla is not attached to the lateral palatal shelves
    b. Prolabium
        i. No orbicularis oris is present
        ii. Diminutive vermillion
    c. Relatively symmetrical lateral lip elements
        i. Orbicularis oris inserts along the alar bases
2. Nose [8]
    a. Symmetry of the nasal ala
    b. Septal deviation is absent or mild in the complete symmetrical cleft
    c. Severe vertical deficiency of the columella
3. Alveolus
    a. Incomplete or complete cleft of the alveolus

Epidemiology

1. Isolated unilateral left lip with and without palate
    a. Most common congenital facial birth defect
        i. General population incidence – ~0.1 to 2.5:1000 births
        ii. Ethnic Breakdown
            - Asian and Native American – 1:450 births
            - Caucasian – 1:1000 births
            - Black – 1:2000 births
    b. Males more likely affected
    c. More common on left side
    d. Risk factors [1, 2, 9]
        i. Genetics
            - Van der Woude syndrome
                - Most common syndrome associated with unilateral cleft lip and palate
                - Characterized by cleft lip and congenital lower lip pits
                - Autosomal dominant, *IRF 6*-linked mutation
            - Other known mutations
                - MSX1
                - TBX22
                - Many genes demonstrate direct relationship to environmental risk factors
        ii. Environmental
            - Maternal folate deficiency
            - Prenatal medications including steroid and antiepileptics
            - Prenatal alcohol and tobacco exposure
        iii. Family history

- Greatest risk factor
- See Table 15.1 for recurrence risk

Table 15.1. Risk of Recurrence: Unilateral Cleft Lip with or without Palate

Affected Family Member(s)	Risk, child (%)
Parent	4%
Parent and Sibling	Up to 15%
Single sibling	4%
Two siblings	9%

2. Bilateral Cleft Lip with and without Palate
    a. Unilateral cleft lip is ~ 9X more common than bilateral cleft lip

Patient Evaluation and Management

Classification

1. Unilateral and Bilateral Cleft Lip Deformity [3, 10]
    a. Complete
        i. Cleft includes the entire lip and may or may not include the nostril floor and sill, alveolus, and palate
    b. Incomplete
        i. Cleft does not include the entire lip and spares the nasal sill and may or may not affect the alveolus and palate
    c. Minor
        i. Cleft with a vermillion notch that is greater than 3 mm
        ii. Vertical depression above the notch into the nasal sill
    d. Microform
        i. Cleft with a vermillion notch that is less than 3 mm
        ii. No nasal deformity
    e. Nasal deformity is variable and typically correlates with cleft lip severity

Presurgical Care

1. Multidisciplinary care with dedicated cleft team is necessary
2. Prenatal consultation, education, and psychological and psychosocial support [11]
3. Cleft lip repair typically done by 6 months of age
4. Can be performed for both unilateral and bilateral cleft lip
5. Presurgical orthopedics
    a. Goal is to optimize surgical outcome by manipulation of alveolar segments and/or nose

b. Options include nasoalveolar molding (NAM), Latham device, taping across the cleft, and isolated nasal molding
   i. NAM - one of the most common forms of presurgical molding in the United States (Figure 15.3)
      - Involves presurgical molding of nasal and alveolar tissue to decrease size of the cleft, align greater and lesser alveolar segments, and shape nose [12]
      - Improves long-term post-operative aesthetic outcomes [13, 14]

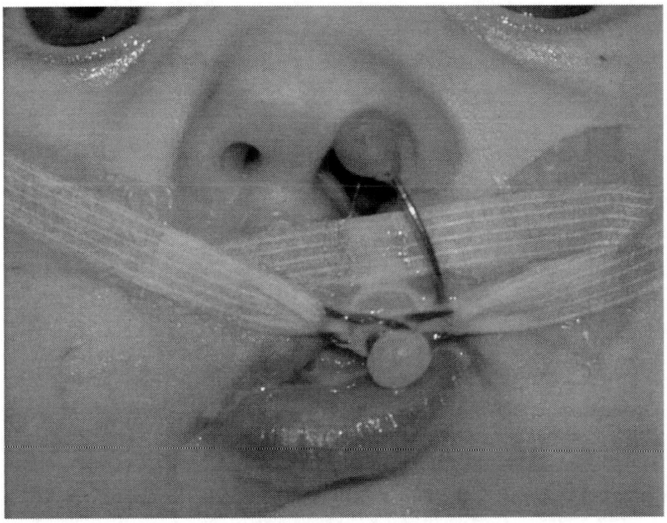

Figure 15.3. 2-month-old patient with a right complete cleft lip undergoing nasoalveolar molding. Note the nasal component that molds or shapes the affected side. An alveolar-palatal splint (not visualized) shapes the alveolar segment to better align the alveolar segments and narrow the cleft.

6. Lip Adhesion
   a. Goal is to optimize final outcome by surgically reapproximating nostril sill and upper aspects of medial and lateral segments (lip and muscle), converting complete cleft to an incomplete morphology
   b. Care should be taken to not disrupt landmarks required for cleft lip repair

Surgical Repair of the Cleft Lip [3, 4, 6]

1. Goals of cleft lip repair
   a. Obliteration of cleft
   b. Establish normal nasolabial anatomy
      i. Muscle sphincter (orbicularis oris)
      ii. Philtral column
      iii. Cupid's bow
      iv. Vermilion shape and height
      v. Inconspicuous post-operative scar

2. Unilateral cleft lip and nasal deformity repair
    a. While multiple repairs have been described, no superior repair has been established
    b. Rotation-Advancement repair is the most common repair [3, 15, 16, 17] (Figure 15.4; Figure 15.5A and B)
        i. Many modifications have been described
        ii. Repair utilizes multiple flaps to reconstruct philtrum, vermilion, cupid's bow, and nasal sill

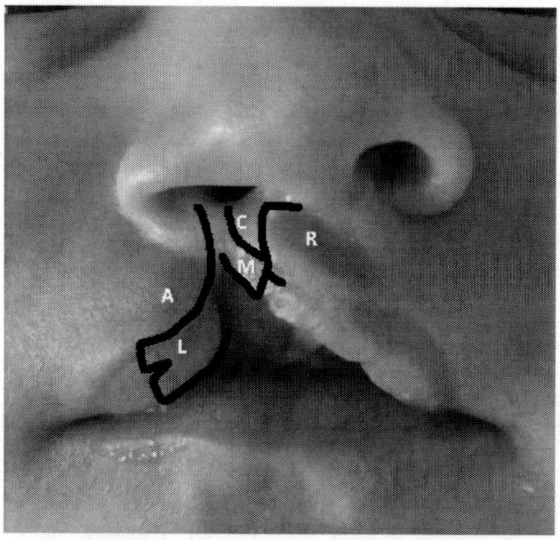

Figure 15.4. Standard rotation-advancement incision markings. A, Advancement flap; C, C-flap; L, L-flap; M, M-flap; N, Noordhoff's point; and R, Rotation flap

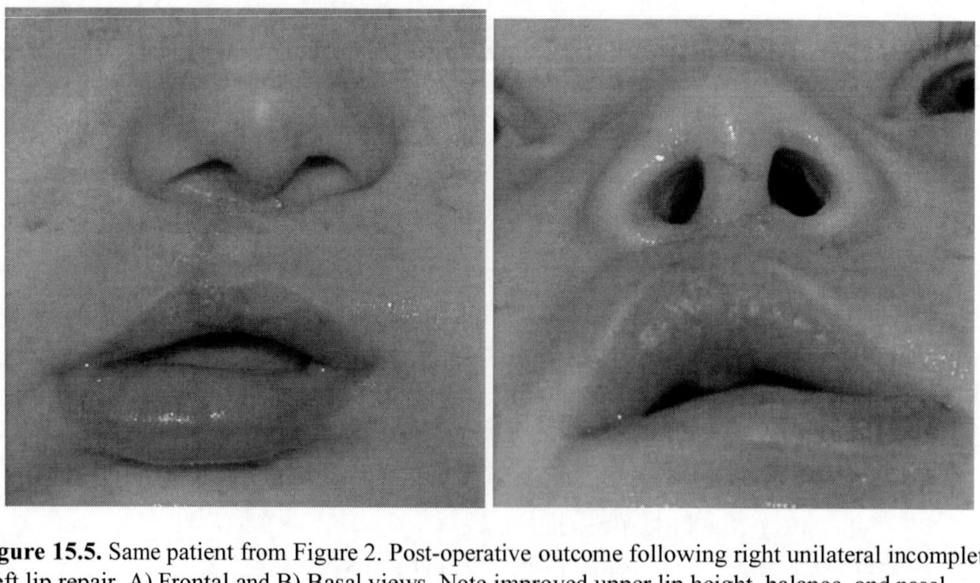

Figure 15.5. Same patient from Figure 2. Post-operative outcome following right unilateral incomplete cleft lip repair. A) Frontal and B) Basal views. Note improved upper lip height, balance, and nasal symmetry.

        iii. Concept
            - Rotation flap

- Medial segment
- Advancement flap
  - Lateral segment
- C-flap
  - Used for columellar augmentation and nasal floor closure
  - Located along base of cleft-side columella
- L-flap
  - Used for nasal mucosa closure
  - Located along lateral segment
- M-flap
  - Used for alveolar/gingivobuccal sulcus reinforcement
  - Located along medial segment

c. Rhinoplasty often performed at time of lip repair [4, 16]
   i. Goals of cleft rhinoplasty
      - Achieve nasal symmetry
      - Columellar lengthening (in bilateral cleft)
      - Minimal disruption of nasal growth
      - Provide foundation for definitive septorhinoplasty
   ii. Semi-open rhinoplasty commonly performed
   iii. Techniques vary but focus on repositioning lower lateral cartilage on cleft side to narrow angle of domal divergence

3. Bilateral cleft lip repair
   a. Millard-Mulliken repair is the most common repair [8, 18]
      i. Philtrum provided by prolabium
      ii. Cupid's bow, white roll, and vermillion reconstructed from bilateral lateral lip advancement flaps

Post-Operative Care

1. Overnight admission for pain control, assistance with feeding, and ensure airway patency
2. Post-operative nasal stenting to mold nasal cartilage commonly employed
3. Aggressive scar precautions:
   a. Silicone taping
   b. Scar massage
   c. Avoidance of sun exposure

Complications

1. Wound dehiscence
   a. Management depends on degree of dehiscence, structures exposed, and time from surgery

2. Infection
    a. Risk of infection is low
3. Excessive scarring [19]
    a. Hypertrophic and keloid formation
        i. Management includes conservative measures (steroid therapy and silicone compression) and lip scar revision
4. Lip asymmetry
    a. Can affect any of the nasolabial components
    b. Vermillion asymmetry frequent
    c. Whistle deformity [20, 21]
        i. Upper and lower lip margins do not touch at repose, giving appearance of one attempting to whistle

Summary Points

1. Dedicated multidisciplinary cleft team is foundational to successful cleft care
2. Detailed understanding of nasolabial embryology and anatomy is essential
3. Cleft lip repair is typically performed between 3 to 6 months of age
4. While no superior approach to cleft lip repair has been established, the rotation-advancement technique is the most commonly performed approach
5. Semi-open rhinoplasty is commonly performed at the time of cleft lip repair
6. Complications following cleft lip repair are rare

Patient Case

A 6-week-old male presents to your clinic with the following congenital deformity:

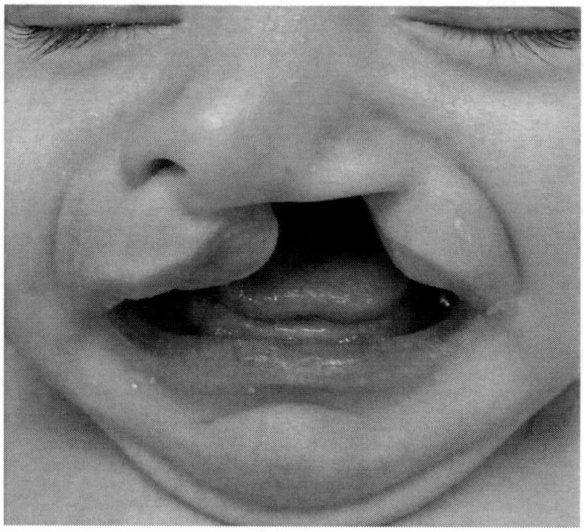

Figure 15.6. Case: Cleft lip.

Q1: How would you classify this cleft?

A1: This is a left unilateral complete cleft lip. A classification system [10] commonly used—L-NS-A-H-S-H-A-NS-L—characterizes the cleft as complete or incomplete, documents laterality, and characterizes the degree of lip, nasal sill, alveolar, and palatal clefting. The complete cleft lip includes a complete cleft of the lip (L) with or without an intact nasal sill (NS), alveolus (A), hard palate (H), and soft palate (S).

Q2: This family's first child was born with a cleft lip, and neither parent has a history of a cleft lip. The parents are considering having another child in the future. What is the probability that their second child will have a cleft lip?

A2: The probability that their next child will have a cleft lip (and palate) is approximately 4%. The probability increases with a family history positive for clefting (see Table 15.1). Cleft lip and palate is more likely to occur in males and presents predominately on the left. Moreover, orofacial clefts occur at a higher frequency in those of Asian and Native American descent.

Q3: You ultimately decide to start presurgical molding, specifically nasoalveolar molding (NAM). What are the goals of NAM?

A3: NAM involves molding the greater and lesser alveolar segments and nasal cleft to align the dental arch and normalize nasal shape. The process is typically overseen by a craniofacial orthodontist and requires frequent visits to the clinic for mold adjustments.

Q4: The cleft patient is now four months-old and you are planning the cleft lip repair. You decide on a modified rotation-advancement repair. The repair entails the creation of multiple flaps, including a C-, M-, and L-flap. What is the purpose of each flap? Which lip segment is rotated, and which segment is advancement?

A4: The rotation-advancement repair, originally described by Millard [15], the creation of several flaps, including a C-flap (used to augment the columella and nasal floor), M-flap (used for alveolar/gingivobuccal sulcus reinforcement), and L-flap (used for nasal mucosa closure). The rotation component is based on the medial lip segment and the advancement flap is based on the lateral lip segment.

Q5: At the time of cleft lip repair, you are also planning on performing a primary rhinoplasty. Describe the typical cleft nasal deformity.

A5: The unilateral cleft nasal deformity is typically corrected at the time of cleft lip repair; however, the majority of patients will benefit from a "definitive" septorhinoplasty once they have achieved skeletal maturity. The cleft nasal deformity is typified by septal deviation (caudal deviation towards the noncleft side and bowing towards the cleft side), nasal tip deviation towards the cleft side, a diminutive and flattened lower lateral cartilage on the cleft side, widened alar base on the cleft side, and vertical height deficiency of the columella. The cleft-side ala is also laterally, posteriorly, and inferiorly displaced.

References

[1] Wantia, N. and Rettinger, G. (2002) 'The current understanding of cleft lip malformations', *Facial plastic surgery: FPS*, 18(3), pp. 147–153. doi:10.1055/s-2002-33061.

[2] Eppley, B.L., van Aalst, J.A., Robey, A., Havlik, R.J. and Sadove, A.M. (2005) 'The spectrum of orofacial clefting', *Plastic and Reconstructive Surgery*, 115(7), pp. 101e–114e. doi:10.1097/01.prs.0000164494.45986.91.

[3] Monson, L.A., Kirschner, R.E. and Losee, J.E. (2013) 'Primary repair of cleft lip and nasal deformity', *Plastic and Reconstructive Surgery*, 132(6), pp. 1040e–1053e. doi:10.1097/PRS.0b013e3182a808e6.

[4] Henry, C., Samson, T. and Mackay, D. (2014) 'Evidence-based medicine: The cleft lip nasal deformity', *Plastic and Reconstructive Surgery*, 133(5), pp. 1276–1288. doi:10.1097/PRS.0000000000000096.

[5] Tse, R.W., Mercan, E., Fisher, D.M., Hopper, R.A., Birgfeld, C.B. and Gruss, J.S. (2019) 'Unilateral Cleft Lip Nasal Deformity: Foundation-Based Approach to Primary Rhinoplasty', *Plastic and Reconstructive Surgery*, 144(5), pp. 1138–1149. doi:10.1097/PRS.0000000000006182.

[6] Xue, A.S., Buchanan, E.P. and Hollier, L.H. (2021) 'Update in Unilateral Cleft Lip Surgery', *Plastic and Reconstructive Surgery*, 148(2), pp. 262e–274e. doi:10.1097/PRS.0000000000008141.

[7] Mulliken, J.B. (2001) 'Primary repair of bilateral cleft lip and nasal deformity', *Plastic and Reconstructive Surgery*, 108(1), pp. 181–194; examination,195-196. doi:10.1097/00006534-200107000-00028.

[8] Mulliken, J.B. (1992) 'Correction of the bilateral cleft lip nasal deformity: evolution of a surgical concept', *The Cleft Palate-Craniofacial Journal: Official Publication of the American Cleft Palate-Craniofacial Association*, 29(6), pp. 540–545. doi:10.1597/1545-1569_1992_029_0540_cpclnd_2.3.co_2.

[9] Stuppia, L., Capogreco, M., Marzo, G., La Rovere, D., Antonucci, I., Gatta, V., Palka, G., Mortellaro, C. andTetè, S. (2011) 'Genetics of syndromic and nonsyndromic cleft lip and palate', *The Journal of Craniofacial Surgery*, 22(5), pp. 1722–1726. doi:10.1097/SCS.0b013e31822e5e4d.

[10] Wang, K.H., Heike, C.L., Clarkson, M.D., Mejino, J.L., Brinkley, J.F., Tse, R.W., Birgfeld, C.B., Fitzsimons, D.A. and Cox, T.C. (2014) 'Evaluation and integration of disparate classification systems for clefts of the lip', *Frontiers in Physiology*, 5, p. 163. doi:10.3389/fphys.2014.00163.

[11] Volpicelli, E.J., Pfaff, M.J., Potemra, H.M.K., De Leon, F.S., Lin, J., Ayeroff, J.R., Bradley, J.P., Wilson, L. and Lee, J.C. (2020) 'Discrepancies in Parent Perceptions and Patient-Reported Psychosocial Function in Children with Craniofacial Anomalies', *Plastic and Reconstructive Surgery*, 145(1), pp. 175–183. doi:10.1097/PRS.0000000000006388.

[12] Grayson, B.H., Santiago, P.E., Brecht, L.E. and Cutting, C.B. (1999) 'Presurgical nasoalveolar molding in infants with cleft lip and palate', *The Cleft Palate-Craniofacial Journal: Official Publication of the American Cleft Palate-Craniofacial Association*, 36(6), pp. 486–498. doi:10.1597/1545-1569_1999_036_0486_pnmiiw_2.3.co_2.

[13] Kurnik, N.M., Calis, M., Sobol, D.L., Kapadia, H., Mercan, E. and Tse, R.W. (2021) 'A Comparative Assessment of Nasal Appearance following Nasoalveolar Molding and Primary Surgical Repair for Treatment of Unilateral Cleft Lip and Palate', *Plastic and Reconstructive Surgery*, 148(5), pp. 1075–1084. doi:10.1097/PRS.0000000000008462.

[14] Nayak, T., Bonanthaya, K., Parmar, R. and Shetty, P.N. (2021) 'Long-Term Comparison of the Aesthetic Outcomes between Nasoalveolar Molding- and Non-Nasoalveolar Molding-Treated Patients with Unilateral Cleft Lip and Palate', *Plastic and Reconstructive Surgery*, 148(5), pp. 775e–784e. doi:10.1097/PRS.0000000000008463.

[15] Millard, D.R. (1958) 'A radical rotation in single harelip', *American Journal of Surgery*, 95(2), pp. 318–322. doi:10.1016/0002-9610(58)90525-7.

[16] Greives, M.R., Camison, L. and Losee, J.E. (2014) 'Evidence-based medicine: Unilateral cleft lip and nose repair', *Plastic and Reconstructive Surgery*, 134(6), pp. 1372–1380. doi:10.1097/PRS.0000000000000721.

[17] Marcus, J.R., Allori, A.C. and Santiago, P.E. (2017) 'Principles of Cleft Lip Repair: Conventions, Commonalities, and Controversies', *Plastic and Reconstructive Surgery*, 139(3), pp. 764e–780e. doi:10.1097/PRS.0000000000003148.

[18] Mulliken, J.B., Wu, J.K. and Padwa, B.L. (2003) 'Repair of bilateral cleft lip: review, revisions, and reflections', *The Journal of Craniofacial Surgery*, 14(5), pp. 609–620. doi:10.1097/00001665-200309000-00003.

[19] Ogawa, R. (2022) 'The Most Current Algorithms for the Treatment and Prevention of Hypertrophic Scars and Keloids: A 2020 Update of the Algorithms Published 10 Years Ago', *Plastic and Reconstructive Surgery*, 149(1), pp. 79e–94e. doi:10.1097/PRS.0000000000008667.

[20] Bhandari, P.S. (2014) 'An algorithmic approach to management of whistle deformity', *Annals of Plastic Surgery*, 72(1), pp. 41–46. doi:10.1097/SAP.0b013e3182583d11.

[21] Garland, K. and Matic, D. (2019) 'Current approaches to cleft lip revision', *Current Opinion in Otolaryngology & Head and Neck Surgery*, 27(4), pp. 287–293. doi:10.1097/MOO.0000000000000556.

Chapter 16

Cleft Palate

Jennifer Grauberger, MD, MS
and Jonathan Y. Lee, MD, MPH

Introduction

Embryology

1. Primary palate:
    a. Comprised of the lip, alveolar process, and hard palate anterior to the incisive foramen
    b. Formed by fusion of the frontonasal and maxillary processes between 4th and 6th week of gestation
2. Secondary palate:
    a. Comprised of the hard palate posterior to the incisive foramen and the soft palate
    b. Formed by midline fusion of the lateral palatal shelves between 7th-8th week of gestation
        i. Shelves rotate from vertical to horizontal orientation to form the palate, right shelf rotates first → higher incidence of left-sided clefts
        ii. Fusion occurs anterior to posterior: all cleft palates include the soft palate

Normal Anatomy (Figure 16.1.A.)

1. Palatal Muscles:
    a. Levator veli palatini
    b. Tensor veli palatini
    c. Palatoglossus
    d. Palatopharyngeus
    e. Musculus uvulae
2. Muscle innervation:
    a. Pharyngeal plexus (primary contributions from cranial nerves IX and X)
    b. TVP innervated by CN V3
3. Palate blood supply:
    a. Hard palate: Greater palatine artery

In: Essential Facial Plastic and Reconstructive Surgery. Volume 1 ISBN: 979-8-89113-306-8
Editors: Yan Ho Lee and Ira Papel © 2024 Nova Science Publishers, Inc.

i. Branch of the descending palatine artery
ii. Artery enters hard palate through the greater palatine foramen
iii. Artery courses anteriorly

b. Soft palate: Lesser palatine artery
i. Branch of the descending palatine artery
ii. Artery enters hard palate through the lesser palatine foramen
iii. Artery courses posteriorly

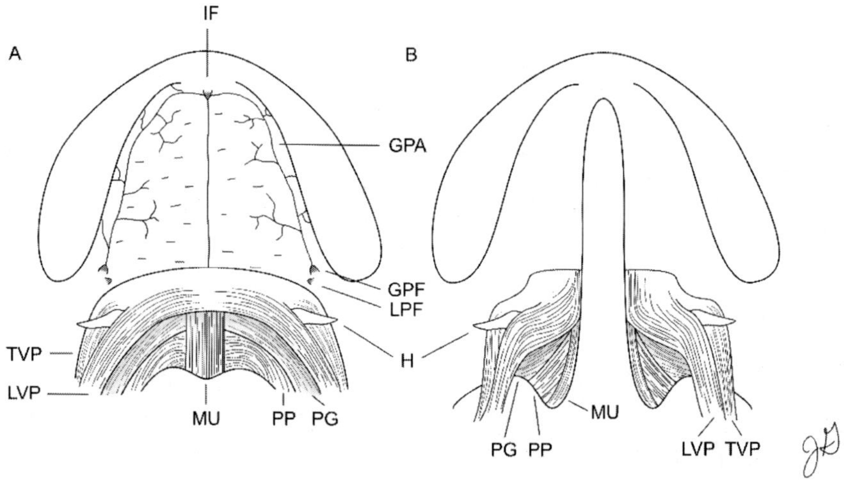

Figure 16.1.A. Normal palate anatomy: The greater palatine artery (GPA) emerges from the greater palatine foramen (GPF) anterior to the lesser palatine foramen (LPF) and travels anteriorly to the incisive foramen (IF). The tensor veli palatini (TVP) muscle and tendon course around the pterygoid hamulus (H). It tenses the soft palate and opens the eustachian tubes. The levator veli palatini (LVP) muscle is the most functionally important muscle for cleft palate repair, forming a transverse sling across the posterior soft palate. It elevates and retracts the soft palate, separating the oral and nasal cavities during swallowing and speech as well as assisting the TVP with eustachian tube opening. The palatoglossus (PG) muscle depresses the soft palate and elevates the posterior tongue. The palatopharyngeus (PP) muscle forms the posterior palatopharyngeal arch and pulls the soft palate superiorly, anteriorly, and medially. The musculus uvulae (MU) muscle forms the uvula. **Figure 16.1.B**. Cleft palate anatomy: The cleft palate defect causes abnormal anterior-posterior positioning of the musculature along the cleft margin with direct insertion into the posterior hard palate. Most significant concern is the loss of the posterior transverse LVP sling.

Cleft Palate Anatomy (Figure 16.1.B.)

1. LVP is oriented longitudinally and inserts into the posterior hard palate
2. Loss of transverse sling prevents effective velopharyngeal closure → hypernasal speech due to air escaping through the nose
3. Abnormal LVP function and fusion with the TVP aponeurosis causes impaired eustachian tube functioning → recurrent or chronic otitis media

Severity and Classification of Cleft Palate

1. Submucous cleft:
    a. Mucosal continuity with misaligned underlying musculature
    b. Calnan's triad: signs of an overt submucous cleft
        i. Bifid uvula
        ii. Palpable notch in the posterior hard palate
        iii. Zona pellucida
    c. Prevalence: unknown given commonality of occult presentations and asymptomatic patients (1:200 for bifid uvulas [1], 1:1,200 to 1:10,000 for submucous clefts [2, 3]
    d. Speech (velopharyngeal insufficiency) and ear pathologies common (45-55%) [2, 3]
2. Secondary palate:
    a. Incomplete cleft palate with variable involvement from soft palate to incisive foramen
    b. Dentition usually normal and symmetric
3. Primary palate:
    a. Complete cleft palate with involvement of hard and soft palate
    b. Alveolar cleft:
        i. Occurs most commonly between lateral incisor and canine
        ii. Maxillary lateral incisor on cleft side most commonly absent (75-90%) or malpositioned/dysmorphic [4, 5, 6, 7]
    c. Unilateral:
        i. Communication between nasal and oral cavities along entire length of palate
        ii. Vomer is connected to one of the lateral maxillary segments
    d. Bilateral:
        i. Premaxillary segment, containing the central and lateral incisor tooth roots, is separated from the alveolar arch
        ii. Vomer remains midline
        iii. Lateral maxillary segments collapse medially
4. Veau classification: categorizes cleft palates into four categories based on location of the defect:
    a. I – isolated soft palate
    b. II – hard and soft palate to the incisive foramen
    c. III – unilateral cleft lip and palate
    d. IV – bilateral cleft lip and palate

Epidemiology

1. Overall orofacial cleft prevalence - 1:690 [8]
    a. Cleft lip versus cleft palate [9]
        i. Cleft lip with or without palate (CL/P) – 1:940

  - ii. Cleft palate only (CPO) – 1:1,574
- b. Laterality (CL/P) [10]
  - i. Unilateral left to right ~ 2:1
  - ii. Unilateral to bilateral ~ 2:1
- c. Race (CL/P) [11]
  - i. Asian/Pacific Islander – 1:500
  - ii. Caucasian – 1:1,000
  - iii. African – 1:2,500
- d. Sex [12, 13, 14, 15]
  - i. Male to female – 2:1 for CL/P
  - ii. Female to male – 2:1 for CPO

2. Genetics
   - a. Etiology likely multifactorial including genetic and environmental factors
   - b. CL/P and CPO have distinctly different genetics
   - c. Risk of cleft based on family history [16, 17, 18]
     - i. No family history – CL/P: 0.1%, CPO: 0.04%
     - ii. One affected child – CL/P: 4%, CPO: 2%
     - iii. One affected parent – CL/P: 4%, CPO: 6%
     - iv. One affected parent and child – CL/P: 17%, CPO 15%
     - v. Two affected children – CL/P: 9%, CPO 1%
3. Environmental risk factors [17]:
   - a. High altitude
   - b. Maternal tobacco use
   - c. Maternal alcohol consumption
   - d. Maternal obesity
   - e. Folic acid deficiency
   - f. Zinc deficiency
   - g. Anti-epileptics exposure
   - h. Isotretinoin exposure
   - i. Stressful events during pregnancy

Syndromes and Sequences Associated with Cleft Palates

1. Cleft palate is highly associated with several syndromes [15, 19, 20]
   - a. 30% of CL/P
   - b. 50% of CPO
2. Common syndromes: Van der Woude syndrome, Stickler syndrome, 22q11 deletion (DiGeorge syndrome, velocardiofacial syndrome), Treacher Collins syndrome, Nager syndrome, oral-facial-digital syndrome
3. Pierre Robin Sequence
   - a. Clinical triad of:
     - i. Congenital micrognathia
     - ii. Glossoptosis
     - iii. Airway obstruction
   - b. 80-90% of patients have concomitant wide, U-shaped cleft palate [21, 22]

Patient Evaluation

1. Multidisciplinary evaluation needed when the defect is identified
    a. Plastic surgery
    b. Speech pathology
    c. Orthodontics
    d. Otolaryngology
    e. Pediatrics
    f. Genetics
    g. Social work
    h. Audiology
2. Feeding and swallowing
    a. Normal feeding requires:
        i. Generation of negative intra-oral pressure (suction)
        ii. Intact swallowing mechanism
    b. Cleft lip and palate causes:
        i. Inability to close lips/oropharynx to create suction
        ii. Poor tongue positioning for moving food boluses posteriorly for swallowing
        iii. Abnormal oral and nasal cavity connection causes irritation, ulceration, and sinusitis
3. Speech
    a. Inability to close off the nasopharynx → hypernasal speech
    b. Development of compensatory and maladaptive speech patterns
4. Ear pathology
    a. Improperly positioned soft palate musculature causes impaired eustachian tube drainage
    b. Eustachian tube dysfunction → chronic obstruction of drainage and serous otitis media
        i. Incidence of otitis media in cleft palate patients: 96-100% [23, 24, 25]
        ii. Incidence of clinically significant hearing loss: 30-70% [24, 26, 27]
5. Overall growth
    a. Cleft palates patients have same average birth weight as unaffected newborns [28]
    b. Decreased growth at time of lip and palate repair [28, 29, 30, 31]
    c. Rate of growth normalizes by age 4 years [32, 33, 34]
    d. May have delayed onset and prolonged duration of puberty with initially slowed skeletal development [35]
    e. Overall same average adult weight/height [36]
6. Maxillary development
    a. Transverse growth of the maxillary arch is narrowed, leading to:
        i. Tooth crowding
        ii. Lateral crossbites
        iii. Open bites

   b. Sagittal deficiency
      i. Development of anterior crossbites common
      ii. 15-20% of patients undergo Le Fort I maxillary advancement [37, 38]
      iii. Controversial whether deficiency is due to intrinsic growth restriction versus scar inhibition after repair

Management

Timing of Cleft Palate Repair

1. Balance between promoting normal speech and maxillary growth
   a. Early repair may improve speech development
   b. Delayed repair may improve maxillary growth as surgical scarring restricts growth
2. Optimal time around 12 months (controversial)

General Principles of Cleft Palate Repair

1. The main goal is to restore intelligible speech via establishing velopharyngeal competency
   a. Restore the LVP muscle sling
   b. Restore separation of the oral and nasal cavities
   c. Restore eustachian tube function to minimize recurrent otitis media and hearing loss
2. All techniques utilize three-layer closure: nasal mucosa, muscle, and oral mucosa
3. Tension-free closure is essential to minimize fistula formation
   a. Dissect nasal layer under the hard palate
   b. Skeletonize neurovascular bundles
4. Careful suturing technique:
   a. Nasal mucosa – simple interrupted stitches
   b. Oral mucosa – mattress stitches
5. Surgical techniques for hard and soft palate repair are combined based on the defect

Operative Techniques for Cleft Palate Repair (Palatoplasty)

1. Hard palate repair
   a. Bipedicled flap (Von Langenbeck technique) (Figure 16.2)
      i. Indications – narrow to moderate-width clefts, Veau 2
      ii. Steps:
         - Medial incision along cleft margin to separate oral and nasal mucosa
         - Bilateral, bipedicled mucoperiosteal flaps raised

  - Dual blood supply:
    - o Anteriorly – nasopalatine artery via the incisive foramen
    - o Posteriorly – greater palatine artery
  - Lateral incision along attached gingiva extended posteriorly lateral to the hamulus
- Layered midline closure

b. Unipedicled flap

i. Veau-Wardill-Kilner V-Y pushback technique

- Indications: palatal lengthening

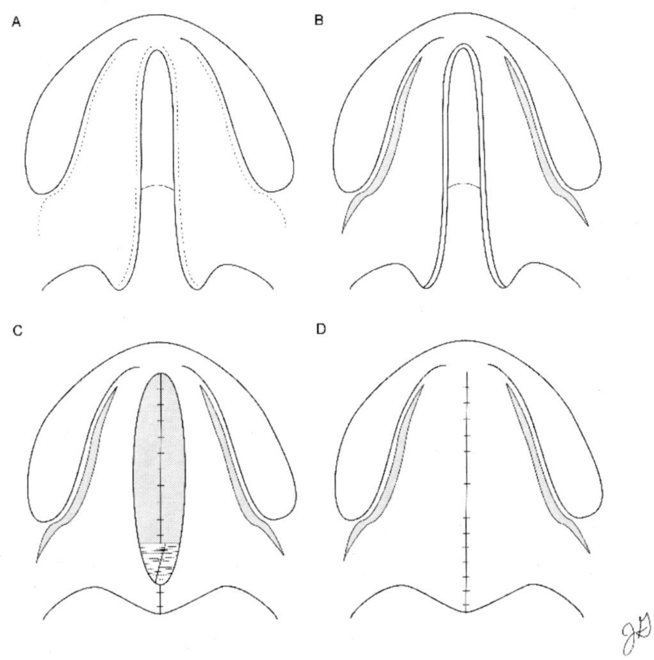

Figure 16.2. Von Langenback repair technique. A. Markings of the medial cleft margin and lateral relaxing incisions. B. Creation of bilateral bipedicled flaps. C. Midline layered closure of the defect including the nasal and oral mucosal layers. The Von Langenback technique is frequently combined with intravelar veloplasty (IVP) to reform the posterior transverse muscular sling. D. Final closure.

- Steps:
  - Central V-shaped incision made on hard palate
  - Bilateral mucoperiosteal island flaps (pedicle: greater palatine artery) raised
  - Y-closure of cleft performed for palatal lengthening
  - Anterolateral areas of hard palate left raw to heal secondarily
  - Single layer closure anteriorly of nasal mucosa
- Not commonly used due to contraction and scarring of raw hard palate, leading to:

- Palatal shortening
- Decreased maxillary width [39, 40]
- Velopharyngeal insufficiency
- Single layer closure → higher anterior fistula rates

ii. Bardach two-flap technique

- Indications:
  - Wide/U-shaped clefts
  - Complete unilateral or bilateral clefts
- Steps:
  - Similar to Von Langenbeck technique, with anterior extension of relaxing lateral incisions to meet medial incision
  - Bilateral mucoperiosteal island flaps raised
  - Midline layered closure
- In complete unilateral clefts, the larger flap can be shifted medially to reduce fistula rate
  - Allows more complete closure anteriorly
  - Off-sets oral mucosal and nasal lining closure

c. Vomer flap

i. Indications:

- Wide anterior clefts
- Bilateral clefts
- Repair of large anterior fistulas

ii. Steps:

- Superiorly based flaps from the vomer are used to close nasal mucosa
- Mucosa from the septum near cleft margin is reflected into defect
- Two layered closure of the hard palate mucosa performed

iii. Advantages:

- Low fistula rates [41]
- No to little impact on maxilla growth [42, 43]

2. Soft palate repair

a. Intra-velar veloplasty (IVV)

i. Used to reform the transverse LVP sling

ii. Term interchangeable with straight-line repair

iii. Steps:

- LVP freed from the posterior hard palate and dissected from nasal and oral mucosa
- LVP is reoriented transversely and posteriorly, then sutured in the midline
- Three-layered closure +/- lateral relaxing incisions

b. Furlow double-opposing Z-plasty (Figure 16.3)

i. Indications:

- Primary cleft repair: same as IVV

- Secondary cleft repair:
  - Previous straight-line repair with inadequate length
  - Previous straight-line repair with small persistent velopharyngeal gapping (5 mm or less)
  - Previous straight-line repair with inverted-V vaulting of the soft palate (inadequate LVP repositioning)

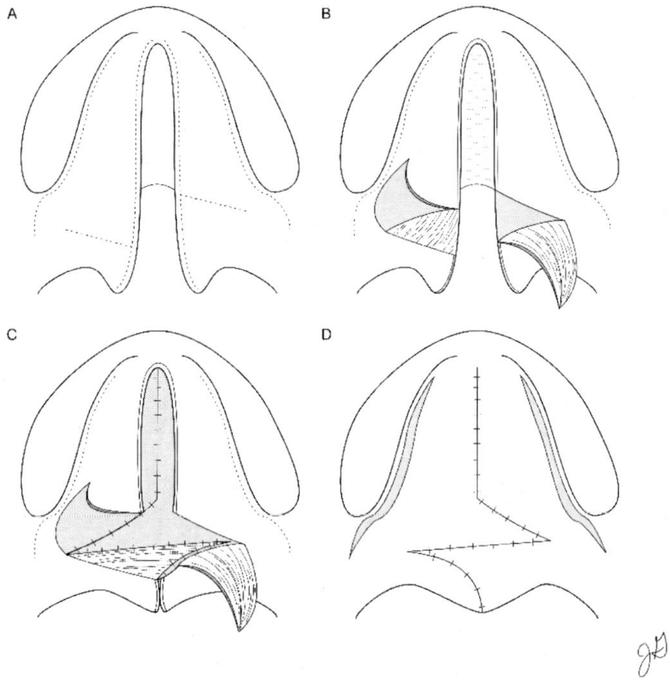

Figure 16.3. Furlow double-opposing Z-plasty technique. A. Markings of the medical cleft margin, lateral relaxing, and opposing Z-plasty incisions (note: opposing Z-plasty incisions of the nasal mucosa not shown). B. Creation of the opposing Z-plasty flaps. In the figure shown, the left oral mucosal flap is raised with the levator muscle whereas the underlying nasal mucosa is raised on its own flap. The opposite is performed on the right side in which the nasal mucosal layer is raised with the LVP and the oral mucosa is raised on its own. C. The flaps are transposed to provide layered closure of nasal and oral mucosa and reform the transverse muscular sling in a posterior position. D. Final closure.

ii. Steps:

- Mucosal incisions along cleft margins and lateral relaxing incisions
- Z-plasty markings are oriented opposite to the underlying Z-plasty
- Bilateral, opposing flaps on each side (nasal and oral) of the cleft, one flap including muscle (i.e. oral mucosa and muscle) and mucosa and the other including mucosa only (i.e. nasal mucosa) are raised

- Flaps including the LVP from both right and left side of cleft margin are transposed posteriorly to reform the levator sling
- Flaps including only mucosa are transposed anterior to close off the communication between the oral and nasal cavities

iii. Advantages:
- Possibly lower rate of velopharyngeal insufficiency development requiring secondary operations compared to intravelar veloplasty [44, 45]
- Lower fistula rate [41, 46, 47]

3. Adjunctive procedures
   a. Buccal fat flap
      i. Indications:
         - Primary cleft palate repair – used as adjunct to primary technique
           - Flap reaches to cover soft palate and posterior third of hard palate
           - Cover areas of exposed bone of the hard palate,
           - Buffer midline incisions under tension
           - Obliterates dead space between LVP repair and posterior edge of hard palate
         - Repair of fistulas after prior palatoplasty
      ii. Steps:
         - Curved scissors are placed in the mucosa of the superior buccal sulcus at the level of the second molar to cause buccal fat pad extrusion
         - Fat pad is teased out gently to preserve delicate blood supply
         - Fat pad is secured laterally to the surrounding gingival mucosa or extended to the midline and placed under mucoperiosteal flaps
      iii. Advantages:
         - Additional vascularized tissue coverage to prevent fistulas
         - Diminishes scar contraction by covering exposed bone in relaxing incision and obliterating dead space
         - Easily accessible autologous tissue without significant additional cost or added operative time
         - Does not require a second surgery for division/inset
   b. Buccal myomucosal flap
      i. Indications:
         - Primary cleft palate repair - assists with closing wide palatal defects
         - Repair of fistulas after previous cleft palate repair
      ii. Steps:
         - 1.5-2 cm wide flaps raised of oral cheek mucosa, including buccinator muscle, ensure wide base at retromolar trigone
         - Flap is tunneled posterior to greater palatine vessels

- Flap is sutured into place alongside the nasal edge of the soft palate defect, with the mucosal side facing the nasal cavity
- Multi-layered closure

iii. Advantages:
- Allows for reformation of the LVP sling without anterior defects
  - Does not displace the sling anteriorly, preserving LVP function
  - No exposed hard palate, leading to minimized scarring
- Lengthens the nasal layer by 1.5-2 cm
- Releases tension on the palate repair in anterior-posterior and transverse directions
- Buccal mucosa is a good match for native palatal mucosa

iv. Outcomes:
- Low rates of fistula formation (0.7-6.1%) when used in primary repair [48, 49, 50]
- Low rates of velopharyngeal insufficiency development (3.5-8.8%) or need for secondary surgery for VPI (6.6%) [48]
- Use of buccal myomucosal flaps associated with interference permanent molar eruption [51]

c. Acellular dermal matrix (ADM, ex: alloderm)

i. Indications:
- Two-layer, tension-free, and watertight cleft palate repair not possible (wider unilateral or bilateral clefts)
- Repair of oronasal fistula

ii. Steps:
- ADM is placed over the nasal closure or persistent defect of the anterior hard palate

iii. Advantages:
- Decreased dehiscence and fistula rate – possibly due to the ADM acting as a hermetic boundary at tenuous areas to prevent progression to fistulation [52]
- Quick epithelialization of ADM in less than four weeks
- No donor site morbidity
- Minimal additional operative time required – faster than autologous flaps

iv. Outcomes:
- Low fistula formation rate (1.5-8.5% using two-flap repair, 0.75% using Furlow double-opposing Z-plasty) [51, 53, 54, 55]

Post-Operative Care

1. Hypoxemia and airway obstruction
    a. Palatoplasty leads to sudden relative decrease in airway size
    b. Prolonged surgeries (over 2 hr) with use of a throat gag puts patients at risk for tongue edema [56, 57, 58]
    c. Significantly airway obstruction occurs in 5.7% of cases [59]
    d. Usually resolves in 24-48 hr post-operatively
    e. Treatment:
        i. Monitor all palatoplasty patients overnight
        ii. Prevent by releasing gag intermittently (ex.: for 5 min every 60 min of surgery)
        iii. Tongue traction suture placement immediately post-op to minimize oral airway device use
        iv. Nasal trumpet (inserted prior to nasal lining repair)
        v. Minimize narcotic use
    f. Patients with syndromic clefts, (i.e. Pierre Robin Sequence) should have closer monitoring, potentially in ICU
2. Bleeding
    a. Oozing for 12-24hr not uncommon
    b. 0.5-2.4% have significant bleeding requiring re-operation [60, 61, 62]
    c. Treatment:
        i. Suturing hemostatic dressings (i.e. surgicel) to raw areas
        ii. Decrease operative time to under 2hrs to allow epinephrine to have ongoing effect during anesthesia emergence
        iii. Direct, light pressure to the hard palate repair at end of case
        iv. Ice packs placed on the posterior neck post-operatively
3. Feeding
    a. Liquid or soft diet for 10-14 days
    b. Use an open/sippy cup, red rubber catheter, or special nipple for feeding
    c. Time meals 30 minutes after pain medication administration
    d. Stop IV fluids post-op day 1 to promote thirst/drinking
4. Immobilization
    a. Arm splints used to prevent damage to repair from fingers or foreign objects

Complications (Table 16.1)

Table 16.1. Complications of Cleft Palate Repair

Complication	Incidence	Presentation	Treatment
Fistula formation	• 2.9-43%, usually ~10% [41, 43, 63, 64, 65] Risk factors: • Wide cleft • High Veau classification • V-Y pushback > von Langenbeck > Furlow	• Pittsburgh Fistula Classification System: based on fistula palate location [66]	• Re-do palatoplasty (Furlow vs IVV) • Buccal mucosal flap • Facial artery musculomucosal flap
Velopharyngeal insufficiency (VPI)	• 6-40% [64, 67, 68] Diagnosis: • Videofluoroscopy • Nasoendoscopy	• Hypernasal speech • Maladaptive speech • Nasal regurgitation/air emission • Pittsburgh Weighted Speech Scale [69]: classifies severity of VPI	• Redo palatoplasty (Furlow) • Posterior pharyngeal flap • Sphincter pharyngoplasty
Maxillary growth restriction	Risk factors: • Early cleft palate repair • Procedures with increased contractures/scarring • Repeated operations	• Midface hypoplasia • Malocclusion: anterior underjet, angle class 3	• Le Fort I maxillary advancement • Le Fort I distraction osteogenesis • Combined Le Fort I maxillary advancement and bilateral sagittal split mandibular setback

Summary Points

1. Patients with cleft palates require multidisciplinary care for work-up and management
2. Ideal timing of cleft palate repair is ~ 1 year of age
3. Hard and soft palate repairs are separate procedures that is simultaneously performed using interchangeable options based on the defect
4. Patients should be admitted overnight for post-operative airway monitoring
5. Cleft palate repair is performed to improve speech, which may require secondary procedures to correct developing or residual velopharnygeal insufficiency

Patient Case

Patient is a 2-month-old male presenting with a complete unilateral left cleft lip and palate. A clinical image of the cleft is shown. (Figure 16.4.)

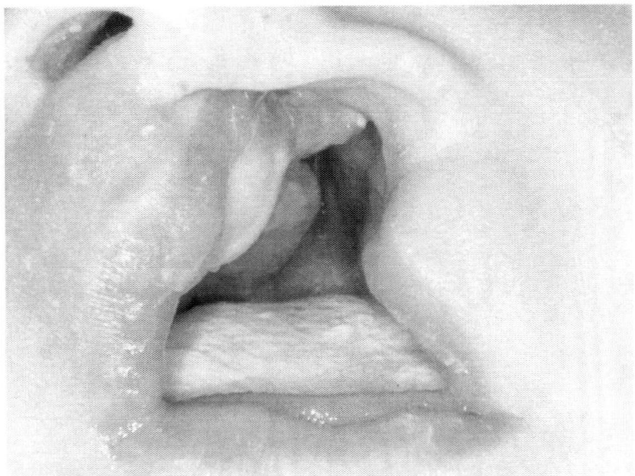

Figure 16.4. Cleft Palate Case Photo.

Q1. In regard to lip repair and palate repair, what should be the sequence and timing of the palate repair?

The lip is generally repaired before the palate in a separate operation. Timing of the palate repair follows the rule of 10's: 10 months of age, hemoglobin 10, weight of 10 pounds. Although the range in timing that is acceptable for repair is controversial, the goal is to balance potential maxillary growth restriction and airway compromise with early repair and potential abnormal speech development with late repair.

Q2. When planning for palate repair, what other intervention is typically indicated and should be coordinated to occur simultaneously?

Cleft palate is always associated with aberrant anatomy of the levator veli palatini muscle, which plays a role in the opening of the Eustachian tube. In turn, nearly all cleft palate patients develop otitis media, resulting in half developing clinically significant hearing loss. Therefore, all cleft palate patients should be assessed for placement of bilateral myringotomy tubes at the time of palate repair to avoid a separate anesthetic event.

Q3. What are the surgical goals in palate repair?

The overall goal of palate repair is to yield intelligible speech, which requires the patient to use the palate to separate the oral and nasal cavities. As such, there are three goals to accomplish in palate repair. 1) Reapproximating the cleft margins in two layers (nasal/oral) under minimal tension. 2) Recreating the levator veli palatini sling by reorienting all the aberrant attachments and posteriorly positioning the muscle to give the best mechanical advantage of action. 3) Provide as much palatal length as possible without compromising anterior closure.

Q4. A year after palate repair, the patient continues to have difficulty with speech, characterized by unintelligible, hypernasal speech with nasal regurgitations and emissions. What are the next steps in evaluation?

This patient appears to have velopharyngeal insufficiency, indicating that the palate is not able to adequately separate the oral and nasal cavities, thus resulting in enough nasal air escape to preclude intelligible speech. The patient is likely indicated for a secondary speech operation; however, the particular operation will largely be determined by pattern of velopharyngeal closure. Closure pattern can be assessed by multi-view videofluoroscopy (Televex) or nasovelopharyngeal endoscopy, either of which should be the next step in evaluation.

References

[1] Shprintzen, R J, R H Schwartz, A Daniller, and L Hoch. 1985. "Morphologic Significance of Bifid Uvula." *Pediatrics* 75 (3): 553–61.

[2] Stewart, J M, M E Ott, and R Lagace. 1971. "Submucous Cleft Palate." *Birth Defects Original Article Series* 7 (7): 64–66.

[3] Ysunza, Antonio, Carmen Pamplona, Mario Mendoza, Fernando Molina, Patricia Martínez, Manuel García-Velasco, and Nicolas Prada. 2001. "Surgical Treatment of Submucous Cleft Palate: A Comparative Trial of Two Modalities for Palatal Closure." *Plastic and Reconstructive Surgery* 107 (1): 9–14. https://doi.org/10.1097/00006534-200101000-00002.

[4] Jordan, R E, B S Kraus, and C M Neptune. 1966. "Dental Abnormalities Associated with Cleft Lip and/or Palate." *The Cleft Palate Journal* 3 (January): 22–55.

[5] Lourenço Ribeiro, Luciana, Lucimara Teixeira Das Neves, Beatriz Costa, and Marcia Ribeiro Gomide. 2003. "Dental Anomalies of the Permanent Lateral Incisors and Prevalence of Hypodontia Outside the Cleft Area in Complete Unilateral Cleft Lip and Palate." *The Cleft Palate-Craniofacial Journal : Official Publication of the American Cleft Palate-Craniofacial Association* 40 (2): 172–75. https://doi.org/10.1597/1545-1569_2003_040_0172_daotpl_2.0.co_2.

[6] Shapira, Y, E Lubit, and M M Kuftinec. 2000. "Hypodontia in Children with Various Types of Clefts." *The Angle Orthodontist* 70 (1): 16–21.

[7] Ranta, R. 1986. "A Review of Tooth Formation in Children with Cleft Lip/Palate." *American Journal of Orthodontics and Dentofacial Orthopedics : Official Publication of the American Association of Orthodontists, Its Constituent Societies, and the American Board of Orthodontics* 90 (1): 11–18. https://doi.org/10.1016/0889-5406(86)90022-3.

[8] Mai, Cara T., Cynthia H. Cassell, Robert E. Meyer, Jennifer Isenburg, Mark A. Canfield, Russel Rickard, Richard S. Olney, Stallings, Erin B., Beck, Meredith, Hashmi, S. Shahrukh, Cho, Sook Ja, Kirby, Russell S. And National Birth Defects Prevention Network. 2014. "Birth Defects Data from Population-Based Birth Defects Surveillance Programs in the United States, 2007 to 2011: Highlighting Orofacial Clefts." *Birth Defects Research. Part A, Clinical and Molecular Teratology* 100 (11): 895. https://doi.org/10.1002/BDRA.23329.

[9] Parker, Samantha E, Cara T Mai, Mark A Canfield, Russel Rickard, Ying Wang, Robert E Meyer, Patrick Anderson, Craig A Mason, Julianne S Collins, Russell S Kirby, Adolfo Correa and National Birth Defects Prevention Network. 2010. "Updated National Birth Prevalence Estimates for Selected Birth Defects in the United States, 2004-2006." *Birth Defects Research. Part A, Clinical and Molecular Teratology* 88 (12): 1008–16. https://doi.org/10.1002/bdra.20735.

[10] Yılmaz, Hanife Nuray, Elvan Önem Özbilen, and Tuğba Üstün. 2019. "The Prevalence of Cleft Lip and Palate Patients: A Single-Center Experience for 17 Years." *Turkish Journal of Orthodontics* 32 (3): 139. https://doi.org/10.5152/TURKJORTHOD.2019.18094.

[11] Dixon, Michael J., Mary L. Marazita, Terri H. Beaty, and Jeffrey C. Murray. 2011. "Cleft Lip and Palate: Synthesizing Genetic and Environmental Influences." *Nature Reviews. Genetics* 12 (3): 167. https://doi.org/10.1038/NRG2933.

[12] Shaw, G M, L A Croen, and C J Curry. 1991. "Isolated Oral Cleft Malformations: Associations with Maternal and Infant Characteristics in a California Population." *Teratology* 43 (3): 225–28. https://doi.org/10.1002/tera.1420430306.

[13] Genisca, Alicia E., Jaime L. Frías, Cheryl S. Broussard, Margaret A. Honein, Edward J. Lammer, Cynthia A. Moore, Gary M. Shaw, Jeffrey C. Murray, Wei Yang, and Sonja A. Rasmussen. 2009. "Orofacial Clefts in the National Birth Defects Prevention Study, 1997-2004." *American Journal of Medical Genetics. Part A* 149A (6): 1149–58. https://doi.org/10.1002/AJMG.A.32854.

[14] Mossey, P A, and B Modell. 2012. "Epidemiology of Oral Clefts 2012: An International Perspective." *Frontiers of Oral Biology* 16: 1–18. https://doi.org/10.1159/000337464.

[15] Wyszynski DF. 2002. *Cleft Lip and Palate: From Origins to Treatment*. New York: Oxford University Press.

[16] Mitchell, L E, and N Risch. 1992. "Mode of Inheritance of Nonsyndromic Cleft Lip with or without Cleft Palate: A Reanalysis." *American Journal of Human Genetics* 51 (2): 323–32.

[17] Kirschner, R E, and D LaRossa. 2000. "Cleft Lip and Palate." *Otolaryngologic Clinics of North America* 33 (6): 1191–1215, v–vi. https://doi.org/10.1016/s0030-6665(05)70277-2.
[18] Mitchell, L E, and K Christensen. 1996. "Analysis of the Recurrence Patterns for Nonsyndromic Cleft Lip with or without Cleft Palate in the Families of 3,073 Danish Probands." *American Journal of Medical Genetics* 61 (4): 371–76. https://doi.org/10.1002/(SICI)1096-8628(19960202)61:4<371::AID-AJMG12>3.0.CO;2-P.
[19] Shi, Min, George L Wehby, and Jeffrey C Murray. 2008. "Review on Genetic Variants and Maternal Smoking in the Etiology of Oral Clefts and Other Birth Defects." *Birth Defects Research. Part C, Embryo Today : Reviews* 84 (1): 16–29. https://doi.org/10.1002/bdrc.20117.
[20] Mossey, Peter A., Julian Little, Ron G. Munger, Mike J. Dixon, and William C. Shaw. 2009. "Cleft Lip and Palate." *Lancet (London, England)* 374 (9703): 1773–85. https://doi.org/10.1016/S0140-6736(09)60695-4.
[21] Vatlach, Scarlet, Christoph Maas, and Christian F. Poets. 2014. "Birth Prevalence and Initial Treatment of Robin Sequence in Germany: A Prospective Epidemiologic Study." *Orphanet Journal of Rare Diseases* 9 (1). https://doi.org/10.1186/1750-1172-9-9.
[22] Caouette-Laberge, L, B Bayet, and Y Larocque. 1994. "The Pierre Robin Sequence: Review of 125 Cases and Evolution of Treatment Modalities." *Plastic and Reconstructive Surgery* 93 (5): 934–42.
[23] Paradise, J L, C D Bluestone, and H Felder. 1969. "The Universality of Otitis Media in 50 Infants with Cleft Palate." *Pediatrics* 44 (1): 35–42.
[24] Sheahan, Patrick, Ian Miller, Jerome N Sheahan, Michael J Earley, and Alexander W Blayney. 2003. "Incidence and Outcome of Middle Ear Disease in Cleft Lip and/or Cleft Palate." *International Journal of Pediatric Otorhinolaryngology* 67 (7): 785–93. https://doi.org/10.1016/s0165-5876(03)00098-3.
[25] Dhillon, R. S. 1988. "The Middle Ear in Cleft Palate Children Pre and Post Palatal Closure." *Journal of the Royal Society of Medicine* 81 (12): 710. https://doi.org/10.1177/014107688808101209.
[26] Kwan, Wendy M.Y., Victor J. Abdullah, Kelvin Liu, C. Andrew van Hasselt, and Michael C.F. Tong. 2011. "Otitis Media with Effusion and Hearing Loss in Chinese Children with Cleft Lip and Palate." *The Cleft Palate-Craniofacial Journal : Official Publication of the American Cleft Palate-Craniofacial Association* 48 (6): 684–89. https://doi.org/10.1597/10-006.
[27] Yules, R B. 1975. "Current Concepts of Treatment of Ear Disease in Cleft Palate Children and Adults." *The Cleft Palate Journal* 12 (July): 315–22.
[28] Seth, A K, and B J McWilliams. 1988. "Weight Gain in Children with Cleft Palate from Birth to Two Years." *The Cleft Palate Journal* 25 (2): 146–50.
[29] Avedian, L v, and R L Ruberg. 1980. "Impaired Weight Gain in Cleft Palate Infants." *The Cleft Palate Journal* 17 (1): 24–26.
[30] Montagnoli, Luiz C., Marco A. Barbieri, Heloisa Bettiol, Ilza Lazarini Marques, and Luiz de Souza. 2005. "Growth Impairment of Children with Different Types of Lip and Palate Clefts in the First 2 Years of Life: A Cross-Sectional Study." *Jornal de Pediatria* 81 (6): 461–65. https://doi.org/10.2223/JPED.1420.
[31] Felix-Schollaart, B, J B Hoeksma, and B Prahl-Andersen. 1992. "Growth Comparison between Children with Cleft Lip and/or Palate and Controls." *The Cleft Palate-Craniofacial Journal : Official Publication of the American Cleft Palate-Craniofacial Association* 29 (5): 475–80. https://doi.org/10.1597/1545-1569_1992_029_0475_gcbcwc_2.3.co_2.
[32] Marques, Ilza Lazarini, John Nackashi, Hilton Coimbra Borgo, Angela Patrícia Menezes Cardoso Martinelli, Luiz de Souza, Jeniffer de Cássia Rillo Dutka, William N. Williams, and Maria Inês Pegoraro-Krook. 2015. "Longitudinal Study of Growth of Children with Unilateral Cleft Lip and Palate: 2 to 10 Years of Age." *The Cleft Palate-Craniofacial Journal : Official Publication of the American Cleft Palate-Craniofacial Association* 52 (2): 192–97. https://doi.org/10.1597/13-161.
[33] Mcheik, Jiad N., and Guillaume Levard. 2010. "Growth in Infants in the First Two Years of Life after Neonatal Repair for Unilateral Cleft Lip and Palate." *International Journal of Pediatric Otorhinolaryngology* 74 (5): 465–68. https://doi.org/10.1016/J.IJPORL.2010.01.020.
[34] Lee, J, J Nunn, and C Wright. 1996. "Height and Weight Achievement in Cleft Lip and Palate." *Archives of Disease in Childhood* 75 (4): 327–29. https://doi.org/10.1136/adc.75.4.327.

[35] Ravi, MS, and S Ravikala. 2013. "Assessment of Skeletal Age in Children with Unilateral Cleft Lip and Palate." *International Journal of Clinical Pediatric Dentistry* 6 (3): 151–55. https://doi.org/10.5005/JP-JOURNALS-10005-1209.

[36] Jensen, B L, E Dahl, and S Kreiborg. 1983. "Longitudinal Study of Body Height, Radius Length and Skeletal Maturity in Danish Boys with Cleft Lip and Palate." *Scandinavian Journal of Dental Research* 91 (6): 473–81. https://doi.org/10.1111/j.1600-0722.1983.tb00848.x.

[37] Lisson, Jörg A., and Catharina Weyrich. 2014. "Extent of Maxillary Deficiency in Patients with Complete UCLP and BCLP." *Head & Face Medicine* 10 (1). https://doi.org/10.1186/1746-160X-10-26.

[38] Good, Phoebe M., John B. Mulliken, and Bonnie L. Padwa. 2007. "Frequency of Le Fort I Osteotomy after Repaired Cleft Lip and Palate or Cleft Palate." *The Cleft Palate-Craniofacial Journal : Official Publication of the American Cleft Palate-Craniofacial Association* 44 (4): 396–401. https://doi.org/10.1597/06-075.1.

[39] Larossa, Don. 2000. "The State of the Art in Cleft Palate Surgery." *The Cleft Palate-Craniofacial Journal : Official Publication of the American Cleft Palate-Craniofacial Association* 37 (3): 225–28. https://doi.org/10.1597/1545-1569_2000_037_0225_TSOTAI_2.3.CO_2.

[40] Pigott, R. W., E. H. Albery, I. S. Hathorn, N. E. Atack, A. Williams, K. Harland, A. Orlando, S. Falder, and B. Coghlan. 2002. "A Comparison of Three Methods of Repairing the Hard Palate." *The Cleft Palate-Craniofacial Journal: Official Publication of the American Cleft Palate-Craniofacial Association* 39 (4): 383–91. https://doi.org/10.1597/1545-1569_2002_039_0383_ACOTMO_2.0.CO_2.

[41] Vandenberg, Katherine, Michael Castle, Fares Qeadan, and Tania Kraai. 2021. "Oronasal Fistula Incidence Associated With Vomer Flap Repair of Cleft Palate: A Systematic Review and Meta-Analysis." *The Cleft Palate-Craniofacial Journal : Official Publication of the American Cleft Palate-Craniofacial Association* 58 (8): 957–65. https://doi.org/10.1177/1055665620974562.

[42] Cohen, S R, J Kalinowski, D LaRossa, and P Randall. 1991. "Cleft Palate Fistulas: A Multivariate Statistical Analysis of Prevalence, Etiology, and Surgical Management." *Plastic and Reconstructive Surgery* 87 (6): 1041–47.

[43] Minatel, Lurian, Jéssica Marcela de Luna Gomes, Cleidiel Aparecido Araújo Lemos, João Pedro Justino de Oliveira Limírio, and Eduardo Piza Pellizzer. 2019. "Influence of Vomer Flap on Craniofacial Growth in Patients with Cleft Lip and Palate: A Systematic Review." *Journal of Cranio-Maxillofacial Surgery* 47 (6): 902–8. https://doi.org/10.1016/J.JCMS.2019.03.011.

[44] Timbang, Mary Roz, Bahar Bassiri Gharb, Antonio Rampazzo, Frank Papay, James Zins, and Gaby Doumit. 2014. "A Systematic Review Comparing Furlow Double-Opposing Z-Plasty and Straight-Line Intravelar Veloplasty Methods of Cleft Palate Repair." *Plastic and Reconstructive Surgery* 134 (5): 1014–22. https://doi.org/10.1097/PRS.0000000000000637.

[45] Anderson, Brady J., Kasra N. Fallah, Austin A. Lignieres, Joseph K. Moffitt, Kim Loan Luu, Alfredo Cepeda, Irene L. Doringo, Phuong D. Nguyen, John F. Teichgraeber, and Matthew R. Greives. 2021. "Predictive Factors for Velopharyngeal Insufficiency Following Primary Cleft Palate Repair." *The Cleft Palate-Craniofacial Journal: Official Publication of the American Cleft Palate-Craniofacial Association*. https://doi.org/10.1177/10556656211026861.

[46] Stein, Michael J., Zach Zhang, Matthew Fell, Nigel Mercer, and Claudia Malic. 2019. "Determining Postoperative Outcomes after Cleft Palate Repair: A Systematic Review and Meta-Analysis." *Journal of Plastic, Reconstructive & Aesthetic Surgery* 72 (1): 85–91. https://doi.org/10.1016/J.BJPS.2018.08.019.

[47] Kara, Murat, Mert Calis, Ilkem Kara, Mavis Emel Kulak Kayikci, Riza Onder Gunaydin, and Figen Ozgur. 2021. "Comparison of Speech Outcomes Using Type 2b Intravelar Veloplasty or Furlow Double-Opposing Z Plasty for Soft Palate Repair of Patients with Unilateral Cleft Lip and Palate." *Journal of Cranio-Maxillo-Facial Surgery : Official Publication of the European Association for Cranio-Maxillo-Facial Surgery* 49 (3): 215–22. https://doi.org/10.1016/J.JCMS.2021.01.003.

[48] Mann, Robert J., and David M. Fisher. 1997. "Bilateral Buccal Flaps with Double Opposing Z-Plasty for Wider Palatal Clefts." *Plastic and Reconstructive Surgery* 100 (5): 1139–45. https://doi.org/10.1097/00006534-199710000-00009.

[49] Mann, Robert J., Matthew D. Martin, Mitchell G. Eichhorn, Keith C. Neaman, Charles G. Sierzant, John W. Polley, and John A. Girotto. 2017. "The Double Opposing Z-Plasty Plus or Minus Buccal Flap Approach for Repair of Cleft Palate: A Review of 505 Consecutive Cases." *Plastic and Reconstructive Surgery* 139 (3): 735e–44. https://doi.org/10.1097/PRS.0000000000003127.

[50] Jackson, Ian T., Andrea A. Moreira-Gonzalez, Amy Rogers, and Barbara J. Beal. 2004. "The Buccal Flap--a Useful Technique in Cleft Palate Repair?" *The Cleft Palate-Craniofacial Journal : Official Publication of the American Cleft Palate-Craniofacial Association* 41 (2): 144–51. https://doi.org/10.1597/02-124.

[51] Freedlander, E, and I T Jackson. 1989. "The Fate of Buccal Mucosal Flaps in Primary Palatal Repair." *The Cleft Palate Journal* 26 (2): 110–12; discussion 112-3.

[52] Gilardino, Mirko S., Salah Aldekhayel, and Alexander Govshievich. 2018. "A Prospective Study Investigating Fistula Rate Following Primary Palatoplasty Using Acellular Dermal Matrix." *Plastic and Reconstructive Surgery. Global Open* 6 (6). https://doi.org/10.1097/GOX.0000000000001826.

[53] Losee, Joseph E., Darren M. Smith, Ahmed M. Afifi, Shao Jiang, Matthew Ford, Lisa Vecchione, Gregory M. Cooper, Sanjay Naran, Mark P. Mooney, and Joseph M. Serletti. 2008. "A Successful Algorithm for Limiting Postoperative Fistulae Following Palatal Procedures in the Patient with Orofacial Clefting." *Plastic and Reconstructive Surgery* 122 (2): 544–54. https://doi.org/10.1097/PRS.0B013E31817D6223.

[54] Aldekhayel, Salah A., Hani Sinno, and Mirko S. Gilardino. 2012. "Acellular Dermal Matrix in Cleft Palate Repair: An Evidence-Based Review." *Plastic and Reconstructive Surgery* 130 (1): 177–82. https://doi.org/10.1097/PRS.0B013E318254B2DC.

[55] Simpson, Andrew, Osama A. Samargandi, Alison Wong, M. Elise Graham, and Michael Bezuhly. 2019. "Repair of Primary Cleft Palate and Oronasal Fistula With Acellular Dermal Matrix: A Systematic Review and Surgeon Survey." *The Cleft Palate-Craniofacial Journal : Official Publication of the American Cleft Palate-Craniofacial Association* 56 (2): 187–95. https://doi.org/10.1177/1055665618774028.

[56] Schettler, Dietrich. 1973. "Intra- and Postoperative Complications in Surgical Repair of Clefts in Infancy." *Journal of Maxillofacial Surgery* 1 (1): 40–44. https://doi.org/10.1016/S0301-0503(73)80011-6.

[57] Senders, Craig W., and John H. Eisele. 1995. "Lingual Pressures Induced by Mouthgags." *International Journal of Pediatric Otorhinolaryngology* 33 (1): 53–60. https://doi.org/10.1016/0165-5876(95)01192-E.

[58] Sherif, Rami D., Paymon Sanati-Mehrizy, and Peter J. Taub. 2018. "Lingual Pressure During Dingman-Assisted Cleft Palate Repair: An Investigatory Case Series." *The Cleft Palate-Craniofacial Journal : Official Publication of the American Cleft Palate-Craniofacial Association* 55 (2): 312–15. https://doi.org/10.1177/1055665617739313.

[59] Antony, Anuja K., and Gerald M. Sloan. 2002. "Airway Obstruction Following Palatoplasty: Analysis of 247 Consecutive Operations." *The Cleft Palate-Craniofacial Journal : Official Publication of the American Cleft Palate-Craniofacial Association* 39 (2): 145–48. https://doi.org/10.1597/1545-1569_2002_039_0145_AOFPAO_2.0.CO_2.

[60] Deshpande, Gaurav Shekhar, Alex Campbell, Rasika Jagtap, Carolina Restrepo, Hannah Dobie, Henry Tait Keenan, and Hiteswar Sarma. 2014. "Early Complications after Cleft Palate Repair: A Multivariate Statistical Analysis of 709 Patients." *The Journal of Craniofacial Surgery* 25 (5): 1614–18. https://doi.org/10.1097/SCS.0000000000001113.

[61] Wheeler, Jonathan S, and Megan Sanders. 2021. "Late Bleeding Following Cleft Palate Repair: An Under-Reported Finding?" *The Journal of Craniofacial Surgery*, September. https://doi.org/10.1097/SCS.0000000000008135.

[62] Moore, M D, W T Lawrence, J J Ptak, and W C Trier. 1988. "Complications of Primary Palatoplasty: A Twenty-One-Year Review." *The Cleft Palate Journal* 25 (2): 156–62.

[63] Wilhelmi, B. J., E. A. Appelt, L. Hill, and S. J. Blackwell. 2001. "Palatal Fistulas: Rare with the Two-Flap Palatoplasty Repair." *Plastic and Reconstructive Surgery* 107 (2): 315–18. https://doi.org/10.1097/00006534-200102000-00002.

[64] Hardwicke, Joseph T., Gabriel Landini, and Bruce M. Richard. 2014. "Fistula Incidence after Primary Cleft Palate Repair: A Systematic Review of the Literature." *Plastic and Reconstructive Surgery* 134 (4): 618e–27. https://doi.org/10.1097/PRS.0000000000000548.

[65] Sullivan, Stephen R., Eileen M. Marrinan, Richard A. Labrie, Gary F. Rogers, and John B. Mulliken. 2009. "Palatoplasty Outcomes in Nonsyndromic Patients with Cleft Palate: A 29-Year Assessment of One Surgeon's Experience." *The Journal of Craniofacial Surgery* 20 Suppl 1 (SUPPL. 1): 612–16. https://doi.org/10.1097/SCS.0B013E318192801B.

[66] Smith, Darren M., Lisa Vecchione, Shao Jiang, Matthew Ford, Frederic W.B. Deleyiannis, Mary Ann Haralam, Sanjay Naran, Christine I Worrall, Jason R Dudas, Ahmed M Afifi, Mary L Marazita and Joseph E Losee. 2007. "The Pittsburgh Fistula Classification System: A Standardized Scheme for the Description of Palatal Fistulas." *The Cleft Palate-Craniofacial Journal : Official Publication of the American Cleft Palate-Craniofacial Association* 44 (6): 590–94. https://doi.org/10.1597/06-204.1.

[67] Steinbacher, Derek M., Jennifer L. McGrath, and David W. Low. 2011. "Is Nasal Mucoperiosteal Closure Necessary in Cleft Palate Repair?" *Plastic and Reconstructive Surgery* 127 (2): 768–73. https://doi.org/10.1097/PRS.0B013E3181FED80A.

[68] Fisher, David M., and Brian C. Sommerlad. 2011. "Cleft Lip, Cleft Palate, and Velopharyngeal Insufficiency." *Plastic and Reconstructive Surgery* 128 (4). https://doi.org/10.1097/PRS.0B013E3182268E1B.

[69] McWilliams, BJ; Phillips, BJ. 1979. "*Velopharyngeal Incompetence: Audio Seminars in Speech Pathology.*" Philadelphia: W. B. Saunders, Inc.

Chapter 17

Craniosynostosis

Donovan Lockwood, MD
and Jonathan Y. Lee, MD, MPH

Introduction

1. Craniosynostosis - premature/pathologic fusion/obliteration of one or more cranial vault sutures
2. Isolated or as part of a genetic syndrome:
    a. Non-syndromic typically involves one suture (simple), 1/2000 births [1]
    b. Syndromic often involves multiple sutures (complex)
3. 92% nonfamilial, 85% nonsyndromic [2]
4. Premature suture obliteration disrupts normal head growth and → abnormal head shape
5. Restricted calvarial growth can restrict brain growth and cause detrimental effects on neurocognitive development

Normal Cranium Physiology

Bone

1. Cranial bones develop through intramembranous ossification – direct conversion of mesenchymal cells into bone
2. Formation begins during 8th week of gestation – thin layer of bone forms between dermis and underlying dura
3. Majority of calvarial growth occurs during gestation and early postnatal period; 85% of total growth by 3 years of age [3]

Sutures

1. Cranial sutures are fibrous-type joints - two bone ends with intervening fibrous tissue
2. Eight major cranial sutures: metopic, sagittal, bilateral coronal, bilateral squamosal, and bilateral lambdoid
3. Junction of three or more sutures forms fontanelles

In: Essential Facial Plastic and Reconstructive Surgery. Volume 1 ISBN: 979-8-89113-306-8
Editors: Yan Ho Lee and Ira Papel © 2024 Nova Science Publishers, Inc.

4. Function of network of sutures – flexibility to accommodate deformation of cranium during birth, increases in intracranial pressures, and mechanical stress [4]
5. Sutures are osteogenic centers - osteoprogenitors proliferate and differentiate to form osteogenic fronts
6. Calvarial growth from sutures occurs perpendicularly
7. Growth can occur appositionally - resorption of endocranial surface and bone deposition on ectocranial surface
    a. Growth can be uneven
    b. Allows for pathological growth disturbances [4, 5]
8. Sutures grow continuously until fusion
9. Initially, open suture is an end-to-end butt joint, but evolves into interlocking joint with increasing interdigitation of bone
10. Obliteration of sutures is pathologic except for the metopic suture, which fuses at 6-8 months of age and is obliterated by year 7
11. Posterior fontanelle closes at 3-6 months of age followed by anterior fontanelle at 9-12 months
12. Normal suture fusion occurs in 3rd decade of life, starting with sagittal at 22 years, coronal at 24 years, and lambdoidal at 26 years [6]
13. Premature suture fusion/obliteration can occur at any time pre/post-natally

Pathogenesis of Craniosynostosis

1. Genetic etiology for both syndromic and nonsyndromic craniosynostosis
2. Multiple theories about pathogenesis:
    a. Some believe craniosynostosis causes changes in cranial base, cerebral spinal fluid (CSF) volume, brain volume, ventricular morphology, and intracranial pressure (ICP)
    b. Some believe alterations in skull base growth (i.e. underdevelopment) will limit normal physiologic stretch at adjacent sutures in cranium, resulting in premature fusion and associated changes in brain development [7-12]

Environmental Factors/Extrinsic Forces

1. Associated with maternal smoking, advanced maternal age, warfarin and nitrofurantoin use during gestation, maternal hyperthyroidism, high altitude gestation, and fertility treatments [13, 14]
2. Associated with prenatal head compression in setting of multiple gestations and uterine constriction [15]
3. Fetal constraint in animal models has also resulted in premature suture fusion with upregulation of FGFR2 and TGF-B [16]
4. Another theory states that craniosynostosis occurs because of lack of expansile force of brain as in cases of microcephaly ventricular shunts [17]

Genetics in Non-Syndromic Synostosis

1. Familial autosomal-dominant (AD) patterns of inheritance account for 8-14% of cases of non-syndromic synotosis [18]
2. Only gene to be identified as a non-syndromic contributor is Ephrin-A4 (EFNA4) [19]

Genetics in Syndromic Synostosis

1. Elevated FGFR2 expression
   a. Target of craniosynostosis research [20]
   b. Tyrosine for cysteine substitution in FGFR2 gene results in dysregulation of FGF signaling and subsequent suture fusion [21]
2. Other growth factors have also been associated with synostosis: TGF-B and BMPs
3. Mutations in FGFR2 gene found in a spectrum of syndromic craniosynostosis including Crouzon's, Pfeiffer's, Apert's, and Jackson-Weiss
4. FGFR3 mutations cause Muenke syndrome
5. TWIST mutations cause Saethre-Chotzen syndrome through upregulation of FGFR expression resulting in premature osteoblast differentiation and early synostosis [22]

Pathologic Cranial Growth

1. Isolated, non-syndromic craniosynostosis - classified by involved suture
2. Syndromic cases - classified by encompassing syndrome (i.e., Crouzon's, Pfeiffer's)
3. In anatomically normal head: anterior-posterior (AP) length is greater than width
4. Cephalic index (CI)
   a. Defined as ratio of transverse width to AP length
   b. Normal CI is between 0.76 and 0.81
   c. CI between 0.71 and 0.76 - classified as scaphocephalic/dolichocephalic
   d. CI < 0.71 - hyperdolichocephalic
5. Trigonocephaly
   a. Describes calvarium in setting of metopic suture obliteration
   b. Typical cases result in high, keel-shaped forehead with bitemporal narrowing and hypotelorism
6. Pathologic scaphocephaly
   a. Associated with sagittal suture obliteration
   b. Features include a midline ridge along obliterated sagittal suture, frontal bossing, occipital bossing, and bitemporal narrowing
7. Brachycephaly
   a. Seen in bicoronal synostosis
   b. AP length is shortened with retrusion of forehead and supraorbital rims
   c. CI typically between 0.81 and 0.85
8. Plagiocephaly
   a. Asymmetric deformity and can be predominantly anterior or posterior

   b. Synostosis-associated plagiocephaly typically arises from unilateral coronal or lambdoid synostosis
9. Unicoronal synostosis
   a. Characteristic anterior plagiocephaly with fronto-facial changes
   b. Ipsilateral orbit has a unique superior-lateral deformity on radiograph termed the harlequin deformity
10. Unilambdoid synostosis
   a. Associated with predominantly posterior plagiocephaly
   b. Characteristic ipsilateral changes include occipital flattening with mastoid bulging, posterior/inferior positioning of ear, and minimal to no forehead bossing
11. Deformational (positional) plagiocephaly
   a. Predominantly posterior
   b. However, ipsilateral occipital flattening does not have a mastoid bulge and oftentimes ipsilateral forehead is bossed
   c. Ear is anteriorly displaced, and fronto-orbital zygomatic complex on contralateral side can be retruded in severe cases
   d. From bird's eye view, deformational plagiocephaly takes on a parallelogram shape whereas unilamboid is trapezoidal
   e. Incidence of deformational plagiocephaly sharply increased with "back to sleep" initiative advocated by American Academy of Pediatrics in early 1990s to reduce incidence of sudden infant death syndrome (SIDS) [23]
12. Turricephaly
   a. Excessive anterior height of cranium with a vertical forehead - frequently observed in untreated brachycephaly
   b. "Volcano sign" describes a widening anterior fontanelle in combination with increased anterior cranial height
13. Oxycephaly
   a. Excessive posterior cranial height in which forehead is retruded, becoming continuous with nasal dorsum
   b. Typically observed in multi-suture synostosis
14. Severe pan-suture synostosis can result in the Kleeblattschädel (clover-leaf) deformity

Syndromic Craniosynostosis

Crouzon's Syndrome

1. Predominantly sporadic
2. In familial cases, linked with mutations in FGFR2 gene with AD inheritance
3. Incidence of 1:60,000 births [24]
4. Bicoronal synostosis with brachycephaly
5. Four key morphological components: exorbitism, retromaxillism, inframaxillism, and paradoxical retrogenia

Apert's Syndrome

1. Predominantly sporadic
2. In familial cases, linked with mutations in FGFR2 gene with AD inheritance
3. Incidence of 1:100,000 to 1:160,000
4. Bicoronal synostosis with turribrachycephaly – a high, prominent forehead – with an enlarged anterior fontanelle, bregmatic bump, and pronounced occipital flattening that distinguishes morphology from Crouzon's
5. Pronounced exorbitism, orbital asymmetry, and hypertelorism, also frequently with nasal deviation with a polly-beak deformity [25-27]

Pfeiffer's Syndrome

1. AD inheritance in familial cases, though sporadic cases are common: overall incidence is 1:100,000 [28]
2. Due to FGFR2 mutations for most patients; however small percentage has a mild form related to FGFR1 mutations
3. Considered a "low Apert" [29,30] - similar degree of midface hypoplasia; however, less severe cranial deformity from bicoronal synostosis

Saethre-Chotzen Syndrome

1. Incidence is 1:25,000 to 1:50,000 with AD inheritance [31]
2. Linked to mutations in TWIST-1 gene (68% of cases) although FGFR2 and FGFR3 mutations have been reported
3. Bicoronal synostosis is common with associated turribrachycephaly; typically asymmetric [28]

Carpenter's Syndrome

1. Autosomal recessive inheritance with incidence 1:1,000,000
2. Linked to mutations in RAB23 gene on chromosome 6 and in MEGF8 gene on chromosome 19 [32]
3. Brachycephalic and asymmetric
4. Typical synostosis of bicoronal sutures, sagittal and lambdoid sutures
5. Most patients have neurodevelopmental delay [33]

Muenke Syndrome

1. Incidence estimated at 1:10,000
2. Linked to mutations in FGFR3 gene with AD inheritance

3. Both unicoronal and bicoronal synostosis are observed
4. Interestingly, sexual dimorphism such that bicoronal synostosis is observed in 58% of female patients and only 37% of male patients

Patient Evaluation

History and Physical Exam

1. Usually first suspected by parents/pediatrician due to head shape
2. Frequent comorbidities that require interdisciplinary team workup
3. Delay in diagnosis can occur when mistaken for positional plagiocephaly
4. Patients with isolated, single suture synostosis have 13% incidence of intracranial hypertension (ICH) (>15mm Hg)
5. As more sutures are involved, incidence of ICH increases
    a. Nonsyndromic multisuture synostosis associated with a 42% incidence of ICH
    b. Syndromic craniosynostosis associated with higher incidence of ICH: 65% with Crouzon's and 83% with Apert's [34, 35]
6. Bulging anterior fontanelle can also be observed with ICH
7. Synostotic sutures will often present with palpable, immobile ridging
8. In contrast, overlapping sutures will also present with ridging; however there is mobility with manipulation
9. CT can be helpful to gauge severity of deformity and establish a baseline
10. Exam revealing multi-suture synostosis should heighten suspicion of syndromic etiology

Assessing Intracranial Pressure

1. ICP can be determined directly or indirectly
2. Direct methods
    a. Include intraventicular and intraparenchymal monitoring
    b. These techniques are invasive with potentially significant morbidity
3. Indirect methods
    a. Structural modalities (dilated fundoscopy, CT, MRI, ocular ultrasound, optical coherence tomography)
    b. Functional modalities (visual evoked potentials (VEPs), transcranial Doppler ultrasound, near-infrared spectroscopy) [36-38]

Imaging

1. High-resolution, 3-dimensional computed tomography (3D CT) - best modality to confirm and assess extent of craniosynostosis

   a. CT can also evaluate ventricular system of brain and identify parenchymal anomalies in corpus callosum and brainstem. (e.g., Type I Chiari, with herniation of cerebellar tonsils into the foramen magnum, frequently observed in syndromic craniosynostosis [39]
   b. Differential resorption of endocranial surface caused by elevated pressure at interface of cranium and brain can be observed as a "thumb-printing" or "copper-beaten" pattern that can result in full thickness defects in severe cases
   c. Loss of gyrification and blunting of subarachnoid and basal cisternae can also be observed with ventricular effacement and midline shift in severe cases
   d. CT can also be used to evaluate optic nerve sheath diameter (ONSD), which is continuous with dura mater; elevated subarachnoid pressure will result in widening of ONSD [40]
2. Magnetic resonance imaging (MRI) - inferior to 3D CT in diagnosis and evaluation of sutures in craniosynostosis
   a. Can be useful in evaluating parenchymal and ventricular abnormalities in patients with established diagnosis
   b. Syndromic craniosynostosis can be complicated with anomalies in venous drainage through scalp with extracranial transverse sinuses [41], so MRI can be useful in planning surgical approach and craniotomies

Surgical Indications and Technique

1. Forty years after pathophysiology of craniosynostosis was first described by Virchow in 1851, first surgical repair of craniosynostosis was performed in 1892 by Lannelongue [42, 43]
2. Modern day techniques evolved from extensive vault reconstructions described in 1980's and 1990's [44-48]
3. Paradigm of "minimally invasive" endoscopic repair began in 1990's and was expanded upon with cranial molding orthotics [49]
4. Spring-mediated cranioplasty was introduced in 1998 to provide dynamic expansion of synostotic sutures [50]
5. Dynamic expansion of cranium was further augmented with application of distraction osteogenesis [51, 52]

Indications for Surgery

1. Patients with craniosynostosis have an elevated risk of psychosocial difficulties throughout life; normalizing aesthetics may help facilitate normal social interactions and improve quality of life
2. Functional concerns include ICH, corneal protection, and upper airway obstruction
   a. ICH

i. Primary functional indication is prevention and treatment of ICH, which if left untreated can result in neurodevelopmental delay, optic atrophy, and blindness [53]
ii. Patients with syndromic diagnosis, multi-suture involvement, and severe plagiocephaly are at higher risk of ICH
iii. Upper airway obstruction, hydrocephalus, and intracranial venous congestion can also cause ICH independent of craniosynostosis

b. Corneal Protection
i. Metopic and coronal synostosis can lead to retraction of superior and inferior orbital rims
ii. Syndromic bicoronal synostosis can result in a more vertically slanting anterior skull base, resulting in a shallow orbit →result in exorbitism with potential lagophthalmos and corneal exposure
iii. Exposure keratopathy can then result in significant visual changes and blindness [54]
iv. Temporary tarsorrhaphy may reduce risk of exposure keratopathy, but can lead to deprivational amblyopia in infants
v. Expanding bony orbit with fronto-orbital advancement or fronto-facial advancement can address oculo-orbital disproportion

c. Upper Airway Obstruction
i. Commonly seen in syndromic craniosynostosis such as Apert's and Couzon's
ii. Likely due to midface hypoplasia with narrowing of pharynx and hypopharynx, which can also be addressed with fronto-facial advancement
iii. There may be multi-level upper airway obstruction in syndromic patients [55]

3. Comprehensive evaluation includes polysomnography and laryngoscopy/bronchoscopy
4. Timing of surgical intervention dependent on severity and is controversial, ranging from several weeks to several years of life
5. Major concern with early intervention is that anticipated blood loss from operation is high in comparison to circulating blood volume (70-80cc/kg) in patients less than 1 year old
6. Early intervention may result in relapse of dysmorphology since much cranial growth is still required [56]; however, operating early arrests deforming pathology in setting of less compensatory growth and greater dural osteogenic potential [57]

Nonsyndromic Surgical Techniques

Metopic

1. Premature metopic craniosynostosis results in trigonocephaly

2. Most common operation to address superior orbital rim retrusion, bitemporal narrowing, and forehead contour is a bilateral fronto-orbital advancement (FOA) [58]
3. Minimally invasive techniques including endoscopic strip craniectomy with cranial orthotic have been described [59]

Unicoronal

1. Unicoronal craniosynostosis (UCS) - defined by ipsilateral superior orbital rim and forehead retrusion and a tall orbit
2. Goal of correction to advance and recontour ipsilateral supraorbital bandeau and anterior cranium
3. In UCS, in addition to anteriorly advancing, ipsilateral bandeau requires lowering in order to:
    a. Shorten height of orbit
    b. Match orientation of vertical orbital plane to contralateral side
4. FOA technique has several modifications in UCS [60]: although a full bifrontal craniectomy and bandeau can be removed as in metopic, a partial (2/3rds) bandeau and full frontal craniectomy is preferred to minimize morbidity since contralateral side has minimal perceivable deformity

Sagittal

1. Scaphocephaly - results in bitemporal and biparietal narrowing as well as varying degrees of frontal and occipital bossing
2. Surgical interventions:
    a. Minimally invasive procedures for early intervention, generally performed between 3-7 months old
    b. More extensive remodeling, performed from 7 months old onward
3. Primary goal of correction: expansion of temporoparietal width, which can result in spontaneous posterior and anterior vault remodeling in patients less than 7 months old [61, 62]
4. Minimally invasive procedures
    a. Initially designed as a bridge to definitive reconstruction but have been found to be effective and with long-lasting results
    b. Now offered as definitive operations
    c. Characterized by decreased blood loss, morbidity, hospital stay, ICU care, and operating room time [63]
    d. 2 main techniques:
        i. Endoscopic strip craniectomy with postoperative cranial molding orthotic
        ii. Spring-assisted surgery
        iii. In both techniques, principal components are 1) removal of obliterated sagittal suture and 2) expansion of midvault to allow brain to grow in coronal plane, limiting further growth in sagittal plane [64]

5. For patients presenting late (>7mo of age) or with severe deformity, a more extensive, open calvarial remodeling operation is required [65]
   a. Variety of techniques
   b. Expansion of midvault is the common principle

Unilateral Lambdoid

1. Plagiocephaly caused by unilambdoid synostosis
   a. Largely posterior, thus surgical techniques focus on posterior vault remodeling
   b. Although minimally invasive techniques, including strip craniectomies [49], have been described, open posterior vault remodeling procedures are currently preferred option
   c. Primary goals of correction are to:
      i. Halt deforming etiology
      ii. Restore cranial symmetry
2. Occipital switch cranioplasty is one technique that has been demonstrated to provide stable long-term results when performed within first year of age [66, 67]

Syndromic Techniques

1. Syndromic patients at high risk for requiring multiple corrective operations throughout their craniofacial development [68]
2. Relative paucity of high-level clinical evidence in treatment pathways has led to significant variability across treatment centers
3. Goals of treatment are: functional optimization of ICP, ocular protection, airway, occlusion, and aesthetics
4. Many techniques used in nonsyndromic synostosis can be applied to syndromic cranium; however, need for earlier and greater degree of cranial expansion and correction of fronto-facial dysmorphology defines differences in both techniques and treatment pathways

Fronto-Facial Surgery

1. *Monobloc* procedure - keystone in fronto-facial surgery
   a. Also referred to as fronto-facial advancement
   b. Describes combination of supraorbital bandeau and subcranial midface as a single unit [69]
   c. Typically performed at 6-8 years of age [70]
2. Other procedures (orbital translocation, facial bipartition, LeFort III) are variations on required exposure and osteotomies

Posterior Vault Distraction Osteogenesis

1. Posterior vault distraction osteogenesis (PVDO) expands cranium and surpasses issues that limit extent of traditional vault expansion techniques
2. When compared to FOA, PVDO provides significantly greater intracranial volume expansion and is associated with subsequent spontaneous remodeling of anterior cranium [71, 72]
3. PVDO is less invasive, preserves vitalization of bone, and can be performed earlier in life due to lower blood loss
4. Treatment pathway for syndromic craniosynostosis in many craniofacial institutions incorporates PVDO as initial intervention at 4-8 months of age [73-77]
5. Earlier distraction may be indicated if signs of ICH are present; however, quality of bone may not be able to support fixation of distractor

Perioperative Care

1. Complications following intracranial interventions for craniosynostosis are relatively rare
2. Historically, blood loss is major contributor to morbidity and mortality in acute perioperative period [78, 79]
3. Therefore, much of perioperative care is centered on reducing blood loss, minimizing blood product transfusions, and maximizing cardiovascular support [80-83]

Summary Points

1. Craniosynostosis has multifactorial etiology, including genetic and environmental factors
2. Compensatory changes in skull growth can result in brain growth restriction and intracranial hypertension, driving need for early diagnosis and appropriate intervention
3. Craniosynostosis can be nonsyndromic or syndromic and thus requires a multi-disciplinary evaluation to thoroughly diagnosis and manage patient
4. Initial evaluation should focus on a full body physical exam as well as non-invasive intracranial pressure assessment and 3D CT imaging of the cranium
5. Syndromic patients require a multi-disciplinary evaluation to optimize timing and type of surgical intervention; however, multiple surgeries are likely throughout development
6. Goals of synostosis surgery focus primarily on expanding intracranial volume and normalizing appearance
7. Relapse and fewer reoperations are associated with surgery at an older age; however, minimally invasive techniques allow intervention at an earlier age, minimizing deformational growth and reducing operative morbidity
8. Complications in acute perioperative period are rare, but can be life-threatening and are usually related to surgical blood loss and cardiopulmonary sequelae
9. Meticulous preparation, communication, and technique are necessary to minimize morbidity and mortality

Patient Case

A 3-month-old male is referred for abnormal head shape. On exam, the head shape demonstrates biparietal narrowing with a cephalic index of 70 (normal 76-81). A palpable ridge is observed spanning anterior to posterior in the cranial midline. No ridge is palpable on the forehead. A clinical image of the head shape taken from above is shown. (Figure 17.1) The parents are interested in "helmet" therapy.

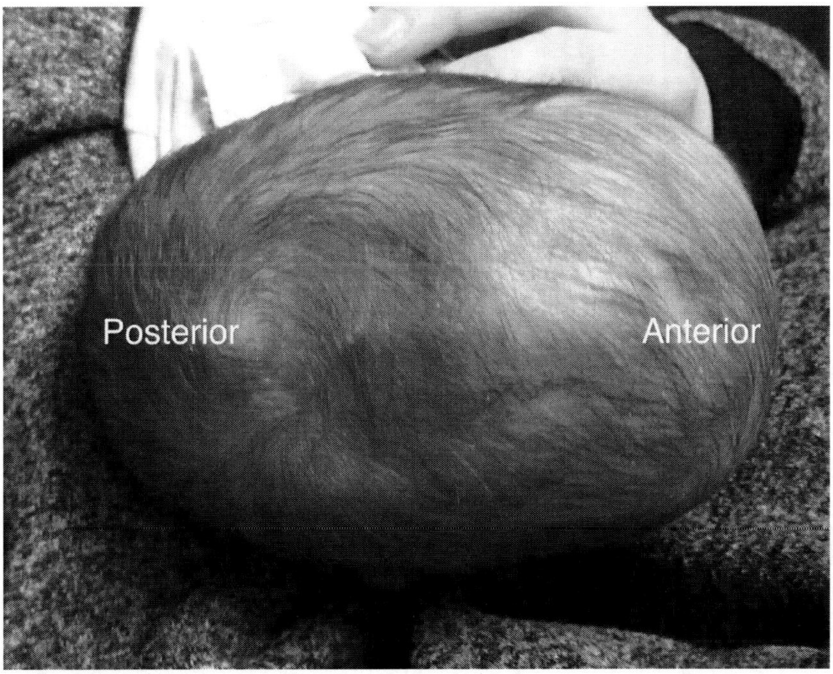

Figure 17.1. Patient case: 3 month old male.

Q1. Based on the exam, what is the likely diagnosis?

A1: The description of the head shape is most consistent with scaphocephaly and the palpable ridge along the sagittal suture strongly suggests a diagnosis of sagittal craniosynostosis.

Q2. Is "helmet" therapy appropriate for this patient?

A2: The indicated treatment is surgical in nature and will not benefit from a cranial molding orthotic alone. Acquired/positional plagiocephaly can benefit from a cranial molding orthotic and can be diagnosed based on physical exam such that the cranial shape from bird's eye view is consistent with a parallelogram without palpable ridging.

Q3. What further evaluations are needed in this patient with suspected craniosynostosis?

A3: Imaging with a CT head and 3D reconstruction will help define the extent of the craniosynostosis and determine if other sutures are involved. The imaging can also be utilized in virtual surgical planning if desired. The patient will also benefit from genetic counseling to rule out a possible associated syndrome, although less likely with sagittal than bicoronal craniosynostosis. Ophthalmology and Neurosurgery evaluation are also indicated to assess concerns of intracranial pressure and to initiate a coordinated surgical plan.

Q4. What are the treatment options for this patient at the current age?

A4: At the 3-6mo age range, patients with sagittal craniosynostosis may be indicated for either strip craniectomy followed cranial molding orthotic or spring assisted surgery. Both procedures can be performed with an endoscopic approach to removal of the sagittal suture and perform barrel staving osteotomies if needed. Cranial springs can then be placed to help with active expansion of the cranium laterally, but will require a second operation for removal. Alternatively, the patient can be placed into cranial molding orthotic to allow the growing brain to passively expand the cranium laterally. Total cranial vault remodeling surgery is also an acceptable alternative surgical option, but is typically performed at an older age of 1 year or older for longer lasting results.

References

[1] Robin NH. Molecular genetic advances in understanding craniosynostosis. *Plast Reconstr Surg.* 1999;103:1060-1070.

[2] Cohen, Meyer Michael. "Craniosynostosis." *Diagnosis, evaluation, and management* (1986): 60-62.

[3] Morriss-Kay GM, Wilkie AO. Growth of the normal skull vault and its alteration in craniosynostosis: Insights from human genetics and experimental studies. *J Anat.* 2005;207:637-653.

[4] Persson M. The role of sutures in normal and abnormal craniofacial growth. *Acta Odontol Scand.* 1995;53:152-161.

[5] Persing JA, Jane JA, Shaffrey M. Virchow and the pathogenesis of craniosynostosis: A translation of his original work. *Plast Reconstr Surg.* 1989;83:738-742.

[6] Cohen MM, Jr. Sutural biology and the correlates of craniosynostosis. *Am J Med Genet.* 1993;47:581-616.

[7] Gunther H. Der Turmschadel als Konstitutionsanomalie und als klinisches Symptom. [The tower skull as a constitutional abnormality and as a clinical symptom.] *Ergebn Med Kinderheilkd.* 1931;40:40.

[8] Moss ML. The pathogenesis of premature cranial synostosis in man. *Acta Anat (Basel).* 1959;37:351-370.

[9] Greenwald JA, Mehrara BJ, Spector JA, Fagenholz PJ, Saadeh PB, Steinbrech DS, Gittes GK, Longaker MT. Immature versus mature dura mater: II. differential expression of genes important to calvarial reossification. *Plast Reconstr Surg.* 2000;106:630-8; discussion 639.

[10] Paige KT, Vega SJ, Kelly CP, Bartlett SP, Zakai E, Jawad AF, Stouffer N, Whitaker LA. Age-dependent closure of bony defects after frontal orbital advancement. *Plast Reconstr Surg.* 2006;118:977-984.

[11] Opperman LA, Sweeney TM, Redmon J, Persing JA, Ogle RC. Tissue interactions with underlying dura mater inhibit osseous obliteration of developing cranial sutures. *Dev Dyn.* 1993;198:312-322.

[12] Fellows-Mayle W, Hitchens TK, Simplaceanu E, Horner J, Barbano T, Losee JE, Losken HW, Siegel MI, Mooney MP. Testing causal mechanisms of nonsyndromic craniosynostosis using path analysis of cranial contents in rabbits with uncorrected craniosynostosis. *Cleft Palate Craniofac J.* 2006;43:524-531.

[13] Alderman BW, Zamudio S, Barón AE, Joshua SC, Fernbach SK, Greene C, Mangione EJ. Increased risk of craniosynostosis with higher antenatal maternal altitude. *Int J Epidemiol.* 1995;24:420-426.

[14] Gardner JS, Guyard-Boileau B, Alderman BW, Fernbach SK, Greene C, Mangione EJ. Maternal exposure to prescription and non-prescription pharmaceuticals or drugs of abuse and risk of craniosynostosis. *Int J Epidemiol.* 1998;27:64-67.

[15] Higginbottom MC, Jones KL, James HE. Intrauterine constraint and craniosynostosis. *Neurosurgery.* 1980;6:39-44.

[16] Hunenko O, Karmacharya J, Ong G, Kirschner RE. Toward an understanding of nonsyndromic craniosynostosis: Altered patterns of TGF-beta receptor and FGF receptor expression induced by intrauterine head constraint. *Ann Plast Surg.* 2001;46:546-53; discussion 553-4.

[17] Kloss JL. Craniosynostosis secondary or ventriculoatrial shunt. *Am J Dis Child.* 1968;116:315-317.

[18] Justice CM, Yagnik G, Kim Y, Peter I, Jabs EW, Erazo M, Ye X, Ainehsazan E, Shi L, Cunningham ML, Kimonis V, Roscioli T, Wall SA, Wilkie AO, Stoler J, Richtsmeier JT, Heuzé Y, Sanchez-Lara PA, Buckley MF, Druschel CM, Mills JL, Caggana M, Romitti PA, Kay DM, Senders C, Taub PJ, Klein OD, Boggan J, Zwienenberg-Lee M, Naydenov C, Kim J, Wilson AF, Boyadjiev SA. A genome-wide association study identifies susceptibility loci for nonsyndromic sagittal craniosynostosis near BMP2 and within BBS9. *Nat Genet.* 2012;44:1360-1364.

[19] Merrill AE, Bochukova EG, Brugger SM, Ishii M, Pilz DT, Wall SA, Lyons KM, Wilkie AO, Maxson RE Jr. Cell mixing at a neural crest-mesoderm boundary and deficient ephrin-eph signaling in the pathogenesis of craniosynostosis. *Hum Mol Genet.* 2006;15:1319-1328.

[20] Delezoide AL, Benoist-Lasselin C, Legeai-Mallet L, Le Merrer M, Munnich A, Vekemans M, Bonaventure J. Spatio-temporal expression of FGFR 1, 2 and 3 genes during human embryo-fetal ossification. *Mech Dev.* 1998;77:19-30.

[21] Mangasarian K, Li Y, Mansukhani A, Basilico C. Mutation associated with crouzon syndrome causes ligand-independent dimerization and activation of FGF receptor-2. *J Cell Physiol.* 1997;172:117-125.

[22] el Ghouzzi V, Le Merrer M, Perrin-Schmitt F, Lajeunie E, Benit P, Renier D, Bourgeois P, Bolcato-Bellemin AL, Munnich A, Bonaventure J. Mutations of the TWIST gene in the saethre-chotzen syndrome. *Nat Genet*. 1997;15:42-46.

[23] American academy of pediatrics AAP task force on infant positioning and SIDS: Positioning and SIDS. *Pediatrics*. 1992;89:1120-1126.

[24] Cohen MM,Jr, Kreiborg S. Birth prevalence studies of the Couzon syndrome: comparison of direct and indirect methods. *Clin Genet*. 1992;41(1):12.

[25] Tessier P. The definitive plastic surgical treatment of the severe facial deformities of craniofacial dysostosis. crouzon's and apert's diseases. *Plast Reconstr Surg*. 1971;48:419-442.

[26] Proudman TW, Moore MH, Abbott AH, David DJ. Noncraniofacial manifestations of crouzon's disease. *J Craniofac Surg*. 1994;5:218-222.

[27] Upton J. Apert syndrome. classification and pathologic anatomy of limb anomalies. *Clin Plast Surg*. 1991;18:321-355.

[28] Schell U, Hehr A, Feldman GJ, Robin NH, Zackai EH, de Die-Smulders C, Viskochil DH, Stewart JM, Wolff G, Ohashi H, Price RA, Cohen MM Jr, Muenke M. Mutations in FGFR1 and FGFR2 cause familial and sporadic pfeiffer syndrome. *Hum Mol Genet*. 1995;4:323-328.

[29] Tessier P: Apert's Syndrome: Acrocephalosyndactyly Type I. In: Caronni EP (ed), *Craniofacial Surgery*. Boston, Little Brown, 1985. Ch 27, pp 280-303.

[30] Cohen MM,Jr. Pfeiffer syndrome update, clinical subtypes, and guidelines for differential diagnosis. *Am J Med Genet*. 1993;45:300-307.

[31] Clauser L, Galie M, Hassanipour A, Calabrese O. Saethre-chotzen syndrome: Review of the literature and report of a case. *J Craniofac Surg*. 2000;11:480-486.

[32] Kadakia S, Helman SN, Healy NJ, Saman M, Wood-Smith D. Carpenter syndrome: A review for the craniofacial surgeon. *J Craniofac Surg*. 2014;25:1653-1657.

[33] 71. Taravath S, Tonsgard JH. Cerebral malformations in carpenter syndrome. *Pediatr Neurol*. 1993;9:230-234.

[34] Doherty ES, Lacbawan F, Hadley DW, Brewer C, Zalewski C, Kim HJ, Solomon B, Rosenbaum K, Domingo DL, Hart TC, Brooks BP, Immken L, Lowry RB, Kimonis V, Shanske AL, Jehee FS, Bueno MR, Knightly C, McDonald-McGinn D, Zackai EH, Muenke M. Muenke syndrome (FGFR3-related craniosynostosis): Expansion of the phenotype and review of the literature. *Am J Med Genet A*. 2007;143A:3204-3215.

[35] Renier D, Sainte-Rose C, Marchac D, Hirsch JF. Intracranial pressure in craniostenosis. *J Neurosurg*. 1982;57:370-377.

[36] Marucci DD, Dunaway DJ, Jones BM, Hayward RD. Raised intracranial pressure in Apert syndrome. *Plast Reconstr Surg*. 2008;122(4):1162-1168.

[37] Padayachy LC. Non-invasive intracranial pressure assessment. *Childs Nerv Syst*. 2016;32:1587-1597.

[38] Tuite GF, Chong WK, Evanson J, Narita A, Taylor D, Harkness WF, Jones BM, Hayward RD. The effectiveness of papilledema as an indicator of raised intracranial pressure in children with craniosynostosis. *Neurosurgery*. 1996;38:272-278.

[39] Desch LW. Longitudinal stability of visual evoked potentials in children and adolescents with hydrocephalus. *Dev Med Child Neurol*. 2001;43:113-117.

[40] Fearon JA, Swift DM, Bruce DA. New methods for the evaluation and treatment of craniofacial dysostosis-associated cerebellar tonsillar herniation. *Plast Reconstr Surg*. 2001;108:1855-1861.

[41] Kimberly HH, Shah S, Marill K, Noble V. Correlation of optic nerve sheath diameter with direct measurement of intracranial pressure. *Acad Emerg Med*. 2008;15:201-204.

[42] Persing JA, Jane JA, Shaffrey M. Virchow and the pathogenesis of craniosynostosis: A translation of his original work. *Plast Reconstr Surg*. 1989;83:738-742.

[43] Lannelongue M. De la craniectomie dans la microcephalie. [Craniectomy in microcephaly.] *CR Acad Sci*. 1890;110:1382–1385.

[44] Mohr G, Hoffman HJ, Munro IR, Hendrick EB, Humphreys RP. Surgical management of unilateral and bilateral coronal craniosynostosis: 21 years of experience. *Neurosurgery*. 1978;2:83-92.

[45] Jane JA, Edgerton MT, Futrell JW, Park TS. Immediate correction of sagittal synostosis. *J Neurosurg*. 1978;49:705-710.

[46] Albright AL. Operative normalization of skull shape in sagittal synostosis. *Neurosurgery*. 1985;17:329-331.

[47] Persing JA, Jane JA, Delashaw JB. Treatment of bilateral coronal synostosis in infancy: A holistic approach. *J Neurosurg*. 1990;72:171-175.

[48] Jimenez DF, Barone CM. The sunrise technique: The correction of occipital plagiocephaly using bandeau occipital plate and radial osteotomies. *Pediatr Neurosurg*. 1995;22:162-5; discussion 166.

[49] Jimenez DF, Barone CM, Cartwright CC, Baker L. Early management of craniosynostosis using endoscopic-assisted strip craniectomies and cranial orthotic molding therapy. *Pediatrics*. 2002;110:97-104.

[50] Lauritzen C, Sugawara Y, Kocabalkan O, Olsson R. Spring mediated dynamic craniofacial reshaping. case report. *Scand J Plast Reconstr Surg Hand Surg*. 1998;32:331-338.

[51] Yonehara Y, Hirabayashi S, Sugawara Y, Sakurai A, Harii K. Complications associated with gradual cranial vault distraction osteogenesis for the treatment of craniofacial synostosis. *J Craniofac Surg*. 2003;14:526-528.

[52] White N, Evans M, Dover MS, Noons P, Solanki G, Nishikawa H. Posterior calvarial vault expansion using distraction osteogenesis. *Childs Nerv Syst*. 2009;25:231-236.

[53] Tamburrini G, Caldarelli M, Massimi L, Santini P, Di Rocco C. Intracranial pressure monitoring in children with single suture and complex craniosynostosis: A review. *Childs Nerv Syst*. 2005;21:913-921.

[54] Tay T, Martin F, Rowe N, Johnson K, Poole M, Tan K, Kennedy I, Gianoutsos M. Prevalence and causes of visual impairment in craniosynostotic syndromes. *Clin Exp Ophthalmol*. 2006;34:434-440.

[55] Inverso G, Brustowicz KA, Katz E, Padwa BL. The prevalence of obstructive sleep apnea in symptomatic patients with syndromic craniosynostosis. *Int J Oral Maxillofac Surg*. 2016;45:167-169.

[56] Posnick JC. Unilateral coronal synostosis (anterior plagiocephaly): Current clinical perspectives. *Ann Plast Surg*. 1996;36:430-447.

[57] Panchal J, Uttchin V. Management of craniosynostosis. *Plast Reconstr Surg*. 2003;111:2032-48.

[58] Selber J, Reid RR, Gershman B, Sonnad SS, Sutton LN, Whitaker LA, Bartlett SP. Evolution of operative techniques for the treatment of single-suture metopic synostosis. *Ann Plast Surg*. 2007;59:6-13.

[59] Jimenez DF, Barone CM. Early treatment of anterior calvarial craniosynostosis using endoscopic-assisted minimally invasive techniques. *Childs Nerv Syst*. 2007;23:1411-1419.

[60] Fearon JA. Beyond the bandeau: 4 variations on fronto-orbital advancements. *J Craniofac Surg*. 2008;19:1180-1182.

[61] David LR, Plikaitis CM, Couture D, Glazier SS, Argenta LC. Outcome analysis of our first 75 spring-assisted surgeries for scaphocephaly. *J Craniofac Surg*. 2010;21:3-9.

[62] Khechoyan D, Schook C, Birgfeld CB, Khosla RK, Saltzman B, Teng CC, Ettinger R, Gruss JS, Ellenbogen R, Hopper RA. hanges in frontal morphology after single-stage open posterior-middle vault expansion for sagittal craniosynostosis. *Plast Reconstr Surg*. 2012;129:504-516.

[63] Garber ST, Karsy M, Kestle JRW, Siddiqi F, Spanos SP, Riva-Cambrin J. Comparing outcomes and cost of 3 surgical treatments for sagittal synostosis: A retrospective study including procedure-related cost analysis. *Neurosurgery*. 2017.

[64] Panchal J, Marsh JL, Park TS, Kaufman B, Pilgram T, Huang SH. Sagittal craniosynostosis outcome assessment for two methods and timings of intervention. *Plast Reconstr Surg*. 1999;103:1574-1584.

[65] Greensmith AL, Holmes AD, Lo P, Maxiner W, Heggie AA, Meara JG. Complete correction of severe scaphocephaly: The melbourne method of total vault remodeling. *Plast Reconstr Surg*. 2008;121:1300-1310.

[66] Taylor JA, Bartlett SP. What's new in syndromic craniosynostosis surgery?. *Plast Reconstr Surg*. 2017;140:82e-93e.

[67] Smartt JM,Jr, Reid RR, Singh DJ, Bartlett SP. True lambdoid craniosynostosis: Long-term results of surgical and conservative therapy. *Plast Reconstr Surg*. 2007;120:993-1003.

[68] Ortiz-Monasterio F, del Campo AF, Carrillo A. Advancement of the orbits and the midface in one piece, combined with frontal repositioning, for the correction of crouzon's deformities. *Plast Reconstr Surg*. 1978;61:507-516.

[69] Bradley JP, Gabbay JS, Taub PJ, Heller JB, O'Hara CM, Benhaim P, Kawamoto HK Jr. Monobloc advancement by distraction osteogenesis decreases morbidity and relapse. *Plast Reconstr Surg*. 2006;118:1585-1597.

[70] Dunaway DJ, Britto JA, Abela C, Evans RD, Jeelani NU. Complications of frontofacial advancement. *Childs Nerv Syst*. 2012;28:1571-1576.

[71] Fearon JA. Halo distraction of the le fort III in syndromic craniosynostosis: A long-term assessment. *Plast Reconstr Surg*. 2005;115:1524-1536.

[72] Britto JA, Greig A, Abela C, Hearst D, Dunaway DJ, Evans RD. Frontofacial surgery in children and adolescents: Techniques, indications, outcomes. *Semin Plast Surg*. 2014;28:121-129.

[73] Derderian CA, Wink JD, McGrath JL, Collinsworth A, Bartlett SP, Taylor JA. Volumetric changes in cranial vault expansion: Comparison of fronto-orbital advancement and posterior cranial vault distraction osteogenesis. *Plast Reconstr Surg*. 2015;135:1665-1672.

[74] Ong J, Harshbarger RJ,3rd, Kelley P, George T. Posterior cranial vault distraction osteogenesis: Evolution of technique. *Semin Plast Surg*. 2014;28:163-178.

[75] Swanson JW, Samra F, Bauder A, Mitchell BT, Taylor JA, Bartlett SP. An algorithm for managing syndromic craniosynostosis using posterior vault distraction osteogenesis. *Plast Reconstr Surg*. 2016;137:829e-41e.

[76] Nguyen C, Hernandez-Boussard T, Khosla RK, Curtin CM. A national study on craniosynostosis surgical repair. *Cleft Palate Craniofac J*. 2013;50:555-560.

[77] Lam S, Fridley J, Desai VR, Srinivasan VM, Jea A, Luerssen TG, Pan IW. Pediatric national surgical quality improvement program: Useful for quality improvement in craniosynostosis surgery?. *J Craniofac Surg*. 2016;27:605-611.

[78] Kang JK, Lee SW, Baik MW, Son BC, Hong YK, Jung CK, Ryu KH. Perioperative specific management of blood volume loss in craniosynostosis surgery. *Childs Nerv Syst*. 1998;14:297-301.

[79] Hansen JK, Lydick AM, Wyatt MM, Andrews BT. Reducing postoperative bleeding after craniosynostosis repair utilizing a low-dose transexamic acid infusion protocol. *J Craniofac Surg*. 2017;28:1255-1259.

[80] Viswanathan R. Techniques to control bleeding from scalp incisions. *J Neurosurg*. 1989;71:630-631.

[81] Fearon JA. Reducing allogenic blood transfusions during pediatric cranial vault surgical procedures: A prospective analysis of blood recycling. *Plast Reconstr Surg*. 2004;113:1126-1130.

[82] Francel PC, Bell A, Jane JA. Operative positioning for patients undergoing repair of craniosynostosis. *Neurosurgery*. 1994;35:304-6; discussion 306.

[83] Kalantar Hormozi A, Mahdavi N, Foroozanfar MM, Razavi SS, Mohajerani R, Eghbali A, Mafi AA, Hashemzadeh H, Mahdavi A. Effect of perioperative management on outcome of patients after craniosynostosis surgery. *World J Plast Surg*. 2017;6:48-53.

Practice Guidelines – Congenital Anomalies

When a particular set of basic criteria is met, then the Qualified Options for treatment, testing, or management below are reasonable and justifiable recommendations.

- When the patient presents with minor ear deformity within a few weeks of life, then ear molding is a qualified option.
- When the patient presents with Microtia Grades 1 or 2, then local flaps, cartilage scoring/resection/grafting are qualified options.
- When the patient presents with Microtia Grades 3 or 4, then Local flaps, cartilage scoring/resection/grafting, total or subtotal ear reconstruction with autologous or homologous cartilage grafts or alloplastic implants, ear prosthesis are qualified options.
- When the patient presents with Cleft Lip (all types), then Multidisciplinary cleft team, speech and language pathology involvement, pediatrics involvement are qualified options.
- When the patient presents with Cleft Lip (unilateral), then Rotation-advancement flap, reconstruction to obliterate cleft and restore form and function are qualified options.
- When the patient presents with Cleft Lip (bilateral), then Millard-Mulliken repair, reconstruction to obliterate clefts and restore form and function are qualified options.
- When the patient presents with Cleft Lip (any type), then Adjunctive procedures including orthopedics, lip adhesion, local flaps, fat/dermal grafts are qualified options.
- When the patient presents with Cleft Nose, then rhinoplasty (nasal reconstruction), grafts, implants are qualified options.
- When the patient presents with Cleft Palate (all types), then Multidisciplinary cleft team, orthodontics/dentistry involvement, speech and language pathology involvement, pediatrics involvement are qualified options.
- When the patient presents with Cleft Palate (hard palate), then reconstruction (e.g., bipedicled flap, unipedicled flap, vomer flap) is a qualified option.
- When the patient presents with Cleft Palate (soft palate), then reconstruction (e.g., intra-velar veloplasty, Furlow double-opposing Z-plasty) is a qualified option.
- When the patient presents with Cleft Palate (any type), then adjunctive procedures (e.g., buccal flat flap, buccal myomucosal flap, acellular dermal matrix, bone grafting) are qualified options.
- When the patient presents with Craniosynostosis (All types), then multi-disciplinary care, intracranial pressure assessment and 3D CT imaging are qualified options.
- When the patient presents with Craniosynostosis (Metopic, trigonocephaly), then reconstruction (e.g., bilateral fronto-orbital advancement, endoscopic strip craniectomy with cranial orthotic) is a qualified option.
- When the patient presents with Craniosynostosis (unicoronal), then reconstruction (e.g., advance and recontour ipsilateral supraorbital bandeau and anterior cranium, ipsilateral bandeau lowering) is a qualified option.

- When the patient presents with Craniosynostosis (Scaphocephaly), then reconstruction (e.g., endoscopic strip craniectomy with postoperative cranial molding orthotic, spring-assisted surgery, open calvarial remodeling operation) is a qualified option.
- When the patient presents with Craniosynostosis (Unilambdoid), then reconstruction (e.g., endoscopic strip craniectomy with postoperative cranial molding orthotic, spring-assisted surgery, open calvarial remodeling operation) is a qualified option.
- When the patient presents with Craniosynostosis (Syndromic), then single or multiple reconstruction(s), Cranial expansion and correction of fronto-facial dysmorphology (e.g., monobloc procedure or fronto-facial advancement, posterior vault distraction osteogenesis) are qualified options.
- When the patient presents with Craniosynostosis (any type), then genetic counseling, eye protection, polysomnography, airway evaluation, laryngoscopy/bronchoscopy are qualified options.
- When the patient presents with Deformational (Positional) Plagiocephaly, then head repositioning, helmet therapy, surgical intervention are qualified options.

Patient Characteristics	**Qualified Option(s)**
Minor ear deformity (within a few weeks of life)	Ear molding
Microtia (Grades 1 or 2)	·Local flaps, cartilage scoring/resection/grafting
Microtia (Grades 3 or 4)	Local flaps, cartilage scoring/resection/grafting, total or subtotal ear reconstruction with autologous or homologous cartilage grafts or alloplastic implants, ear prosthesis
Cleft Lip (All types)	Multidisciplinary cleft team, speech and language pathology involvement, pediatrics involvement
Cleft Lip (Unilateral)	Rotation-advancement flap, reconstruction to obliterate cleft and restore form and function
Cleft Lip (Bilateral)	Millard-Mulliken repair, reconstruction to obliterate clefts and restore form and function
Cleft Lip (Any type)	Adjunctive procedures including orthopedics, lip adhesion, local flaps, fat/dermal grafts
Cleft Nose	Septorhinoplasty (single or multiple) for pediatric or adult patient Graft(s): skin/mucosal/composite/cartilage/bone Autologous, homologous, or alloplastic implants
Cleft Palate (All types)	Multidisciplinary cleft team, orthodontics/dentistry involvement, speech and language pathology involvement, pediatrics involvement
Cleft Palate (Hard palate)	Reconstruction (e.g., bipedicled flap, unipedicled flap, vomer flap)
Cleft Palate (Soft palate)	Reconstruction (e.g., intra-velar veloplasty, Furlow double-opposing Z-plasty)
Cleft Palate (Any type)	Adjunctive procedures (e.g., buccal flat flap, buccal myomucosal flap, acellular dermal matrix, bone grafting)

Craniosynostosis (All types)	Multi-disciplinary care, intracranial pressure assessment and 3D CT imaging
Craniosynostosis (Metopic, trigonocephaly)	Reconstruction (e.g., bilateral fronto-orbital advancement, endoscopic strip craniectomy with cranial orthotic)
Craniosynostosis (Unicoronal)	Reconstruction (e.g., advance and recontour ipsilateral supraorbital bandeau and anterior cranium, ipsilateral bandeau lowering)
Craniosynostosis (Scaphocephaly)	Reconstruction (e.g., endoscopic strip craniectomy with postoperative cranial molding orthotic, spring-assisted surgery, open calvarial remodeling operation)
Craniosynostosis (Unilambdoid)	Reconstruction (e.g., open posterior vault remodeling including occipital switch cranioplasty, minimally invasive techniques including strip craniectomies)
Craniosynostosis (Syndromic)	Single or multiple reconstruction(s) Cranial expansion and correction of fronto-facial dysmorphology (e.g., monobloc procedure or fronto-facial advancement, posterior vault distraction osteogenesis)
Craniosynostosis (Any type)	Genetic counseling, eye protection, polysomnography, airway evaluation, laryngoscopy/bronchoscopy
Deformational (Positional) Plagiocephaly	Head repositioning, helmet therapy, surgical intervention

Part 4. Trauma

Chapter 18

Mandibular Fractures

Alan Wellington Johnson, MD, MS

Introduction

Mandible fractures present unique challenges due to multiple complicating aspects: strong forces from associated muscles, intricate dental interactions, multi-focal and comminuted fracture patterns, varied fracture locations, etc. This chapter reviews the pertinent mandibular anatomy, fracture considerations, and management options. The facial trauma surgeon needs a thorough understanding of these principles to match the approach and fixation strategies to the trauma complexity.

Anatomy

1. The mandible constitutes the lower third of the facial skeleton and articulates with the cranium by the two temporomandibular joints (TMJs).
2. The mobility of the mandible enables mastication (chewing) as it opposes the maxilla, which is part of the middle third of the facial skeleton.
3. The mandible and maxilla each contain 16 teeth, totaling 32; they are counted from 1 to 32 starting with the right posterior maxillary molar; 16 is the left posterior maxillary molar; 17 the left posterior mandibular molar; 32 the right posterior mandibular molar. (note: other terminology for dentition includes: “distal” which is further from the midline, “mesial” which is closer to the midline, “buccal” which is the side closer to the cheek aka buccal mucosa, and “lingual” which is the side closer to the tongue)
4. Fracture sites by location (Figure 18.1):
    a. *Condyle* - articulates with the skull base at the glenoid fossa forming the TMJ. This joint, containing synovial fluid and a cartilage disk, enables opening, closing, protrusion, retrusion, and translation of the mandible to the left or right.
    b. *Coronoid* - bony prominence providing strong insertion of the temporalis muscle for mastication.
    c. *Ramus and angle* - receive muscle insertions from the masseter laterally and the medial pterygoid medially.
    d. *Body, parasymphysis, and symphysis* - support the dentition in a U-shaped arch upon which the mylohyoid, anterior belly of digastric, genioglossus, and geniohyoid insert

In: Essential Facial Plastic and Reconstructive Surgery. Volume 1 ISBN: 979-8-89113-306-8
Editors: Yan Ho Lee and Ira Papel

© 2024 Nova Science Publishers, Inc.

e. *Alveolus* - constitutes the bone investing the tooth roots of this U-shaped arch
5. The mandibular branch of the trigeminal nerve (V3) provides motor fibers to the mylohyoid and anterior belly of digastric muscles before entering the mandible. Upon entering, it becomes the inferior alveolar nerve providing sensation to the teeth and terminates giving sensation to the lower lip and chin as the mental nerve.
6. Surgical dissection tip: The mental nerve resides inferior to the second mandibular premolar. Plan intra-oral incisions accordingly, and approach this region with caution.

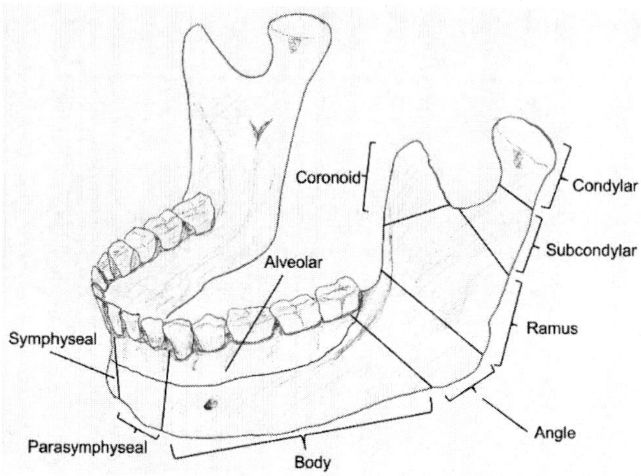

Figure 18.1. Mandible fracture location classification.

Epidemiology

1. Men in the U.S. are 4 times more likely than women to sustain a mandible fracture. [1]
2. Causes: Assault (49%M, 15%F) and motor vehicle accidents (25%M, 54%F) constitute the majority of fractures. Falls are also a common cause and predominate in seniors. [1]
3. Mandibular segments show varying incidence of fracture: symphysis/parasymphyseal (19%), body (18%), angle (16%), condyle (15%), subcondyle (13%), ramus (11%), alveolus (5%), coronoid process (3%). [1]
4. Bilateral fractures of the mandible are more common than isolated unilateral mandible fractures.

Patient Evaluation

Presentation and Work-Up

1. Emergency room (common site of presentation) vs clinic
   a. Always assess ABCs first (airway, breathing, circulation)
   b. Critical: Assess for cervical spine injury and neurologic status
2. History - Assess the following:

a. Mechanism of injury determines extent and type of injuries – blunt vs penetrating, low/moderate/high energy
b. Pain, numbness, difficulty chewing, altered bite, loose teeth
c. Past medical/social history: diabetes, airway/respiratory concerns, prior trauma/surgery, anticoagulation, drug use/withdrawal, allergies, medications

3. Physical examination
   a. Observation:
      i. General: soft tissue tears, edema, avulsion, bleeding, and additional head and neck trauma
      ii. Oral cavity: missing/loose/avulsed/chipped teeth, bleeding, lacerations, dental hygiene, presence of 3rd molars
      iii. Dentition/occlusion:
         - Premature contact, open bite, cross bite, fractured/missing teeth
         - Type I occlusion (normal):
            - The mesiobuccal cusp of the first maxillary molar aligns with the buccal groove of the first mandibular molar.
         - Type II occlusion: Overbite (mandible relatively posterior to maxilla)
         - Type III occlusion: Underbite (mandible relatively anterior to maxilla)
   b. Palpation:
      i. Feel for tenderness to palpation, bony irregularities/step-offs, mental nerve numbness, foreign bodies, penetrating wounds, TMJ crepitus, mobility of dentition.

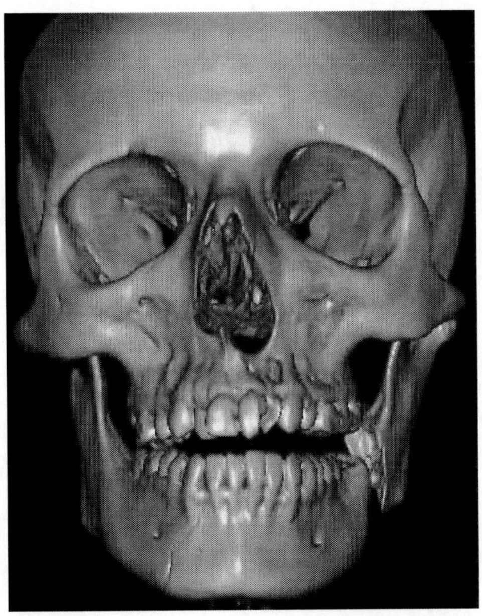

Figure 18.2. Facial CT scan 3D reconstruction showing displaced left angle and right non-displaced body fractures.

4. Imaging
    a. CT scan (most common): with axial, coronal, and sagittal views; enables 3D evaluation (Figure 18.2)
    b. Alternative - orthopantomogram (brand name: "Panorex"): incurs low radiation, lower cost, displays mandible on 1 film, but lacks 3D evaluation; more accurate for the symphysis, parasymphysis, body, angle, and ramus, but less detail on the condyle

Fracture Classifications

1. Closed vs open
2. Unilateral vs bilateral
3. Incomplete vs complete vs. green-stick vs. comminuted
4. Location: symphysis, parasymphyseal, angle, ramus, subcondylar, coronoid, condyle, alveolar (see figure 1)
5. Dentition status: dentulous, partially dentulous, edentulous, mixed dentition (pediatric)
6. Favorable vs non-favorable: depending on vectors placed on bony fragments by muscles of mastication

Management

Medical Considerations

1. Consider comorbidities:
    a. Airway assessment:
        i. Simultaneous midface fractures or multiple mandibular fractures may necessitate a surgical airway (tracheostomy)
        ii. Septal deviation or skull base injury may complicate trans-nasal intubation
        iii. Obstructive sleep apnea: Management may prevent CPAP use
    b. Concomitant injuries: may need to prioritize other injuries including neurosurgical, ocular, orthopedic, thoracic injuries
    c. Diabetes: uncontrolled diabetes can increase infection and complication risk
    d. Substance use/abuse: withdrawal can complicate timing, compliance and outcomes
    e. Bleeding diathesis or anticoagulation use: may increase bleeding risk
2. Pain control: consider pain medications, fracture reduction, jaw sling/support, ice application
3. Infection control: Fractures in the dentate mandible involve gingival tears, resulting in oral cavity contamination. Consensus historically has been to provide oral flora coverage with antibiotics (i.e., amoxicillin/clavulanic acid or clindamycin); chlorhexidine mouth rinse commonly employed

Fracture Considerations

1. Priority: restoring dental occlusion to pre-morbid state
    a. If possible, assess if patient had type I, II, or III occlusion previously
2. Maxillomandibular fixation (MMF) is typically necessary to stabilize dentition for fracture immobilization. MMF involves securing the dentition into its premorbid occlusion, traditionally with arch bars, so that the fracture fragments are reduced. This is also known as closed reduction or closed management.
    a. Fracture management with MMF by itself is an option for immobilization that can preclude open reduction with internal fixation (ORIF)
        i. Limitations: MMF management without ORIF typically requires longer immobilization increasing risk of post-treatment trismus.
3. Force analysis: Distraction, compression, and torsional forces can be applied to fractures of the mandible when chewing.
    a. Fractures in the tooth-bearing mandible will typically distract (pull apart) at the alveolar border of the fracture when chewing. These same fractures will be in compression on the lower border.
    b. Applying techniques to halt distraction, such as a bridle wire, an arch bar, a tension band plate, or a plate along the line of osteosynthesis for an angle or body fracture, will provide stability for the fracture to heal.
4. Plating techniques/types
    a. A tension band plate is 1.5-2.0mm and utilizes 4mm screws to minimize potential tooth root/nerve injury (monocortical). These are used in "load-sharing" situations where the reduced fracture fragments retain some inherent stability.
    b. A mandibular reconstruction plate is 2+ mm thick and can be applied along the mandibular border with bi-cortical screws. These are used in "load-bearing" situations such as comminuted fracture or edentulous mandible fractures that do not have any inherent stability upon fracture reduction.

Treatment Ladder: Treatment Interventions Need to Match Severity of the Fracture(s)

1. Non-operative:
    a. Soft diet - This is reserved for non-displaced pediatric "green stick" or mono-cortical fractures, minimal to nondisplaced condylar or subcondylar fractures, or pathologic fractures in a frail patient
2. Closed reduction/management:
    a. Indications:
        i. Non-displaced or incomplete or greenstick fractures
        ii. Grossly comminuted fractures (not amenable to plate fixation)
        iii. Pediatric fractures with developing dentition
        iv. Edentulous fractures not amenable to open fixation
        v. Coronoid fractures

   vi. Non- or minimally-displaced condylar or subcondylar fractures
  b. MMF techniques (can be applied in OR or clinic):
   i. Arch bars (2 to 6 weeks of immobility)
   ii. Other wire techniques
    - Bridle wires, Ivy loops, Ernst ligatures, Risdon wire
   iii. Intermaxillary fixation (IMF) screws
   iv. Hybrid (or bone-anchored) arch bars
   v. Embrasure wires (intra-operative use only)
   vi. Dental occlusion ties (up to 3 weeks)
   vii. Note: arch bars, hybrid arch bars, and IMF screws enable post-op guiding elastics
3. Open reduction with internal fixation +/- MMF: ORIF is typically employed after stabilizing a reduced fracture pattern with MMF. Surgeon should be satisfied with the MMF and dental occlusion prior to rigid ORIF.
  a. Plating/internal fixation
   i. Titanium mini-plates for favorable fractures (with inherent stability)
    - Single vs two-plate techniques, depending on location
   ii. Load-bearing plates for unfavorable fractures (inherent instability)
  b. Surgical approaches
   i. Intra-oral (majority managed with incisions in gingivobuccal sulcus)
    - Ensure adequate soft tissue for closure by incising with a wide cuff of mucosa on the gingival side of the incision
    - Anticipate the location of the mental nerve inferior to the second premolar
    - Endoscopy can be used to assist with visualization
   ii. Extra-oral/transcutaneous: Submandibular, submental, retromandibular (Risdon – 2cm below the angle of the mandible), pre-auricular, peri-lobular, endaural
    - Proceed cautiously, aware of facial nerve/branch locations.
    - Use of a trocar can enable transcutaneous access with negligible facial nerve risk

Treatment Options by Mandibular Segment

1. Unilateral: Most will have some inherent stability from the contralateral side which provides for some versatility in management options such as avoiding post-operative MMF or limited MMF.
  a. Condyle – closed management predominates (see MMF techniques above)
   i. Open treatment - commonly described absolute indications:
  - Displacement into middle cranial fossa
  - Inability to establish dental occlusion
  - Lateral extracapsular displacement of the condyle
  - Presence of foreign body
  - Open fracture with potential for fibrosis [2]

   b. Subcondylar region – ORIF indicated if there is substantial loss of vertical height; options commonly based upon surgeon familiarity: closed management with MMF, endoscopic trans-oral ORIF, open/transcutaneous ORIF
   c. Ramus – ORIF (transoral +/- with percutaneous trocar access), 1-2 plates
   d. Angle – ORIF (transoral) with 1 plate (Champy technique) or 2 plate technique
      i. *Champy technique* – placement of a single plate along the ideal lines of osteosynthesis (the tension bands of the mandible) from the lingual ramus to the buccal body (superior Champy line) or just lateral to the angle (lateral Champy line). [3]
   e. Body, parasymphysis – typically ORIF with 2 mini-plates, 1 mandibular reconstruction plate, or 1 reconstructive plate with 1 miniplate, with additional post-operative MMF if needed for stability
   f. Symphysis – ORIF with 2 plates or lag screw technique
      i. *Lag screw technique* – placement of 2 parallel screws through the anterior mandible, oriented perpendicular to the vertical fracture line. The distal end of the screw engages the distal bone fragment and upon tightening the screw head engages the proximal bone, achieving compression at the fracture line. This technique can be used in any overlapping bones, such as a bicortical oblique fracture in the mandibular body.
   g. Coronoid – rare, typically managed conservatively without fixation/plating
2. Bilateral fractures: essentially all fractures will require a means of intra-operative MMF. Most will have some inherent instability which will favor ORIF and post-operative MMF management.
3. Multiple/comminuted fractures
   a. Need to provide prolonged dental stabilization to provide fracture immobility for healing to counteract strong forces involved with jaw muscles and movements
   b. Large mandible reconstruction plate (load-bearing) + post-operative MMF
4. Edentulous mandible
   a. Consider closed techniques such as a hybrid arch bar while incorporating dentures or Gunning splints (can be made by dentist or oral surgery team) to establish fracture reduction, pre-morbid alignment, and immobilization
   b. ORIF typically warrants a mandibular reconstruction plate (load bearing), as mandible is commonly atrophic
5. Pediatric fractures
   a. Uncommon, but present unique challenges:
      i. Un-erupted teeth can be injured and growth can be potentially altered with titanium plates and screws (consider using resorbable plates/screws)
      ii. Consider using closed reduction with wire techniques, splints, or circum-mandibular wires.

Post-Operative Assessment

1. For patients with post-operative MMF:
   a. Assess MMF stability; if MMF has relaxed, wires may be cautiously tightened in clinic
   b. Remove wires or elastics holding occlusion and assess bite alignment; reapply fixation or elastics with intent of guiding occlusion
   c. Examine gingiva and buccal mucosa for ulcerations/abrasions; consider bending/repositioning wires or applying dental wax for patient comfort
2. For all Patients:
   a. Occlusion and dentition assessment
      i. Consider revision surgery or orthodontia if significant malocclusion
      ii. Palpate for teeth mobility, color-change, sensitivity
   b. Incision healing – assess for dehiscence
      i. Prevent dehiscence with a tension-free double-layered closure; leaving a wide mucosal cuff when making intra-oral incision to facilitate closure
      ii. Encourage good oral hygiene (brush teeth with small tooth brush, mouth rinse), good nutritional status (consider liquid nutritional supplements), control of diabetes and other co-morbidities
   c. Trismus/jaw opening
      i. Early mobilization and physiotherapy help prevent trismus (jaw stiffness); this is particularly helpful in condylar/subcondylar fractures
   d. Mental nerve assessment
      i. Injury can occur from initial fracture or from fracture reduction or screw placement resulting in tooth or lip/chin numbness
3. Imaging: Consider CT scan for malocclusion or suspicion of suboptimal ORIF (i.e. malunion, or nonunion)

Complications

1. Malocclusion:
   a. CT imaging is typically helpful to guide decision-making. CT images can help determine need for guiding elastics, revision surgery, or orthodontia.
2. Malunion: This is defined as fully healed without proper occlusion. This complication is rare, as close follow-up assessment can identify post-op malocclusion prompting appropriate adjustments.
3. Nonunion: Fracture that has not healed/ossified; likely requires revision surgery while identifying and treating any underlying causes (poor nutritional status, poor wound healing, improper reduction, etc)
4. Infection:
   a. May require incision/drainage, washout, debridement (higher suspicion in contaminated wounds)

   b. May require hardware removal, as hardware (especially loose plates/screws) can be seeded with causative organism(s)
5. Trismus: Defined as limited jaw range of motion related to scarring and immobility of the temporomandibular joint during healing. Common in condylar and subcondylar fractures. Early jaw mobilization and physiotherapy can limit/counteract trismus.
6. Incision dehiscence: Typically managed with emphasis on oral hygiene and secondary intention healing
7. Nerve injury (inferior alveolar) and tooth root injury: Avoid by gentle retraction, identification of the nerve, and strategic placement of screws or avoidance of screw-based techniques
8. Gingivitis/poor dental hygiene: Manage with oral rinses, gentle tooth brushing, and water pick
9. Scars: Typically avoided by using trans-oral techniques aided with endoscopes or trans-cutaneous trocar approaches; recommend massage with sun protection and silicone scar products
10. Chin mal-positioning: ptosis of chin ("witch's chin") – usually due to failure to resuspend mentalis; prevent this by making sure the mentalis is approximated

Summary Points

1. Mandible fractures entail many variables including differences in dentition, fracture severity, and comorbidities.
2. Management requires a thorough understanding of these diverse concerns to construct a comprehensive treatment plan.

Patient Case

A 27-year-old male was assaulted with a single punch to the face. He presents to the ER with pain in the right pre-auricular area, left jaw, and with the complaint that he can't close his jaw.

Q1. What important questions should be asked in the history?

A1.

1. History of present illness:
   What was the mechanism of injury?
   How do your teeth feel/align? Did you lose any teeth?
   Do you feel numb in for face/lip/teeth?
2. Medical/Surgical History including allergies/medications
3. Social History

Q2. The patient complains of premature contact with his right dentition and inability to make contact on the left without effort and pain. What does this indicate?

A2.

1. Right-sided displaced fracture with a loss of mandibular height

Q3. Examining his occlusion, it appears that his mesiobuccal cusp of his first maxillary molar aligns with the buccal groove of the first mandibular molar. What occlusion does this indicate?

A3.

1. Class I occlusion

Q4. What imaging is indicated at this time?

A4.

1. Orthopantomogram ("Panorex")
2. Mandible CT scan

Q5. The CT reveals bilateral mandible fractures – left angle and right subcondylar with loss of vertical height. What is the appropriate operative strategy?

A5.

1. MMF using surgeon's preferred method
2. Trans-oral approach to the left angle fracture employing a 1-plate Champy technique or a 2-plate technique (can also do transcutaneous recon plate)
3. Transcutaneous or endoscopic approach to subcondylar fracture
4. Likely post-operative MMF

Q6. In the case that you decided to perform the intraoral 1-plate Champy technique, what are your operative steps?

A6.

1. With or without a bite block on the other side, make a 3-4cm incision along the gingivobuccal sulcus either lateral to the mandible or curvilinear along the molars ascending across the anterior ramus.

2. Dissect down to the subperiosteal plane (elevate subperiosteal layer with molt number 9 or freer) until the fracture is exposed.
3. Clean off callus or debris.
4. Use toe-in or toe-out retractors and manually reduce the fracture.
5. Bend a 4-hole or 6-hole miniplate until it contours to the ideal lines of osteosynthesis (Champy lines, either lateral or superior).
6. Place monocortical screws to secure plate into plate into bone (at least 2 screws on either side of the fracture).
7. Consider taking patient out of MMF if screw placement is difficult.
8. Close mucosa meticulously as plate exposure can be problematic in the retromolar trigone region (2 layers if possible).

Q7. You choose to apply 2 to 3 weeks of post-operative MMF for increased fracture stability and immobilization. What are some MMF options?

A7.

1. Arch bars with wire occlusion or elastics
2. Hybrid arch bar with wire occlusion or elastics
3. Intermaxillary fixation screws with wire occlusion or elastics
4. Dental occlusion ties

Q8. The patient's post-operative course was unremarkable and his MMF was removed post-op day 16. Had his post-operative MMF remained in place for 5 weeks, what complications would have been more likely?

A8.

1. Trismus
2. TMJ ankylosis

Conflict of Interest Statement

Dr. Johnson is the lead inventor of dental occlusion ties, an FDA-cleared maxillomandibular fixation technology.

References

[1] Afrooz, Paul N., Michael R. Bykowski, Isaac B. James, Lily N. Daniali, and Julio A. Clavijo-Alvarez. "The Epidemiology of Mandibular Fractures in the United States, Part 1: A Review of 13,142 Cases from the US National Trauma Data Bank." *Journal of Oral and Maxillofacial Surgery* 73, no. 12 (December 2015): 2361–66. https://doi.org/10.1016/j.joms.2015.04.032.

[2] Stacey, D. Heath, John F. Doyle, Delora L. Mount, Mary C. Snyder, and Karol A. Gutowski. "Management of Mandible Fractures." *Plastic and Reconstructive Surgery* 117, no. 3 (March 2006): 48e–60e. https://doi.org/10.1097/01.prs.0000209392.85221.0b.

[3] Champy, Maxime, J.P. Loddé, R. Schmitt, J.H. Jaeger, and D. Muster. "Mandibular Osteosynthesis by Miniature Screwed Plates via a Buccal Approach." *Journal of Maxillofacial Surgery* 6 (January 1978): 14–21. https://doi.org/10.1016/S0301-0503(78)80062-9.

Additional Resources

Chung, William, Shah, Gaurav A. "Fractures of the Mandible." In *Operative Otolaryngology E-Book: Head and Neck Surgery*. Edited by Carl H. Snyderman. 1292-1298. Netherlands: Elsevier Health Sciences, 2017.

Kellman, Robert. "Maxillofacial Trauma." In *Cummings Otolaryngology: Head and Neck Surgery, 3-Volume Set.* edited by Paul W. Flint, Bruce H. Haughey, Valerie J. Lund, K. Thomas Robbins, J. Regan Thomas, Marci M. Lesperance, and Howard W. Francis, eds., 286-310. United States: Elsevier, 2020.

Odono, Lauren T., Brady, Colin M., Urata, Mark. "Mandible Fractures." In *Facial Trauma Surgery: From Primary Repair to Reconstruction.* Edited by Amir H. Dorafshar, Eduardo D. Rodriguez, and Paul N. Manson. 168-185. United Kingdom: Elsevier, 2019.

Smith, Brian M, Deshmukh, Atul M., Barber, H. Dexter, Fonseca, Raymond J. "Mandibular Fractures." in *Oral and Maxillofacial Trauma.* Edited by H. Dexter Barber, Raymond J. Fonseca, David E. Frost, Michael E. Powers. 293-330. United Kingdom: Elsevier Health Sciences, 2013.

Chapter 19

Zygomaticomaxillary Complex Fractures

Francis D. Graziano, MD
and Peter J. Taub, MD, MS

Introduction

Causes

1. Fractures of the zygoma are almost always the result of high-impact trauma. Most common mechanisms:
    a. Assault
    b. Motor vehicle collisions
    c. Falls
    d. Sporting injuries [1]
2. Most zygomatic fractures occur in men between the ages of 20 and 29 [1]

Anatomy

1. Bones
    a. Zygomaticomaxillary complex (ZMC) is a tetrapod, creating a quadrangular shape
    b. Zygoma has four articulations:
    c. Frontal
        i. Maxillary
        ii. Sphenoid
        iii. Temporal
    d. The four legs of the zygoma:
        i. Stabilize the position of the face with respect to the cranium
        ii. Provide both midface projection and facial width.
    e. Note: a ZMC fracture may mistakenly be referred to as "tripod fracture", though the correct terminology is "tetrapod fracture"
2. Muscular attachments
    a. Inferior border of the zygomatic arch is the origin of the masseter muscle (masseter is the main deforming force that acts on a ZMC fracture,pulling the zygoma inferiorly)

In: Essential Facial Plastic and Reconstructive Surgery. Volume 1 ISBN: 979-8-89113-306-8
Editors: Yan Ho Lee and Ira Papel © 2024 Nova Science Publishers, Inc.

   b. Superficial musculoaponeurotic system (SMAS) and temporoparietal fascia both insert into superior surface of zygomatic arch (the SMAS resists inferior force from masseter)
   c. Zygoma provides origin attachments of: zygomatic head of the quadratus labii superioris which includes zygomaticus major and minor muscles
3. Vascular supply
   a. Zygoma mainly supplied by a combination of the maxillary and facial arteries [2]
4. Nervous innervation
   a. Infraorbital nerve (V2) courses within or just beneath orbital floor, exits the zygoma through the infraorbital foramen, travels inferiorly as it courses anteriorly towards the orbital rim, ultimately exits the maxilla approximately 10 mm inferior to orbital rim.
   b. ZMC fractures frequently associated with ipsilateral anesthesia of the cheek, upper lip and maxillary dentition; typically self-limited and represents a neuropraxia injury, however may vary depending on the degree of trauma

Diagnosis

1. History
   a. Assess timing and mechanism of injury
   b. Ascertain if blunt or penetrating trauma (penetrating trauma is more likely to be associated with deep neurovascular injuries)
   c. Ask about history of prior facial trauma or facial surgeries
   d. Always consider abuse, especially in pediatric and elderly patients.
2. Physical examination
   a. Presentation may include any or all of the following:
      i. Periorbital hematoma and subconjunctival hemorrhage
      ii. Malar flattening
      iii. Palpable step offs (i.e. zygomatic arch, orbital rim)
      iv. Infraorbital paresthesia
      v. Trismus - medial displacement of the zygomatic arch may compress the temporalis muscle between the coronoid process of the mandible, thus decreasing mandibular excursion; assess maximal incisor opening (MIO) usually 45-55mm in adults; <35mm considered trismus
      vi. Enophthalmos, hypoglobus, or diplopia – orbital floor fractures may be associated with ZMC fractures; leads to increased orbital volume and herniation of orbital soft tissue into maxillary sinus
      vii. Downward-sloping palpebral fissure - the Tubercle of Whitnall is located on themedial surface of the frontal process of the zygoma and is where the lateral canthal tendon attaches, therefore ZMC fractures that displace the zygoma inferiorly can result in a downward slant of the palpebral fissure

viii. Consider associated cervical spine injury

3. Imaging studies
   a. Computed tomography (CT) is diagnostic and is the gold standard imaging study; 3D reconstruction can be useful for preoperative planning
   b. On CT, assess for:
      i. Degree of comminution
      ii. Medial/lateral rotation
      iii. Anteroposterior displacement
      iv. Associated fractures, including orbital floor

Classification

Numerous classification systems have been proposed to predict which fractures would remain stable after reduction. Knight and North [3] proposed a classification scheme in 1961 that was based on the direction of the anatomic displacement and fracture pattern (Table 19.1). In 1973, Yanagisawa [4] presented a modification to the Rowe and Killey classification (Table 19.2), which emphasized rotation in both the vertical and horizontal aspects in addition to displacement. More recently, Zingg [5] proposed a classification in 1992 that groups fractures based on surgical implications (Table 19.3). While the three classification schemes are slightly different, they all address the degree of comminution and displacement and favor open reduction and internal fixation with higher degrees.

Table 19.1. Knight and North classification (1961) [3]

Group I	No significant displacement of fracture
Group II	Arch fracture
Group III	Unrotated body fracture
Group IV	Medially rotated body fracture
Group V	Laterally rotated body fracture
Group VI	Complex fracture

Table 19.2. Yanagisawa (1973) [4]

Type I	Non-displaced fracture
Type II	Zygomatic arch fracture
Type III	Rotation around the vertical axis
Type IV	Rotation around the longitudinal axis
Type V	Displacement without rotation
Type VI	Rim fractures
Type VII	Complex fractures

Table 19.3. Zingg (1992) [5]

A1	Isolated zygomatic arch fracture
A2	Isolated lateral orbital fractures
A3	Isolated orbital rim fractures
B	Monofragment zygomatic fractures (tetrapod fracture)
C	Multifragment zygomatic fracture

Management

1. Exposure - depends on which buttresses require reduction and fixation
    a. Anterior approach: Consists of 3 incisions that provide exposure of the critical zygomaticarticulations.
        i. Lateral extension of upper blepharoplasty or lateral brow incision: provides access tozygomaticofrontal (ZF) buttress and lateral orbital wall
        ii. Lower eyelid incision: provides exposure of the infraorbital rim and orbital floor (surgeon preference)
            - Subciliary – increased risk of ectropion
            - Subtarsal – scar slightly more noticeable, less risk of ectropion
            - Transconjunctival (preseptal) – no external scar, less risk of ectropion; less orbital contents in the way but less direct access to the orbital rim
            - Transconjunctival (postseptal) - no external scar, less risk of ectropion; more orbital contents/fat in the way but more direct access to orbital rim
        iii. Note: can be extended with lateral canthotomy for access to lateral orbital rim or wall
    b. Upper gingivobuccal sulcus incision: provides exposure of the maxilla for reduction and fixation of the zygomaticomaxillary (ZM) buttress.
    c. Posterior approach: coronal incision used in cases of severe posterior displacement ofthe zygoma and cases of medially or laterally displaced zygomatic arch fractures
2. Reduction
    a. Open reduction and internal fixation
        i. Mainstay treatment for displaced fractures
        ii. Traditionally, ZMC fractures required fixation at 3 buttresses (ZF, ZM, and infraorbitalrim), however is a trend towards fixation at fewer buttresses [6]
        iii. An elevator or malar hook can be placed under the malar eminence and used to apply anteriorly-based pressure to reposition the zygoma
        iv. The segment can also be repositioned by insertion of a Carroll-Girard screw (placed percutaneously or via the sulcus incision), which acts

as a joystick and allows for more controlled manipulation of the fracture segment

v. Malleable, low profile miniplate fixation is most commonly used at suture articulations

vi. The typical order of fixation starts with the ZF articulation, as this sets the vertical height while also allowing for additional manipulation of the fracture segment. Next, the ZM articulation is fixated. Lastly, the infraorbital rim is fixated

vii. Orbital floor implants may be placed if concomitant orbital floor fractures are present (forced duction test should be performed before and after implant placement)

viii. After ORIF, soft tissue suspension should be performed to resuspend degloved midface tissues (sutures can be placed from the deep soft tissue of the cheek to temporalis fascia, zygomatic periosteum and/or infraorbital plate)

ix. A lateral canthopexy or canthoplasty may be required if taken down for exposure

x. At the conclusion of the case, a Frost suture can be placed along the gray line of the lower lid at the lateral limbus to help minimize postoperative ectropion

Pre-Operative Care

1. Preoperative medications:
    a. Peri-operative steroids may help reduce swelling
    b. Peri-operative antibiotic use may be considered; currently not enough high-level evidence to guide antibiotic usage

Post-Operative Care

1. Vision
    a. Evaluation of patient's vision is performed once the patient is awakened from anesthesia and then at regular intervals until discharge.
    b. The patient may only be able to see light through a swollen eyelid or Frost suture, and may not identify objects
2. Postoperative positioning
    a. Head of bed elevation (roughly 30 degrees) may significantly improve periorbitaledema and pain.
3. Nose-blowing
    a. Patients should be instructed to avoid blowing their nose for at least 10 days after surgery in order to prevent orbital emphysema.
4. Medications

a. Post-operative medications are subject to debate and are subject to individual surgeon preferences.
b. Antibiotics - there is no clear advantage to using antibiotics, type of antibiotic orduration.
c. Analgesia as needed
d. Steroids can be used in cases of severe edema
e. Antibiotic or steroid eyedrops can be used depending on surgeon preference
f. No aspirin or nonsteroidal anti-inflammatory medications for at least 7 days post-operatively
g. Perioral and oral wound care if intraoral incision is used

Complications

1. Lower eyelid malposition
    a. Overall incidence of lower lid malposition (ectropion, lower lid retraction or entropion) occurs around 5% after periorbital trauma [7]
    b. Causes include lack of midface soft tissue resuspension after degloving of the ZMC, hematoma, orbital septum adhesion, scar contracture and paralysis of the orbicularoculi muscle
    c. Intraoperative techniques to avoid lower lid malposition include canthopexy, canthoplasty, resuspension of degloved midface soft tissue, and Frost suture
    d. Nonoperative treatment includes scar massage and taping, whereas surgical treatmentincludes middle or posterior lamellar spacer grafts
2. Infraorbital nerve anesthesia
    a. Roughly a quarter of patients with ZMC fracture will experience infraorbital nerve paresthesia. [8] Fracture lines through the nerve foramen are common. Neuropraxia ofthe infraorbital nerve manifests as decreased sensation of the cheek, upper lip and maxillary dentition.
    b. Typically, the neuropraxia is transient, however if anesthesia exists for over 6 months,then it is likely that the nerve is severely damaged or transected; sometimes may take 12-18 months to fully recover
    c. If the nerve is impinged by bone fragments (particularly in medially and posteriorly displaced fractures) then reduction or decompression of the infraorbital canal and neurolysis is indicated
3. Orbital complications
    a. Include diplopia, visual loss, globe injury, enophthalmos and exophthalmos
4. Plate complications
    a. Hardware complications include screw loosening, plate exposure, plate contamination/infection requiring removal; plates can be become prominent and palpable, most commonly at the orbital rim, zygomatic arch and at the zygomaticofrontal suture

Summary Points

1. ZMC fractures can be complex fractures to reduce and fixate due to propensity for displacement in 3 planes of orientation. Accurate reduction is further complicated by the challenge of intraoperative assessment of reduction of all 4 articulations, along with concurrent orbital floor fractures.
2. Preoperatively, a thorough history/physical, imaging and planning are critical to optimize fracture reduction and minimize intraoperative and postoperative complications.
3. Indications for proceeding to surgical intervention are based on degree of displacement and comminution.
4. Majority of fractures can be accessed with gingivobuccal sulcus incision combined with upper and lower eyelid incisions.
5. Lower eyelid malposition should be assessed postoperatively. Frost suture and resuspension of midface soft tissues can be utilized intraoperatively to decrease the incidence of malposition. If patient has malposition postoperatively, frequent follow up and massage are used to address scar contraction.

Patient Case

A 63 year-old male patient came into the ED after a mechanical fall onto the dresser. His left cheek and periorbital area are edematous and left eye is swollen shut.

Question 1: What would you like to ask him?

A1:

1. Timing of injury
2. Any vision changes or changes to his occlusion/dentition
3. History of prior facial trauma or facial surgeries
4. Always consider abuse, especially in pediatric and elderly patients; ask about history of other injuries
5. Full medical/surgical/social history including allergies and medication (blood thinners, etc.)

Question 2: On exam, his left eye is edematous and has significant chemosis and subconjunctival hemorrhage. When opening his eyelids manually, his extraocular movements are full, his vision is intact. On palpation, there is a step-off and depression of his left maxilla. Oral cavity exam was normal, occlusion was normal. There is mild trismus to 30mm maximal incisor opening. He does have numbness along left cheek and right upper lip. What would you like to do next?

A2.

1. Imaging: CT of the facial bones (fine cuts) with axial, sagittal, and coronal views, and if possible, 3D reconstruction

Question 3: CT facial bones shows the following selected images. Please describe.

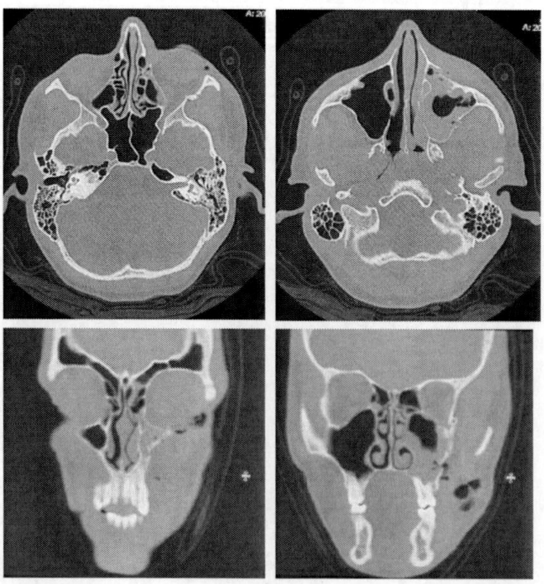

Figure 19.1. Case - CT facial bones.

A3.

1. CT Facial bones shows left depressed ZMC fracture including fractures of zygomaticomaxillary, zygomatico-sphenoidal, and (minimally displaced) zygomaticofrontal articulations. There is a small orbital floor component laterally. There is emphysema of the soft tissues around the left eye and cheek.

Question 4: What are the options for treatment for this pt? What are the advantages/disadvantages for each?

A4.

1. To OR for ORIF of left ZMC fractures immediately
   a. Adv: pt would not have to return for surgery
   b. Adv: may resolve trismus sooner or if there is compression of V2, may be able to decompress sooner
   c. Disadv: edema may make surgical approach slightly more challenging (may need bigger incision or may not be able to perform transconjunctival incisions)
2. Observation for 2 weeks for possible ORIF of left ZMC fractures
   a. Adv: If no external deformity or functional deficits may be able to avoid surgery
   b. Adv: Allows time for edema to resolve to facilitate approaches (esp transconjunctival incisions) during surgery
   c. Disadv: Patient may be lost to follow-up

Question 5: What are the possible approaches to these fractures?

A5.

1. Lateral extension of upper blepharoplasty or lateral brow incision: zygomaticofrontal (ZF) buttress
2. Lower eyelid incision (subciliary, subtarsal or transconjunctival): the infraorbital rim and orbital floor
3. Upper gingivobuccal sulcus incision: the maxilla and the zygomaticomaxillary (ZM) buttress

Question 6: Patient returns 1 week after surgery complaining of continued numbness of the left upper lip and cheek. What should you tell him?

A6.

It is still early in the healing process. The nerve may have been traumatized during the initial injury or stretched during the surgery (transient neuropraxia), and may take days, weeks, or even months to heal. By 12 months to 18 months, full healing would have occurred.

References

[1] Erdmann D, Follmar KE, Debruijn M, Bruno AD, Jung SH, Edelman D, Mukundan S, Marcus JR. A retrospective analysis of facial fracture etiologies. *Ann Plast Surg.* 2008;60(4):398-403.

[2] Otake I, Kageyama I, Mataga I. Clinical anatomy of the maxillary artery. *Okajimas Folia Anat Jpn.* 2011;87(4):155-64.

[3] Knight JS, North JF. The classification of malar fractures: an analysis of displacement as aguide to treatment. *Br J Plast Surg.* 1961;13:325-39.

[4] Yanagisawa E. Symposium on maxillo-facial trauma. 3. Pitfalls in the management of zygomatic fractures. *Laryngoscope.* 1973;83(4):527-46.

[5] Zingg M, Laedrach K, Chen J, Chowdhury K, Vuillemin T, Sutter F, Raveh J. Classification and treatment of zygomatic fractures: a review of 1,025 cases. *J Oral Maxillofac Surg.* 1992;50(8):778-90.

[6] Hollier LH, Thornton J, Pazmino P, Stal S. The management of orbitozygomatic fractures.*Plast Reconstr Surg.* 2003;111(7):2386-92, quiz 93.

[7] Ridgway EB, Chen C, Colakoglu S, Gautam S, Lee BT. The incidence of lower eyelid malposition afterfacial fracture repair: a retrospective study and meta-analysis comparing subtarsal, subciliary, and transconjunctival incisions. *Plast Reconstr Surg.* 2009;124(5):1578-86.

[8] Marcus JR, Erdmann D, Rodriguez ED. *Essentials of craniomaxillofacial trauma.* St. Louis,Mo.: Quality Medical Pub.; 2012.

Chapter 20

Naso-Orbital-Ethmoid Complex Fractures

Sydney C. Butts, MD, FACS
and David Hamlar, MD, DDS

Introduction

Definition and Anatomy

1. Skeletal Anatomy
    a. Naso-orbital-ethmoid (NOE) fractures involve a region of the midface that results in injury to several adjoining bones. The disruption of this area can result in significant impacts on orbital, nasal and paranasal sinus function and may involve intracranial extension
    b. The NOE region is the space between the orbits, inferior to the anterior skull base [1]
    c. Bones that constitute the NOE complex include [1-3]:
        i. Ascending (frontal) process of the *maxilla* (contributes to the infraorbital rim and nasal sidewall)
        ii. Angular process of the *frontal bone* - articulates with the ascending process of the maxilla, forming the *nasomaxillary (medial) buttress* of the midface *(*one of the three vertical buttresses of the craniomaxillofacial skeleton) [1]
        iii. *Lacrimal bone* - posterior to the ascending process of maxilla*;* houses the lacrimal sac; one of the bony attachments for the *medial canthal tendon (MCT)*.
        iv. The *ethmoid bone*[1] - contributes to the anterior skull base (the roof of the NOE region) specifically the *fovea ethmoidalis* and the *cribiform* plate and the medial oirbital wall
    d. *Nasal bones* may also be fractured but are anterior to the NOE complex, articulating with the ascending process of maxilla. Concomitant nasal bone and septal fractures can worsen nasal skeletal collapse
2. Soft Tissue Anatomy
    a. *Medial Canthal Region* - anchoring of the medial eyelids and functioning of the naso-lacrimal drainage system relies on the MCT, which consists of three limbs that are extensions of the pretarsal orbicularis oculi muscle [2, 3]:
        i. Anterior limb attaches to the frontal process of maxilla where it joins with thennasal bones

In: Essential Facial Plastic and Reconstructive Surgery. Volume 1 ISBN: 979-8-89113-306-8
Editors: Yan Ho Lee and Ira Papel © 2024 Nova Science Publishers, Inc.

ii. Superior limb attaches to the junction of maxilla and frontal bone
iii. Posterior limb anchors to the posterior crest of the lacrimal bone [3]

b. NOE fractures cause muscular, ligamentous and bony injury that de- stabilizes the MCT
   i. In comminuted fractures, the tendon is avulsed from its bony attachments; rounding or inferior displacement of the medial canthal angle and *telecanthus* (increased distance between the medial canthi) can result
   ii. MCT attachment to bone is maintained in less severe fractures but displacement of the bone may alter the position of the medial canthus [1]
c. Proper drainage of tears can also be affected by fractures and/or disruption of the muscle and ligaments of the medial canthal region which is responsible for pumping of the lacrimal sac [2, 3]
   i. Tears are collected through small puncta located at the medial inferior and superior eyelids leading to the inferior and superior canaliculi which drain into the lacrimal sac.
   ii. Soft tissue injury can disrupt the canaliculi and impair tear collection and drainage by the lacrimal system, resulting in *epiphora* (leakage of tears)
   iii. Epiphora may present immediately but also may develop in a delayed fashion. All patients should be monitored for epiphora [5]
   iv. Suspicion for any disruption of the tear drainage system warrants an ophthalmologic evaluation

Mechanism

1. Significant forces are usually involved in development of NOE fractures [6]
2. Common causes: blunt trauma from motor vehicle accidents (MVA), falls and interpersonal violence/assault [7, 8]

Demographics/Epidemiology

1. NOE fractures represent *5-15%* of all facial fractures [6] - range accounts for underdiagnosis (NOE fractures are sometimes isolated but often associated with other facial fractures) [4-8]
2. Men more frequently injured than women; adults more frequently injured than children, young adults more often injured than the elderly [5, 8, 9]
3. Craniofacial anatomical differences between adults and young children influence fracture patterns. The skull to facial ratio in infants is 8:1, early childhood it is 4:1, adulthood 2.5:1 [5, 10]
4. Significantly higher proportion of associated skull and skull base fractures in children with NOE fractures due to prominence of cranium in children and incomplete paranasal sinus development until adolescence [5, 9, 10]

5. Status of dentition impacts fracture patterns [5, 9]

Fracture Classification Systems

Depends on the extent of attachment of the MCT to the fractured bone of the NOE complex and the status of the bone (single fragment, moderate or severe comminution).

1. *Gruss 1985* - 5 subtypes of fractures which are differentiated by the regional involvement of other areas of the midface [7]
2. *Markowitz 1991* (Figure 20.1) - introduced the term "central fragment" to define the tendon-bearing bone fragment; has three subtypes (unilateral or bilateral) [4]:
    a. Type I - single fragment injury with the MCT insertion undisturbed; may be incomplete or complete
    b. Type II - comminuted with the MCT attached to a bone fragment that can be stabilized
    c. Type III - comminuted with avulsion of the MCT from its bony insertion.
3. *Burstein 1997* - applicable to the pediatric population, accounts for the lack of frontal sinus development and prominence of the cranium
    a. Type I (central) - includes the superior NOE, central frontal bone, medial to the supraorbital foramen
    b. Type II (lateral) - fractures are unilateral and encompass the entirety of the supraorbital rim, extending to the lateral orbital wall and may involve the temporal and frontal bones
    c. Type III - includes both Type I and II and are bilateral fractures [5, 10, 11]

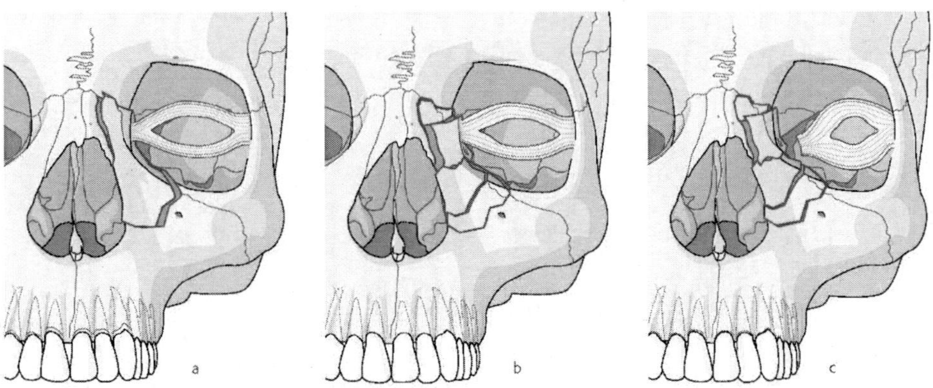

Figure 20.1. Markowitz classification of NOE fractures. From Antonyshyn O. 2012. Nasoorbitoethmoidal (NOE) fractures. In *Principles of Internal Fixation of the Craniomaxillofacial Skeleton: Trauma and Orthognathic* Surgery edited by Michael Ehrenfeld, Paul Manson and Joachim Prein, 235-245. New York: Thieme (Reprinted **with** permission).

Patient Evaluation [2, 6, 10]

1. ATLS protocols to address airway, breathing and circulation (ABCs) and other systems must be performed initially
2. Facial trauma assessment may not be the first priority
3. Patients may already be intubated and/or have a low Glasgow Coma Score (GCS), making the initial assessment limited
4. Evaluation should be repeated over several days (marked edema may mask certain physical findings, neurologic status may improve for patients with head injuries)
5. Patients must have radiographic or clinical clearance of the cervical spine. Until this time, the patient should have cervical spine stabilization (i.e. c-spine collar)

Physical Examination Findings (Signs and Symptoms)

1. Ecchymosis and edema of upper 1/3 of the face, especially peri-orbital region
2. Palpable step-offs at the infra-orbital rim and lateral nasal sidewall
3. Lacerations: nasal skin, forehead, medial cheek, peri-orbital region
4. Nasal region: flattening of nasal dorsum (telescoping), widening of bony base, deviation of upper 1/3 of the nasal skeleton, septal hematoma, septal fracture with deviation, nasal obstructive symptoms, hyposmia, rhinorrhea
5. Ocular and Peri-Ocular region: chemosis, subconjunctival hemorrhage, diplopia, limitation of extra-ocular movements, injury to canalicular system, immediate or delayed epiphora, lower eyelid displacement, lacerations of eyelids, enophthalmos, hypoglobus, telecanthus (see below), proptosis/signs of retrobulbar hematoma (especially patients on aspirin or other blood thinners), vision loss (afferent pupillary defect, diminished visual acuity)
6. Cranial nerve findings: hypesthesia of V1 or V2
7. Full facial trauma assessment to rule out other associated fractures, especially frontal sinus, skull base, LeFort and zygomaticomaxillary complex (ZMC) fractures

Specific Testing and Laboratory Tests

1. *Bimanual Palpation* -a clamp is placed in the nasal cavity, pushing laterally against the nasal sidewall; mobility of the bone in this region suggests NOE fracture [3, 5, 10]
2. *Bowstring Test* - one finger palpates the region of the medial canthus while the lower eyelid is pulled laterally. In a positive (abnormal) test, the area of the medial canthus is mobile and will be felt to move during distraction (Figure 20.2) [5, 10, 12]
3. *Intercanthal Distance (Telecanthus)* - normal distance between the right and left medial canthi is roughly 35mm in adults; when the central fragment is laterally displaced or the canthal tendon is avulsed from the bone, the intercanthal distance increases. The interpupillary distance is normal (Figure 20.3) [2, 5, 10]

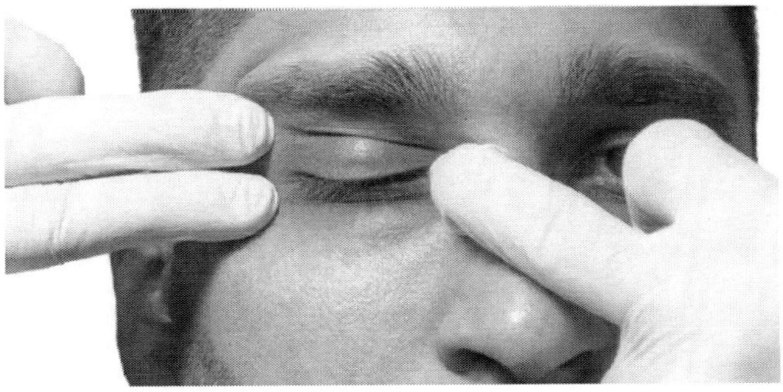

Figure 20.2. The bowstring test detects mobility of the bone anchoring the MCT. From Balaraman K. 2021. Frontal and Naso-Orbito-Ethmoid Complex Fractures. In *Oral and Maxillofacial Surgery for the Clinician* edited by Krishnamurthy Bonanthaya, Elavenil Panneerselvam, Suvy Manuel, Vinay V. Kumar, Anshul Rai, 1251-1266.Singapor: Springer. (Reprinted with permission).

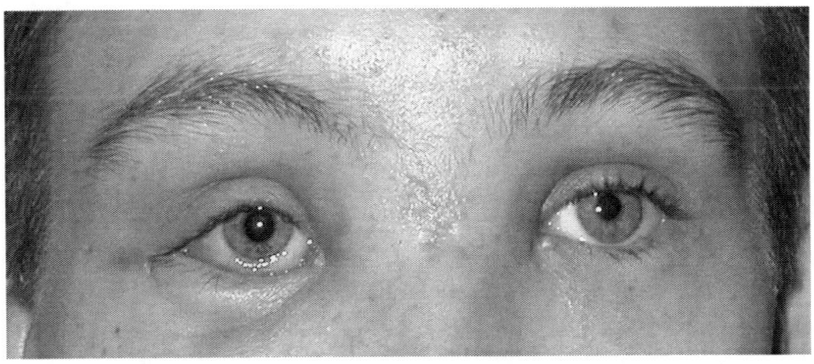

Figure 20.3. Right telecanthus.

4. *Pseudotelecanthus* - in patients with depression of the nasal dorsum, the intercanthal distance appears widened
5. *Exophthalmometry* - NOE fractures can result in change in orbital volume (because of fractures of the orbit). Change in globe position may be observed immediately but often becomes apparent after resolution of edema several days following the injury. Exophthalmometer used to measure globe protrusion or retrusion [13, 14]
    a. *Exophthalmos (*increased protrusion of the globe)
    b. *Enophthalmos* (decreased protrusion of the globe)
    c. *Hypoglobus* (inferior displacement of the globe)
6. *Forced duction testing* - muscle entrapment or tethering may result in extra ocular motion restriction.
    a. Used to distinguish between entrapment or tethering vs edema, contusion, or nerve injury
    b. Bulbar conjunctiva topically anesthetized with anesthetic eye drops and grasped with fine forceps to move the globe in all directions
    c. Resistance to movement in the plane of the muscle in question is a positive (abnormal) test [14]
    d. Note: usually an entrapped muscle is pinched between a trapdoor or minimally-displaced fracture, and a tethered muscle will have a larger, displaced bony defect

7. Clear rhinorrhea - may be elicited when the patient tilts the head forward in the setting of an anterior skull base fracture (cribriform plate or posterior table of the frontal sinus). This liquid should be collected and sent for *B2 transferrin* to rule out a cerebrospinal fluid (CSF) leak [6]

Consultations to Request

1. *Ophthalmology* – can perform dilated funduscopic examination, examination of the anterior chamber, measuring intraocular pressure, assess canalicular system and nasolacrimal duct function and manage associated eyelid lacerations
2. *Neurosurgery* - should be requested if fractures of anterior skull base or posterior table of frontal sinus, confirmed or suspected CSF leak, pneumocephalus, intracranial bleed

Imaging

1. Fine cut CT scans in all three planes (axial, coronal and sagittal)
2. Structures visualized well in the *coronal* plane - frontal sinus outflow tract, height of the nasomaxillary buttress, medial orbital wall, infraorbital nerve foramen, nasal bones, nasal septum [1] (Figure 20.4a)

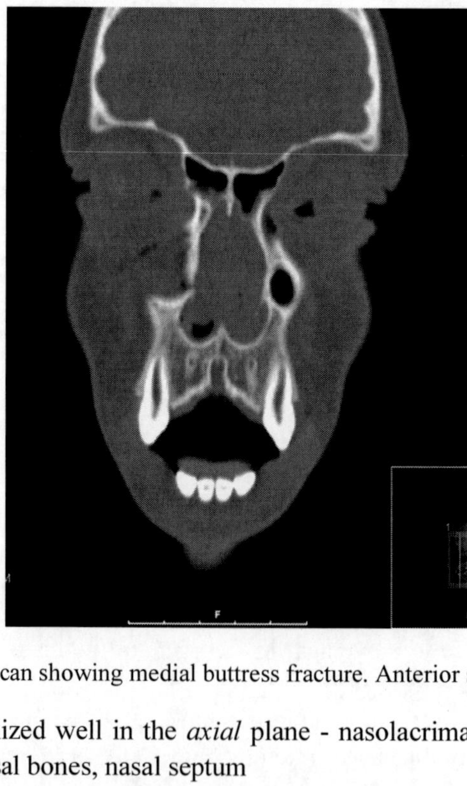

Figure 20.4a. Coronal CT scan showing medial buttress fracture. Anterior skull base intact.

3. Structures visualized well in the *axial* plane - nasolacrimal duct, medial and lateral orbital walls, nasal bones, nasal septum
4. Structures visualized well in the *sagittal* plane - slope of the orbital floor, posterior extent of orbital floor fracture, frontal sinus, nasal bones [13]

5. Request 3D reconstruction when available - demonstrates degree of displacement of the central segment [1, 15] (Figure 20.4b)
6. Other facial fractures may be present; critical to systematically review all films and discuss with radiology when complex injuries are present
7. NOE fractures have been reported in up to 1/3 of ZMC fractures which may be missed by operating surgeons and reviewing radiologists [8]
8. Recommend photographic documentation of pre-injury examination and post-operative outcomes

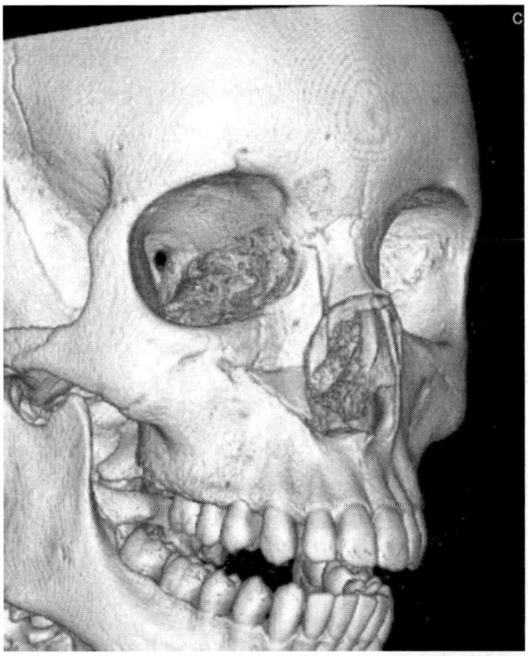

Figure 20.4b. 3D reconstruction CT of the same patient showing a right NOE fracture (Markowitz Type I). Mild dislocation and infra-orbital rim, large central segment with a second inferior fracture involving the lower aspect of the nasomaxillary (medial) buttress.

Management [1, 5, 10, 16]

1. Repair involves restoration of bony and soft tissue structures; securing the bone enables soft tissue, muscle, subcutaneous tissues, and skin to settle in the correct anatomical positions
2. Surgical approaches for exposure of NOE fractures:
    a. *Coronal incision* - provides exposure of the frontal bone, supraorbital rims, frontomaxillary articulation, nasal bones, superior medial buttress; access to parietal bone for split calvarial bone harvest if needed (Figure 20.5)
    b. *Eyelid incisions* (transconjunctival, transcutaneous, transcaruncular) - provide exposure of infraorbital rim, orbital floor, and medial orbital wall, respectively
    c. *Upper gingivobuccal sulcus (vestibular) incision* - allows access to the nasomaxillary buttress

d. *Lacerations* - provide direct access. Avoid lengthening lacerations

3. Type I fractures:
   a. *Approaches:* upper vestibular incision and eyelid incision to access nasomaxillary buttress, infraorbital rim and orbital floor; if superior aspect of NOE displaced, include coronal incision
   b. *Fixation*: nasomaxillary, infraorbital rim +/- nasofrontal articulation (Figure 20.5)
4. Type II fractures:
   a. Approaches: coronal, eyelid incisions, upper vestibular incision
   b. Fixation:
      i. As for Type I fracture
      ii. Plate bone pieces (stable to unstable)
      iii. Trans-nasal wiring may be required to stabilize canthal bearing segment (Figure 20.6)
5. Type III fractures:
   a. Approaches:
      i. Same exposures as used for Type II fractures
      ii. Repair orbital rims first
      iii. May need to reconstruct medial orbital wall/floor
   b. Fixation:
      i. Trans-nasal canthopexy utilizing wiring and possibly canthal barb/anchor
      ii. Consider nasal dorsum support: depends on septal and mid-vault nasal support
6. Trans-nasal wiring
   a. Utilizes stainless steel wire to medialize the MCT
   b. Many available techniques but the vector of fixation should be posterior and superior to posterior lacrimal crest
   c. Wire placed through the avulsed medial canthal tendon, passed through the medial orbit (at superior aspect of posterior lacrimal crest) across the nasal cavity to the contralateral medial orbit, anchored to a screw on the contralateral frontal bone (Figure 20.5)
7. Nasal reconstruction with calvarial bone graft
   a. Primary bone grafting for dorsal nasal support may be necessary due to severe nasal dorsal deformity
   b. Split-calvarial bone harvested from lateral parietal bones (avoid sagittal sinus)
   c. Onlay graft placed as a cantilever suspended from frontal bone (Figure 20.6)
8. Bone grafts may be needed to reconstruct the medial orbital wall, orbital floor or critical defects of the medial buttress [1, 2]
9. Postoperative nasal bolster for splinting:
   a. Helps with soft tissue adaptation to the underlying skeletal framework
   b. Avoid over-tightening of bolsters to prevent underlying skin necrosis
   c. Does not address the canthal position—purely to address soft-tissue re-draping

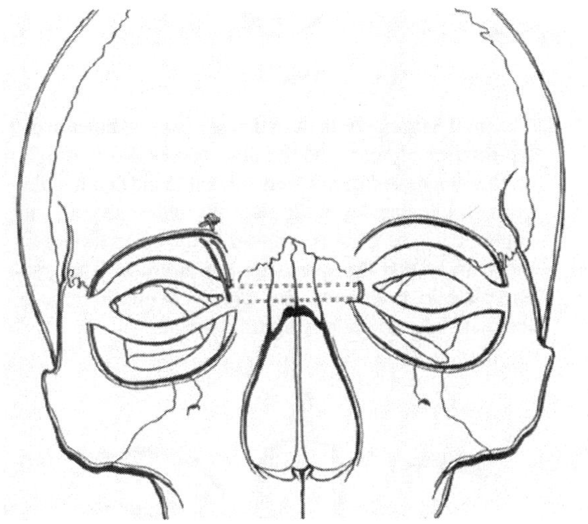

Figure 20.5. Trans-nasal wiring.

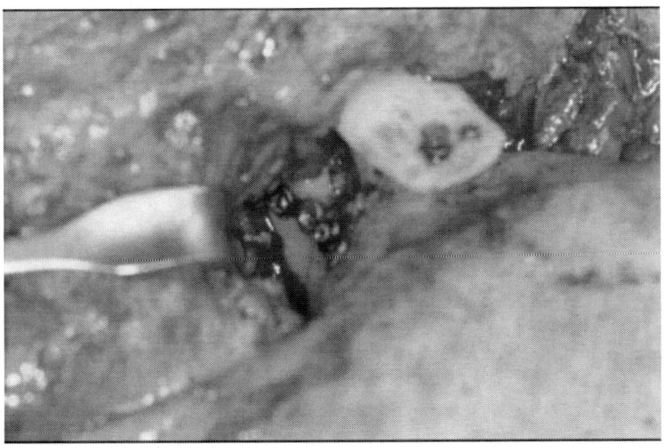

Figure 20.6. ORIF of nasofrontal articulation, dorsal nasal onlay graft, exposure via coronal approach.

Complications

1. Primary complication: improper repositioning of the medial canthal tendon
2. Other complications:
    a. Nasal obstruction
    b. Nasolacrimal duct dysfunction (with epiphora)
    c. Lower eyelid malposition
    d. V1 or V2 hypesthesia
    e. Diplopia
    f. Vision loss
    g. Persistent post-traumatic nasal deformity
    h. Medial canthal soft tissue deformity

Summary Points

1. NOE complex fractures are unilateral or bilateral, simple or comminuted
2. Classification is based on status of the medial canthal tendon bearing bone
3. Inadequate treatment leads to telecanthus
4. Medial canthal tendon repair is key for success
5. Bone graft for dorsal nasal support
6. External nasal splints aid soft-tissue adaptation

Patient Case

A 20-year-old male patient presents to the emergency room after being assaulted with fists during an altercation outside of a bar. He has significant periorbital edema and the right eye is swollen shut, with edema involving the medial cheek. He does not remember all of the events around the attack.

Q1:What would be your initial steps in the evaluation of this patient?

A1:

1. ATLS protocol, full evaluation by trauma team.
2. Cervical spine collar.
3. Obtain thorough history of the event from the patient and/or any bystanders.
4. Focused questions regarding: eye pain, vision changes, facial numbness or pain, epistaxis, nasal obstruction/drainage, headache, nausea, and lightheadedness
5. Review past medical history including: contact lenses, eyeglasses, last check of visual acuity, history of eye disease.
6. Ask about prior facial or head trauma or surgery, current medications and allergies, smoking history, alcohol use, illicit drug use.
7. Take note of patient's profession, as the injury may cause significant limitations for certain occupations that have high visual demands.

Q2: Describe the focused facial trauma assessment/examination in a patient like this.

A2:

1. Examination of cranial nerves with focus on the sensory exam of upper and midface, extraocular movements, pupil reaction to light and facial nerve function.
2. Document lacerations.
3. Palpate maxillofacial skeleton for step-offs, crepitus, hematoma.
4. Assess the nasal dorsal height to rule out depression or widening.
5. Anterior rhinoscopy (possibly nasal endoscopy) to exclude septal fracture or hematoma.
6. Head tilt exam for suspected CSF leak; if clear rhinorrhea ⍰ send for beta-2-transferrin.
7. Measure intercanthal distance to rule out telecanthus.

Q3: What imaging and tests would you order?

A3:

1. Cervical Spine CT
2. Head CT
3. Maxillofacial CT with thin cuts (1-1.5mm) with 3D reconstruction
4. Pre-operative labs if anticipate operative reconstruction: complete blood count, basic or complete metabolic panel, urine toxicology, Beta-hCG for women of child-bearing age and other specific tests if appropriate

Q4: What consultants should the Emergency Department contact to evaluate the patient?

A4:

1. Ophthalmology - for patients whose fractures have an orbital component.

2. Neurosurgery - for patients with a skull base fracture (anterior skull base, posterior table of frontal sinus).
3. Neurology - can be considered for outpatient follow-up given likelihood of concussion. [17-20] Patients suffering facial fractures may have additional closed head injuries with higher rates of concussion than previously appreciated. Signs and symptoms of concussion may evolve over days with vertigo, memory loss, headache and problems sleeping. In many patients, concussion symptoms are self-limited with improvement in 7-10 days. If symptoms do not improve or worsen, should provide outpatient referral to neurology. [20]

Q5: The CT scan images for the patient are shown. (Figure 20.7) Please describe the findings.
A5:
1. There is a large central segment with displacement of the infra-orbital rim. The medial (nasomaxillary) buttress is medially displaced into the nasal airway.

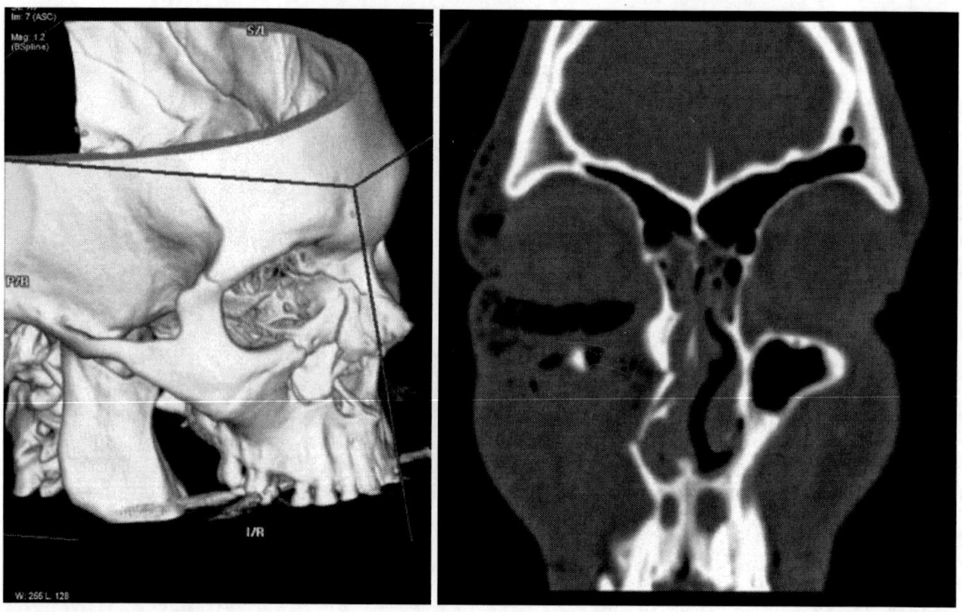

Figure 20.7. Case study imaging.

Q6: How would you classify this fracture?
A6:
1. Type 1 unilateral (right) NOE fracture (Markowitz). [21]

Q7: What treatment plan would you discuss with this patient? What are the risks and benefits?
A7:
1. Given comminution and displacement of the fracture at the infraorbital rim with medial displacement of lateral nasal wall, open reduction and internal fixation should be discussed.
2. Approach [22]:
   a. Upper gingivobuccal sulcus incision

b. Transconjunctival incision (+/-lateral canthotomy) to approach the orbital rim
c. Straight or curvilinear plate (1.7mm) used to span the nasomaxillary buttress (at least 2 screws on each side of the fracture and screws within the fractured segment)
d. Low profile (1.2mm) plate used to span infraorbital rim

3. Benefits of treatment:
   a. Relieve nasal obstruction from displacement of the nasomaxillary buttress.
   b. Restores the ability of this buttress to absorb masticatory forces.
   c. Restore contour or infraorbital rim, re-establish pre-morbid lower eyelid position.
   d. Fixation of the infra-orbital nerve(V2) bearing segment of the orbital rim can allow recovery of sensory function in patients with hypesthesia.
4. Risks of the surgery:
   a. Infection
   b. Bleeding
   c. Scar, chronic pain
   d. Hardware failure (loosening and extrusion of screws)
   e. Malunion, nonunion
   f. Persistent V2 hypesthesia or dysesthesia
   g. Orbital complications: ectropion, entropion, epiphora, corneal abrasion, vision loss
   h. Persistent nasal obstruction

Q8: The patient is cleared by the trauma team (cervical spine CT and head CT are negative) and his fractures have been fully evaluated with recommendations for outpatient surgery. What medications would you discharge the patient home on—specifically address: need for antibiotics, analgesia.

A8:

1. Need for antibiotics

   Strong evidence suggests that in trauma of the midface and upper face, the risk of postoperative infection is best reduced with *perioperative antibiotics only* (prophylactic antibiotics with gram positive and anaerobic coverage given within 30-60 minutes of the incision and repeat dosing for up to, but not exceeding the first 24 hours after surgery).

   No reduction in infection has been seen in prescribing antibiotics from the time of the injury to the time of surgery (this differs from the published recommendations for mandibular fractures) or beyond 24 hours after surgery. [23]
2. Analgesia

   Perioperative analgesia regimens should begin with over the counter (OTC) pain medications (acetaminophen, NSAIDs). Opioids may be added for breakthrough pain. It is advised that surgeons discuss the analgesia regimen with patients, focusing on prior experiences with opioids or other agents, any chronic use of such medications or any adverse reactions to such agents in the past. Many hospitals have instituted opioid risk screening tools that must be completed prior to the processing of an opioid prescription. In states where this is applicable, the opioid prescribing monitoring program should be reviewed to determine if the patient has recently received prescriptions for other controlled substances. n. [24]

Q9: Six weeks following surgery, the patient reports having excessive tearing from the right eye. What could explain this? What should the next steps be?

A9:

1. The patient has epiphora that could have developed from any injury of the tear collecting system (from the punctum-canaliculi-nasolacrimal sac-nasolacrimal duct). The obstruction to tear drainage could be from soft tissue, bony, or both causes. The patient should be referred to ophthalmology for testing of the nasolacrimal drainage system to determine the level and site of obstruction and help determine management [22].

References

[1] Antonyshyn O. 2012. Nasoorbitoethmoidal (NOE) fractures. In *Principles of Internal Fixation of the Craniomaxillofacial Skeleton: Trauma and Orthognathic Surgery* edited by Michael Ehrenfeld, Paul Manson and Joachim Prein, 235-245. New York: Thieme.

[2] Birgfeld C. 2020. Naso-Orbito-Ethmoid (NOE) Fractures. In *Facial Trauma Surgery: From Primary Repair to Reconstruction* edited by Amir H.Dorafshar, Eduardo D. Rodriguez and Paul N Manson, 129-136. Philadelphia: Elsevier.

[3] Sargent LA. 2006. Acute Management of Nasoethmoid Orbital Fractures. In *Evaluation and Treatment of Orbital Fractures: A Multidisciplinary Approach* edited by David E. E. Holck and John D. Ng, 163-182. Philadelphia: Elsevier.

[4] Markowitz BL, Manson PN, Sargent L, Vander Kolk CA, Yaremchuk M, Glassman D, Crawley WA.(1991) Management of the medial canthal tendon in nasoethmoid orbital fractures: the importance of the central fragment in classification and treatment. *Plast Reconstr Surg.* 87(5):843-53.

[5] Liau JY, Woodlief J, van Aalst JA. (2011) Pediatric nasoorbitoethmoid fractures. *J Craniofac Surg.* 22(5):1834-8.

[6] Rosenberger E, Kriet JD, Humphrey C.(2013) Management of nasoethmoidal fractures. *Curr Opin Otolaryngol Head Neck Surg.* 21(4):410-6.

[7] Gruss JS.(1985) Naso-ethmoid-orbital fractures: classification and role of primary bone grafting. *Plast Reconstr Surg.* 75(3):303-17.

[8] Nissen NJ, Okhah ZI, Basta MN, Hsieh S, Crozier JW, Jehle CC, Rao V, Woo AS.(2020) Underdiagnosis of Nasoorbitoethmoid Fractures in Patients with Zygoma Injury. *Plast Reconstr Surg.* 145(4):1001-1008.

[9] Lopez J, Luck JD, Faateh M, Macmillan A, Yang R, Siegel G, Susarla SM, Wang H, Nam AJ, Milton J, Grant MP, Redett R, Tufaro AP, Kumar AR, Manson PN, Dorafshar AH. (2019) Pediatric Nasoorbitoethmoid Fractures: Cause, Classification, and Management. *Plast Reconstr Surg.* 143(1):211-222.

[10] Pawar SS, Rhee JS. (2014) Frontal sinus and naso-orbital-ethmoid fractures. *JAMA Facial Plast Surg.* 16(4):284-9.

[11] Burstein F, Cohen S, Hudgins R, Boydston W. (1997) Frontal basilar trauma: classification and treatment. *Plast Reconstr Surg.* 99(5):1314-21.

[12] Balaraman K. 2021. Frontal and Naso-Orbito-Ethmoid Complex Fractures. In *Oral and Maxillofacial Surgery for the Clinician* edited by Krishnamurthy Bonanthaya, Elavenil Panneerselvam, Suvy Manuel, Vinay V. Kumar, Anshul Rai, 1251-1266. Singapore: Springer

[13] Kikkawa DO and Korn BS. 2017. Orbital Fracture Repair. In *Video Atlas of Oculofacial Plastic and Reconstructive Surgery*, 2nd edition. Edited by Bobby S. Korn and Don O. Kikkawa, 468-475. Philadelphia: Elsevier.

[14] Chang A, Carter KD and Nerad JA. 2006. Orbital Floor Fractures. In *Evaluation and Treatment of Orbital Fractures: A Multidisciplinary Approach* edited by David E. E. Holck and John D. Ng, 93-102. Philadelphia: Elsevier.

[15] Remmler D, Denny A, Gosain A, Subichin S.(2000) Role of three-dimensional computed tomography in the assessment of nasoorbitoethmoidal fractures. *Ann Plast Surg.* 44(5):553-62.

[16] Hollier, LH, Koshy, JC, Ngyuen. (2010) Pearls of Nasoorbitoethmoid Trauma Management. *Semin Plast Surg.* 24(4): 383–388.

[17] Davidoff G, Jakubowski M, Thomas D, Alpert M. (1988) The spectrum of closed-head injuries in facial trauma victims: incidence and impact. *Ann Emerg Med* 17:6-9

[18] Pappachan B, Alexander M. (2006) Correlating Facial Fractures and Cranial Injuries. *J Oral Maxillofac Surg* 64:1023-1029.

[19] Martin RC 2nd, Spain DA, Richardson JD.(2002) Do facial fractures protect the brain or are they a marker for severe head injury? *Am Surg* 68:477-481

[20] Sobin L, Kopp R, Walsh R, Kellman RM, Harris T. (2016) Incidence of Concussion in Patients With Isolated Mandible Fractures. *JAMA Facial Plast Surg.* 18(1):15-18.

[21] Markowitz BL, Manson PN, Sargent L, Vander Kolk CA, Yaremchuk M, Glassman D,Crawley WA.(1991) Management of the medial canthal tendon in nasoethmoid orbital fractures: the importance of the central fragment in classification and treatment. *Plast Reconstr Surg.* 87(5):843-53.

[22] Rosenberger E, Kriet JD, Humphrey C.(2013) Management of nasoethmoid fractures. *Curr Opin Otolaryngol Head Neck Surg*. 21(4):410-6.

[23] Mundinger GS, Borsuk DE, Okhah Z, Christy MR, Bojovic B, Dorafshar AH, Rodriguez ED.(2015) Antibiotics and facial fractures: evidence-based recommendations compared with experience-based practice. *Craniomaxillofac Trauma Reconstr.* 8(1):64-78.

[24] Anne S, Mims JW, Tunkel DE, Rosenfeld RM, Boisoneau DS, Brenner MJ, Cramer JD, Dickerson D, Finestone SA, Folbe AJ, Galaiya DJ, Messner AH, Paisley A, Sedaghat AR, Stenson KM, Sturm AK, Lambie EM, Dhepyasuwan N, Monjur TM. (2021) Clinical Practice Guideline: Opioid Prescribing for Analgesia After Common Otolaryngology Operations Executive Summary. *Otolaryngol Head Neck Surg.* 164(4):687-703.

Chapter 21

Orbital Fractures

Larissa Habib, MD

Introduction

1. Orbital fractures account for about 30-40% of all facial fractures, of those 10% are isolated orbital fractures
2. Range from small non-displaced fractures to large, multiwall fractures
3. Fractures defined by location and involvement of surrounding orbital tissue
4. Two theories on pathophysiology: buckling theory and hydraulic theory [1]
    a. Buckling theory states that there is a blow to orbital rim which is transmitted to floor causing a fracture
    b. Hydraulic theory states that force transmitted to floor is from orbit and soft tissue

Orbital Anatomy

1. Volume of orbit is $30cm^3$
2. Anteriorly, width is 45mm and height is 35mm on average
3. Widest dimension is 1cm behind anterior rim
4. On Axial view:
    a. Angle between lateral walls is 90°
    b. Angle between medial and lateral walls is 45°
5. Orbital roof:
    a. Composed of orbital plate of frontal bone and lesser wing of sphenoid posteriorly at apex
    b. Separates orbit from frontal sinus anteriorly and from anterior cranial fossa posteriorly
    c. Lacrimal gland fossa can be found within roof anterolaterally.
    d. Anteromedially is site of trochlea, a pulley-like structure for superior oblique muscle
6. Medial wall:
    a. Composed of ethmoid bone (lamina papyracea), lacrimal bone, frontal bone and sphenoid bone posteriorly
    b. Thinnest orbital wall: 0.2-0.4mm in thickness
    c. Medial walls are parallel to each another

In: Essential Facial Plastic and Reconstructive Surgery. Volume 1 ISBN: 979-8-89113-306-8
Editors: Yan Ho Lee and Ira Papel © 2024 Nova Science Publishers, Inc.

d. Distance from anterior to apex is 45mm on average
e. Medial wall meets with roof at frontoethmoidal suture line
f. Anterior and posterior ethmoidal foramina are located along frontoethmoidal suture line (24-12-6 rule)
    i. Anterior ethmoidal neurovascular bundle is 24-25mm from the anterior lacrimal crest
    ii. Posterior bundle is 12mm posterior to anterior ethmoidal bundle
    iii. Optic canal is 6 mm posterior to posterior bundle
    iv. These lie at level of cribriform plate and are important surgical landmarks

7. Orbital floor:
    a. Made up of maxillary bone, zygomatic bone anterolaterally and palatine bone posteriorly
    b. Shortest wall; 40mm from rim
    c. Ends at posteriorly limit of the maxillary sinus, inferior orbital fissure; does not extend to apex
    d. Infraorbital canal: thinnest area and most common site for fracture
    e. Inferior orbital fissure (IOF) separates floor from lateral wall
        i. Maxillary division of trigeminal nerve, maxillary artery, inferior ophthalmic vein branches and postganglionic parasympathetic fibers travel through the IOF
    f. Inferior oblique muscle originates from medial portion of floor just lateral to nasolacrimal canal
8. Lateral wall:
    a. Formed by greater wing of sphenoid posteriorly and zygomatic process of frontal bone and orbital process of zygomatic bone anteriorly
    b. Strongest wall
    c. Thinnest portion is at zygomaticosphenoid suture line
    d. Superior orbital fissure (SOF) lies between greater and lesser wings of sphenoid
        i. Lies between optic foramen and foramen rotundum
        ii. Oculomotor nerve (CNIII), trochlear nerve (CNIV), abducens nerve (CNVI), ophthalmic division of trigeminal nerve (V1), and superior ophthalmic vein pass travel through SOF
    e. Whitnall's tubercle:
        i. 10mm inferior to frontozygomatic suture
        ii. Attachment site for lateral canthal tendon, Lockwood's ligament, lateral horn of levator aponeurosis and check ligament of lateral rectus
    f. Zygomaticofacial and zygomaticotemporal neurovascular bundles perforate near anterior end of IOF
9. Important orbital landmarks:
    a. Infraorbital nerve
        i. Anteriorly, it runs in a canal along medial floor
        ii. Posteriorly, it is more superficial and lies immediately beneath periosteum of floor.

- iii. *With a large fracture the nerve serves a guide to depth of dissection*
- iv. Before exiting orbit, it bisects inferior orbital fissure and then turns medially to cross pterygopalantine fossa to enter skullbase at foramen rotundum

b. Inferior orbital fissure
- i. Separates lateral wall and floor
- ii. 2mm long, runs posteromedially
- iii. Communicates with intratemporal fossa anteriorly and pterygopalatine fossa posteriorly

c. Greater wing of sphenoid
- i. Important landmark of lateral orbital wall
- ii. Orbital plate of greater wing varies in thickness
  - Anterolaterally, where it articulates with zygoma, it is thin and can fracture along with zygoma fractures
  - Centrally, known as trigone, it is thicker
- iii. This separates orbit from middle cranial fossa
- iv. Fractures of trigone are very rare and is often associated with sudden vision loss

d. Orbital plate of palatine bone
- i. Reliable landmark of medial floor
- ii. Located at posteromedial floor, medial to junction of infraorbital nerve and infraorbital fissure
- iii. Stronger than portion of floor composed of maxilla and rarely disrupted
- iv. With large fractures this may be the only part of floor not disrupted

Presentation

1. Swelling and ecchymosis of eyelids
2. Periocular emphysema due to connection with sinuses
3. Diplopia (most commonly associated with floor fractures)
4. Hypesthesia associated with infraorbital nerve injury
5. Children may present with minimal signs of trauma, "white-eyed blowout fracture"
6. Bradycardia with vertical eye movement due to oculocardiac reflex

Evaluation

1. Complete ophthalmic examination should be performed in any patient with periorbital, orbital or facial trauma
   - a. Assessment for globe and/or optic injury
   - b. Visual acuity, pupil response and extraocular motility
   - c. Hypesthesia in V2 pattern (infraorbital injury and frequently associated with floor fracture)

    d. Globe position
        i. Proptosis due to orbital edema, hemorrhage
        ii. Enophthalmos typically manifests after edema resolves
    e. Examine for: palpable step-offs, telecanthus in midface trauma, pulsatile proptosis in roof fractures
2. Extraocular motility
    a. An increase of intraocular pressure greater than 4mm when attempting to look into field of diplopia indicates restriction
    b. Forced ductions should be performed to assess for entrapment
3. Differential diagnoses for limitation of extraocular motility
    a. Edema or hemorrhage of extraocular muscle may limit its function
    b. Entrapment of muscle or perimuscular tissue can lead to restriction
    c. With head trauma there can be a neurogenic cause of diplopia
        i. Involvement of cranial nerves III, IV or VI
        ii. On exam there would be no increase in pressure with attempt to move eye in that gaze and no pain with eye movement
    d. An acute retrobulbar hematoma can result in frozen globe, elevated intraocular pressure, periorbital edema, retinal artery pulsations
        i. This is a vision threatening compartment syndrome
        ii. Requires immediate canthotomy and cantholysis
4. CT imaging is gold standard for orbital trauma
    a. Orbital CT has fine cuts of 1-2.5mm
    b. Able to evaluate for orbital foreign body, fractures, integrity of globe and optic nerve, and for retrobulbar hemorrhage
    c. Some limitation in delineating degree of soft tissue herniation
    d. Good correlation between entrapment on CT imaging and operative findings in adults but correlation is not as strong in children [3]
    e. A good clinical examination remains important, particularly in children, at detecting entrapment
5. MRI
    a. MRI shows better soft tissue definition and may aid in determining entrapment
    b. However, exam time is much longer and patients with implanted devices or possible foreign body may not be able to undergo MRI in a trauma setting

Classification

1. Classification systems have been developed to aid in surgical management and timing
2. Most urgent type of fracture is trapdoor fracture with muscle entrapment
    a. Particularly important to consider in pediatric population given flexibility of their bones
    b. Pediatric patients can present with “white-eye blowout fracture” and therefore should always be on differential in children with orbital trauma

c. On exam these children will have upgaze restriction in setting of otherwise normal exam as well as nausea, vomiting or bradycardia on upgaze due to oculocardiac reflex
d. Compartment syndrome and ischemia may occur if not released in 1-3 days
e. This is a clinical diagnosis as bone fragment may swing back into position trapping muscle and evading a radiologic diagnosis
f. CT evidence includes hemorrhage in adjacent sinus and tenting of muscle or soft tissue at fracture site

Management [4]

1. Caution patient to avoid nose blowing to prevent forced air into orbit
2. No evidence to support use of prophylactic antibiotics but are commonly given
3. If significant edema, consider short course of steroids
4. Surgical indications remain controversial with evidence varying widely
5. General principles regarding when to consider surgical intervention
    a. Involving more than 50% of floor and/or medial wall
    b. Evidence of soft tissue involvement
    c. Diplopia with motility limitation within 30 degrees of primary
    d. Early enophthalmos of more than 2mm
6. Trapdoor fractures with muscle incarceration
    a. Consensus that should be performed within 48 hours but earlier the better
7. Trapdoor fracture with incarceration of soft tissue
    a. No consensus, most sources recommend repair within 2 weeks for:
        i. Symptomatic diplopia (with positive forced ductions)
        ii. CT evidence of entrapment
8. Outcomes at various time points remains controversial:
    a. Some sources report that 1) entrapped soft tissue or 2) large fractures likely to cause enophthalmos both will benefit from intervention within two weeks [5]
    b. A study advocated for early (within 2 months) repair citing better outcomes for extraocular movement as well as enophthalmos [6]
    c. Other sources report no difference before two weeks versus after [7, 8, 9, 10]
    d. Others report improvement in diplopia and enophthalmos at 6 weeks post injury [11]
    e. In a study of 72 blowout fractures who did not undergo surgical intervention, only 1 patient had persistent diplopia at 6 months [12]

Surgical Technique [13]

1. Goals of surgery:
    a. Reduction of herniated orbital tissue
    b. Restoration of orbital volume
    c. Resolution of diplopia

2. Forced duction testing should be performed prior to incision and repeated after implant is placed
3. Approaches
    a. Transorbital
        i. Conjunctival "transconjunctival" incision
            - Incision placed 3mm below tarsus
                - If placed too high: risk of post-operative eyelid malposition
                - If placed too low: orbital fat prolapse can make dissection more challenging
            - Preseptal dissection to orbital rim where periosteum is incised and elevated along floor/medial wall to locate fracture
            - There must be stable bone around fracture to support implant
            - Elevate prolapsed tissue into orbit and place implant on bare bone
            - If fracture is large, consider using combination titanium/porous polyethylene plate that can be fixated
            - If combined medial wall and floor, preformed right and left implant can be used
            - Take care to place implant under inferior oblique muscle to avoid diplopia
            - Can be combined with lateral canthotomy, inferior cantholysis to increase exposure
        ii. Subciliary incision
            - 2mm beneath lash line
            - Dissection deep to orbicularis to inferior orbital rim and then proceed as above
        iii. Subtarsal
            - Not usually used unless there is an existing laceration
            - Results in visible scar, risk of ectropion
        iv. Infraorbital
            - Not usually used unless there is an existing laceration
            - Results in visible scar
            - Direct access to orbital rim/floor
    b. Transantral [14]
        i. Allows access to floor from maxillary sinus
        ii. Maxilla exposed through upper buccal sulcus incision and subperiosteal dissection
        iii. Antrostomy made with osteotome/drill, 2x1.5cm, with upper osteotomy just inferior to infraorbital foramen
        iv. Periorbita dissected free to allow reduction of orbital contents;
        v. Implant is placed
        vi. If no posterior edge available for stabilization of implant, titanium micromesh is used for stabilization rather than porous polyethylene
        vii. Avoids potential eyelid complications

viii. Particularly useful in cases where globe manipulation needs to be kept to minimum, as with concurrent ruptured globe

ix. Endoscopy can also be used with this approach to improve visualization [15]

x. Limitations: longer operating time, paresthesia of upper lid and cheek from retraction

4. Implant [16]
   a. Should be easy to manipulate, have sufficient strength to support orbital contents, easily anchored, and inert
   b. Titanium:
      i. Allows for osteointegration, inert, porous, can be easily manipulated to follow contour of orbit, easily anchored, available in various sizes, can be used for rim reconstruction as well
      ii. Have been shown to lead to adhesion syndrome and can be difficult to remove
   c. Porous polyethylene [17]
      i. Material is inert, easily manipulated and allows for tissue integration
      ii. Reports of late exposure or hematoma
      iii. Not visible on radiography
   d. Poly L/DL Lactide
      i. Material is thermolabile and can be customized and shaped to fit defect
      ii. Absorbed in 15-24 months and allows for bony healing
      iii. May not adequately restore anatomy in large defects
   e. Polydioxanone (PDS)
      i. Readily available and inexpensive
      ii. Useful for small-medium fractures but does not have the support for larger fractures
      iii. Risk of pseudocapsule formation
   f. Autogenous bone grafts
      i. Donor site morbidity
      ii. Increases surgery time
      iii. Unpredictable reabsorption
   g. Patient specific implants
      i. Use of CT imaging to mirror unaffected side; some with algorithms to also account for late orbital fat loss
      ii. Wide variety of materials have been used including titanium, methylmethacrylate, hydroxyapatite, porous polyethylene, and polyetheretherketone (PEEK)
      iii. Particularly useful in revision surgery, late presentations, large and complex defects

Challenges

1. Operating within orbit can lead to difficulties with intraoperative visualization necessitating a thorough understanding of anatomy [18]
2. Large fracture may have limited remaining bone for fixation
3. Oftentimes, volume loss is related not only to bony displacement but also due to orbital fat loss; with recent development of patient specific implants that are able to account for fat loss based on volumetric analysis of contralateral side, this can be addressed as needed [19]

Complications [20]

1. Eyelid malposition: ectropion, retraction, entropion
2. Scar
3. Retrobulbar hematoma
4. Implant migration
5. Infection of implanted material
6. Diplopia
7. Enophthalmos/Exophthalmos
8. Need for revision surgery [21]

Summary Points

1. Thorough understanding of orbital anatomy is crucial for proper repair of orbital fractures
2. Approaches to the repair have advantages and disadvantages, and should be chosen with these in mind
3. Various implant materials are utilized to repair the orbital floor; usually chosen based on surgeon preference and comfort with material

Patient Case

28 year-old male patient comes in after assault and presents with left eye swelling.

Q1. What would a focused history and physical include?

A1. Complete ophthalmic examination should be performed:

1. globe and/or optic injury, hyphema
2. Visual acuity, pupil response and extraocular motility
3. Hypesthesia in V2 pattern
4. Globe position (proptosis, enophthamos, hypoglobus)
5. Look for palpable step-offs, telecanthus in midface trauma, pulsatile proptosis

Q2. He has diplopia. How would you assess gaze restriction?

A2. Have patient look to all directions. May have to manually open eyelids due to edema. Forced ductions should be performed to assess for entrapment. An increase of intraocular pressure greater than 4mm when attempting to look into field of diplopia indicates restriction.

Q3. His CT scan shows the following images. Please describe.

A3. His CT face on coronal and sagittal views shows a large inferiorly displaced orbital floor fragment with herniation of orbital contents into the left maxillary sinus. Also involved the full length of the orbital floor.

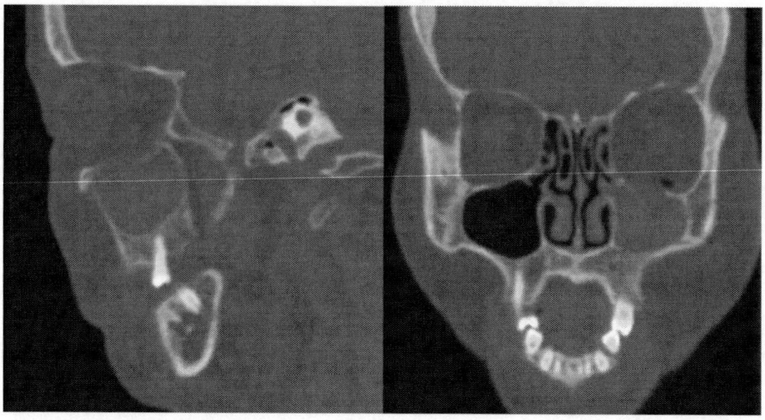

Figure 21.1. CT images of patient.

Q4. How would you manage this patient?

A4. Operative repair with implant within 2 weeks to allow for edema to improve. More urgent if there is any sign of oculocardiac reflex.

Q5. What incisions can be utilized for surgical repair of this type of fracture and what are the advantages/disadvantages?

A5.

1. Transorbital
    a. Conjunctival "transconjunctival" incision: pre-septal or post-septal
        i. Pre-septal: less fat herniation into the field but longer route to the orbital rim

   ii. Post-septal: closed to the rim, but orbital fat prolapse can make dissection more challenging
 b. Subcilliary incision – higher risk of ectropion, visible scar, may be easier if there is significant edema of the eyelid.
 c. Can be combined with lateral canthotomy, inferior cantholysis to increase exposure

2. Transantral
   a. Allows access to floor from maxillary sinus
      i. Avoids potential eyelid complications
      ii. Particularly useful in cases where globe manipulation needs to be kept to minimum, as with concurrent ruptured globe
      iii. Endoscopy can also be used with this approach to improve visualization
      iv. Limitations: longer operating time, paresthesia of upper lid and cheek from retraction
3. Infraorbital
   a. not usually used unless there is an existing laceration
   b. visible scar
   c. direct access to the orbital rim/floor

Q6. Patient comes back post-operative day 1 and reports that he has significant pain on the left eye and vision went from being normal after surgery to being increasingly blurry. How would you manage him?

A6. Immediate canthotomy/cantholysis. Consult to ophthalmology to help measure IOP and to monitor. Consider antibiotics, steroids, eyedrops for decreasing IOP, head of bed elevation.

References

[1] Smith B, Regan WF. Blow-out fracture of the orbit; mechanism and correction of internal orbital fracture. *Am J Ophthalmol* 1957;44:733–9.

[2] Parameswaran, A., Marimuthu, M., Panwar, S., Hammer, B. (2021). Orbital Fractures. In: Bonanthaya, K., Panneerselvam, E., Manuel, S., Kumar, V.V., Rai, A. (eds) *Oral and Maxillofacial Surgery for the Clinician.* Springer, Singapore. https://doi.org/10.1007/978-981-15-1346-6_57.

[3] Parbhu KC, Galler KE, Li C, Mawn LA. Underestimation of soft tissue entrapment by computed tomography in orbital floor fractures in the pediatric population. *Ophthalmology*. 2008;115(9):1620-1625.

[4] El Toukhy EA, ed. *Oculoplastic Surgery: A Practical Guide to Common Disorders*. Springer; 2021.

[5] Burnstine MA. Clinical recommendations for repair of isolated orbital floor fractures: an evidence based analysis. *Ophthalmology* 2002; 109: 1207–1210.

[6] Hawes MJ, Dortzbach RK. Surgery on orbital floor fractures. Influence of time of repair and fracture size. *Ophthalmology* 1983; 90: 1066–1070.

[7] Simon GJ, Syed HM, McCann JD, Goldberg RA. Early versus late repair of orbital blowout fractures. *Ophthalmic Surg Lasers Imaging* 2009; 40: 141–148.

[8] Dal Canto AJ, Linberg JV. Comparison of orbital fracture repair performed within 14 days versus 15 to 29 days after trauma. *Ophthal Plast Reconstr Surg* 2008; 24: 437–443.

[9] Shin KH, Baek SH, Chi M. Comparison of the outcomes of non-trapdoor type blowout fracture repair according to the time of surgery. *J Craniofac Surg* 2011; 22: 1426–1429.

[10] Beigi B, Khandwala M, Gupta D. Management of pure orbital floor fractures: a proposed protocol to prevent unnecessary or early surgery. *Orbit* 2014;33:336–42.

[11] Scawn RL, Lim LH, Whipple KM, Dolmetsch A, Priel A, Korn B, Kikkawa DO. Outcomes of orbital blow-out fracture repair performed beyond 6 weeks after injury. *Ophthal Plast Reconstr Surg* 2016; 32: 296–301.

[12] Kasaee A, Mirmohammadsadeghi A, Kazemnezhad F, Eshraghi B, Akbari MR. The predictive factors of diplopia and extraocular movement limitations in isolated pure blow-out fracture. *J Curr Ophthalmol.* 2016 Sep 25;29(1):54-58. doi: 10.1016/j.joco.2016.09.001. PMID: 28367528; PMCID: PMC5362382.

[13] Nerad JA. *Oculoplastic Surgery*. Mosby; 2007.

[14] Pankratov AS, Gotsiridze ZP, Kondrat AN, Karalkin AV. Repair of orbital floor fractures via the transantral approach with osteosynthesis plate. *Oral Maxillofac Surg*. 2020;24(3):309-316.

[15] Cheong EC, Chen CT, Chen YR (2010) Broad application of the endoscope for orbital floor reconstruction: long-term follow-up results. *Plast Reconstr Surg.* 125(3):969–978.

[16] Balaji SM, Balaji P (2019) Surgical Correction of diplopia in orbital fracture: influence of material and design. *Ann Maxillofac Surg*. 9(1):129–134.

[17] Song X, Li L, Sun Y, Fan X, Li Z (2016) Long-term infectious complications of using porous polyethylene mesh for orbital fracture reconstruction. *Medicine*. 95(25):e3819.

[18] Evans BT, Webb AAC. Post-traumatic orbital reconstruction: anatomical landmarks and the concept of the deep orbit. *Br J Oral Maxillofac Surg*. 2007;45(3):183-189.

[19] Kim SM, Jeong YS, Lee IJ, Park MC, Park DH. Prediction of the development of late enophthalmos in pure blowout fractures: delayed orbital tissue atrophy plays a major role. *Eur J Ophthalmol*. 2017;27(1):104-108.

[20] Brucoli M, Arcuri F, Cavenaghi R, Benech A. Analysis of complications after surgical repair of orbital fractures. *J Craniofac Surg* 2011; 22: 1387–1390.

[21] Kim JS, Lee BW, Scawn RL, Korn BS, Kikkawa DO. Secondary orbital reconstruction in patients with prior orbital fracture repair. *Ophthalmic Plast Reconstr Surg*. 2016;32(6):447-451.

Chapter 22

Frontal Sinus Fractures

Eliezer Kinberg, MD
and William Lawson, MD, DDS

Introduction

1. Frontal sinus development - forms as anterior ethmoid cells expand into the frontal bone separating inner and outer tables of the frontal bone [1-3]
    a. Forms as early as age 2 but generally appears radiographically at age 6
    b. 96% of people have a fully-formed frontal sinus by age 14; for others, stops growing by age 20 after the medullary bone is fully resorbed [4]
2. Frontal sinus anatomy
    a. Drains via the frontal sinus outflow tract (FSOT, nasofrontal duct) into middle meatus
        i. In most patients, FSOT is an ostium (The "nasofrontal duct" is a true duct in only 15% of population)
        ii. The FSOT is bordered anteriorly by the agger nasi cell, laterally by the orbit, and medially by the middle turbinate
    b. Lined with pseudostratified ciliated columnar epithelium that acts as a humidifier to warm air [4]
    c. Thickness of outer table is 4-12mm [5], posterior table 0.1-4.8mm [5]
3. Frontal sinus fractures:
    a. 5-15% of maxillofacial trauma
    b. 1/3 isolated to anterior table, 2/3 involve both tables and/or the FSOT
    c. Force required to fracture frontal sinus is high (800-1600 pounds of force) [5]
    d. Trend towards minimally invasive surgery with endoscopic techniques [6]
    e. Etiology of frontal sinus fractures [7]:
        i. Fall: 37%
        ii. Motor Vehicle Accident 31%
        iii. Pedestrian: 10%
        iv. Sports: 5%
        v. Assault: 3%
        vi. Other: 13%

In: Essential Facial Plastic and Reconstructive Surgery. Volume 1 ISBN: 979-8-89113-306-8
Editors: Yan Ho Lee and Ira Papel © 2024 Nova Science Publishers, Inc.

Patient Evaluation

As there is no randomized controlled trial on frontal sinus fracture management, the guidelines listed in this chapter are based on available literature and are to be used as a guide rather than absolute indications.

1. Initial factors to consider:
    a. The primary goal for sinus function is patency of the FSOT and continued sinus aeration [8].
        i. Patency of the FSOT is challenging to achieve [9]
        ii. A variety of mucosal grafts, flaps, and stents can be used [10, 11]
        iii. Operative management can involve endoscopic enlargement via Draf II (unilateral) or Draf III (bilateral) via drillout of frontal sinus floor and conjoining the two sinuses
        iv. Past experience has taught us that the tendency of the FSOT to obliterate (by fibrosis and osteoneogenesis) is an idiosyncratic feature which can limit endoscopic success. Draf stated that this led him to go from unilateral enlargement (Draf II) with 30% failure rate to the bilateral (Draf III) which decreased the failure rate to 7% (personal communication with the author)
2. Frontal sinus fractures can be subdivided into those involving the anterior table, the FSOT, and the posterior table. Fractures involving multiple sites have the greatest incidence of injury to contiguous structures, require a more complex operative management, and carry increased complication rates. [12] Questions to consider:
    a. Which table is injured?
    b. Is the fracture displaced?
    c. Is there CSF leakage?
    d. Is there FSOT injury?
    e. Is there an existing laceration/scar allowing for trans-cutaneous access?
    f. Are there concordant indications for neurosurgical intervention [7]?
        i. Focal neurologic symptoms
        ii. Increasing intra-cranial pressures or cerebral compression
        iii. Persistent CSF leak or hygroma
        iv. Dural laceration or pneumocephalus
3. Concordant injuries to be expected [5]:
    a. Skull base: cribriform plate, CSF leak 11%
    b. Intracranial: pneumocephalus 26%, cerebral contusion 18%, dural tear 14%, subdural, epidural, and intra-parenchymal hematomas
    c. Ophthalmologic: orbital apex syndrome; post-traumatic volume discrepancy, muscle entrapment, diplopia, retinal detachment, lens displacement, blindness
    d. Maxillofacial: nasorbitoethmoid (NOE) complex, orbital wall, midface, zygomatic complex (ZMC), panfacial fractures
4. Fracture features that pre-dispose to meningitis: fracture of the cribriform or fronto-ethmoid region, >1cm displacement, CSF rhinorrhea lasting > 8 days [13]
5. Determination of FSOT injury [5]

a. Difficult to assess extent of injury on imaging
b. Fractures presumed to involve the FSOT are:
    i. Fractures of the floor of the sinus
    ii. Depressed naso-ethmoid complex fractures
    iii. Inferior fractures of the posterior wall
    iv. Depressed fractures of the posterior table
    v. Persistent air-fluid levels 7-10 days post-injury

Management

1. Considerations in Management of Anterior Table Fractures:
    a. Depends on size of the fracture, displacement, and degree of comminution; displaced fractures generally require surgery, non-displaced fractures may be managed expectantly [14]
    b. General indications for expectant management
        i. Non-displaced fracture with no FSOT injury and no cosmetic deformity
        ii. Minimal FSOT injury with a well-ventilated sinus
    c. Fractures displaced greater than the thickness of anterior wall (average thickness 4 mm) require elevation to restore forehead contour.
    d. General indications for open reduction of anterior table [15]:
        i. Fracture of the supra-orbital rim
        ii. Greater extent of fractures and degree of comminution
        iii. Consider open approach if the injury has already exposed the sinus trans-cutaneously [16]
        iv. FSOT injury
    e. ORIF should be performed within 7-10 days to correct contour deformity and release entrapped mucosa to decrease risk of mucocele formation and chronic sinusitis
    f. The authors' preferred approach to anterior table fractures:
        i. Trephine at junction of the superior and medial walls of the orbit along supraorbital ridge through a 2 -2 1/2 cm incision
        ii. Sinus walls and FSOT can be examined with angled endoscopes
        iii. Depressed segment elevated with a thin curved instrument, and if necessary, supported by the balloon of a small pediatric Foley catheter that is left in place for 5 to 7 days
    g. Extensively comminuted fractures of the anterior table:
        i. Removal and reassembly of the fractures with miniplates, then re-insertion and fixation
        ii. Exposure through direct brow, pretricheal or coronal incision (depending on location and hairline)
        iii. Cover area with fascia or a sheet of acellular dermal matrix to smooth hardware and bony irregularities
2. Considerations in Management of Posterior Table Fractures [5, 14]:

a. Isolated posterior wall fractures (3-5% of cases) can result from a contrecoup injury by the brain from trauma to the back of the head; should monitor for CSF leak, intracranial injury, bleeding
b. Majority of fractures involving anterior and posterior tables will have injury of FSOT
c. Surgical repair has controversy involving the procedure of choice; need to consider status of the FSOT, extent of posterior wall comminution, presence of intracranial penetration or concomitant intracranial damage
d. Endoscopic management of FSOT usually involves a Draf IIb or III procedure, with repositioning of the bony fragments and coverage with a soft tissue graft.
e. Open management employs the osteoplastic flap with obliteration or cranialization
    i. Lesser injuries involves an osteoplastic flap through a laceration with a compound fracture, or a coronal flap
    ii. Severe injuries require cranialization performed by a bifrontal craniotomy
    iii. Due to risk of meningitis and even death with untreated posterior wall fractures, many favor an "isolation" type procedure to separate intracranial contents and the sinus with soft tissue
    iv. Reconstructed FSOT should be carefully monitored as silent obstruction can result in chronic sinusitis, osteomyelitis or mucopyocele years or decades later
f. General management of minimally displaced (<25%) fractures:
    i. No CSF leak → Observe
    ii. CSF leak:
        - Initial observation for 5-7 days with IV antibiotics, bed rest, head elevation
        - Consider lumbar drain with drainage of 10cc/hr of CSF
        - Consider obliteration if the leak persists beyond 8-10 days
        - If no intra-cranial injury, consider endoscopic management
g. General management of displaced (>25%) fractures: cranialization (with dural repair as indicated)

3. Protocol for frontal sinus fracture management has been proposed with good clinical outcomes [17, 18]:
    a. Immediate repair if patient undergoing frontal craniotomy for neurosurgical indications
    b. Delayed repair for other surgical indications: persistent CSF leak, intra-cranial infection, operative facial fractures
    c. Remaining patients observes with repeat CT scans at 3 months
        i. Normal cosmesis and aeration → observe
        ii. Partial aeration or minor deformity → Repeat CT scan at 6 months
        iii. Complete opacification and/or deformity → endoscopic or open repair
4. Operative Methods

a. Layers of the soft tissue covering of the cranium (SCALP)
   i. Skin
   ii. SubCutaneous tissue
   iii. Aponeurosis and muscle
   iv. Loose areolar tissue - contains rich blood supply from surrounding vessels (supra-orbital, supra-trochlear, occipital, posterior auricular, and superficial temporal) and penetrating vessels from the galea
   v. Pericranium
b. Open approach to the frontal sinus [19]
   i. Coronal incision well behind hairline; extend inferiorly to the helix
   ii. Dissection in either a sub-galeal or sub-periosteal plane
   iii. Dissection must be deep to the temporoparietal fascia at the temporalis muscle to avoid injury to frontal branch of the facial nerve
   iv. Transition to a sub-periosteal plane no closer than 2-3cm from the orbital rim to avoid injury to supratrochlear and supra-orbital neurovascular bundles
c. Open vs endoscopic approach [20]:
   i. To date, there is no randomized controlled trial comparing endoscopic vs open outcomes
   ii. Post-surgical mucocele rate appears higher after open repair (4%) than after endoscopic intervention (<1%)
   iii. No difference in post-operative CSF leak, meningitis, or sinusitis rates
   iv. Headache rates are lower after endoscopic approach, likely due to avoidance of supratrochlear/supraorbital nerve injury [21]
   v. Post-operative monitoring easier after endoscopic surgery than after obliterative surgery due to difficulties in endoscopic examination and non-specific post-obliteration radiologic findings (i.e., differentiating granulations from mucocele or graft material is challenging) [22]
d. Pericranial flap:
   i. Pericranial flaps are composite flaps of the pericranium and overlying loose areolar tissue to ensure excellent flap vascularity and appropriate bulk to obliterate the dead space [23]
   ii. Can be axial or random
   iii. Axial pericranial flap designs:
      - Anteriorly-based: based on supraorbital and supratrochlear arteries
      - Laterally-based: based on anterior branch of superficial temporal artery
e. Obliteration
   i. There are four forms of frontal sinus obliteration:
      - Riedel procedure (1750): removal of the anterior table, collapsing the skin into the defect [24]; led to extreme deformity [25]

- Macbeth procedure: auto-obliteration based on osteoneogenesis, through hinged osteoperiosteal flap and removal of sinus contents (unreliable, no longer performed) [26]
- Obliteration with graft (autogenous (bone, muscle, fascia, free and pedicled tissue) or alloplastic (acrylic, polypropylene, hydroxyapatite) materials); preferred materials: abdominal adipose tissue, muscle
- Cranialization – can be considered a form of obliteration

ii. The goals are:
- Block communication between the frontal sinus and nasal cavity
- Minimize dead space in the frontal sinus
- Reduce the risk of infection by preventing accumulation of blood and fluid
- Reduce risk of mucocele or mucopyocele formation

iii. Disadvantages are:
- Materials used can be re-absorbed
- Open spaces fill with granulation, can become infected, leaving the sinus empty and relying on auto-obliteration
- Secondary frontal mucocele may develop from residual respiratory epithelium secreting mucous in a now closed cavity

iv. The choice of material may be less critical than ensuring complete mucosal removal and occlusion of the FSOT [27]

v. Synthetic materials (i.e., polytetrafluoroethylene and methylmethacrylate) were previously used but did not vascularize or integrate into native tissue, resulting in high infection and extrusion rates

vi. Hydroxyapatite contours readily, is osteo-conductive (allows for bone growth along its surface), and resists mucosal ingrowth making it an option when obliteration is indicated [27, 28]. However, chronic infection may require removal of material [29-31] (Avoid hydroxyapatite in an infected sinus)

vii. Curette all of the mucosal lining of sinus and ensure that the FSOT is fully stripped of mucosa; all of the walls of the sinus are drilled to remove mucosal tags and mucosa along the veins of Breschet [32]

viii. Obliterate FSOT with autogenous bone graft, temporalis muscle and fascia plugs, or pericranial or galeal flaps

ix. A recent review of osteoplastic flap outcomes by Lee et al. concluded that frontal sinus fractures generally warrant open management, and if obliteration is required abdominal fat is the procedure of choice [33]. There was insufficient evidence to comment on a non-obliterative approach in conjunction with an endoscopic dissection of the FSOT [26].

f. Cranialization
   i. Role in posterior table fractures with a high degree of comminution and/or persistent CSF leakage [34]
   ii. Eliminates frontal sinus by removing the posterior wall permitting the brain and dura to herniate forward. This is often combined with a pericranial flap
g. Trephination - can be utilized to assess posterior table fractures and explore for presence of CSF leak
   i. The supra-trochlear and supra-orbital neurovascular bundles are located 1.7 and 2.2cm from the midline respectively [35]
   ii. Trephination should be performed 1cm from midline at the medial aspect of the brow, aiming above the orbital rim (Figure 22.1). The presence of a frontal sinus should be confirmed on imaging pre-operatively
   iii. A mini-trephination may be performed for drainage of an abscess of an infection, while a full-trephination (4mm) may be performed to allow insertion of an endoscope [36]; can be used to reduce simple anterior table fracture by inserting a curved instrument. If fracture is unstable, a pediatric foley can be inserted and inflated to reduce the fracture.
   iv. FSOT patency can be confirmed by demonstrating drainage of saline or methylene blue dye into the nose via the trephination [5]

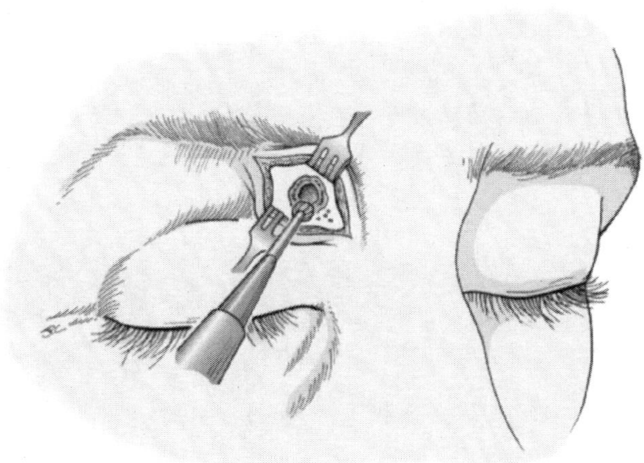

Figure 22.1. Demonstration of frontal sinus trephination. [37]

Complications

1. Rates of headache after frontal sinus fracture appear higher in surgically treated groups than non-treated groups [6]
   a. May result from supra-orbital nerve injury
   b. Overall headache rate is roughly 30% [38]

2. Failed obliteration can present any time after surgery, including after many years, with indistinct imaging features
    a. Etiologies of failure include: retained sinus mucosa, mucosal ingrowth via the FSOT into sinus, granulation tissue in retained dead space
    b. Consider surgical exploration (open or endoscopic) for any patient with persistent symptoms after prior obliteration [14]
3. Mucocele formation [39]:
    a. Mucoceles are expansile mucus filled cysts; may erode through frontal sinus table or into orbit
    b. Can become infected and result in a mucopyocele, with intra-cranial and intra-orbital complications
    c. Intra-cranial spread may occur via:
        i. Necrotic bone, resulting in extra-dural empyema
        ii. Valveless diploic veins connecting sinus mucosa to the intra-cranial venous system, resulting in septic thrombophlebitis
4. Irregular forehead contour from [39]:
    a. Failure to recognize a displaced fracture due to overlying soft tissue edema
    b. Poor stabilization of bony fragments
    c. Cicatricial contracture of overlying skin revealing underlying hardware or regions of poor bony contact
    d. Failure to restore orbital roof, resulting in downward displacement of the globe

Summary Points

1. The management of frontal sinus fractures is evolving as endoscopic approaches take root and expand in their versatility.
2. Non-displaced frontal sinus fractures can generally be safely managed non-operatively, while surgical intervention is indicated in cases of displaced fractures or CSF leakage that persists at least 8-10 days after the initial fracture.
3. The selection of open versus endoscopic approach will be dictated by the severity of the injury and by the surgeon's comfort level and clinical judgement.
4. A more extensive body of literature is needed for evidence-based guidance in the management of frontal sinus trauma.

Patient Case

You are called in to evaluate a patient who sustained a motor vehicle accident with a radiology report indicating the presence of a frontal sinus fracture (details are unavailable). Look at Case Figure 22.2.

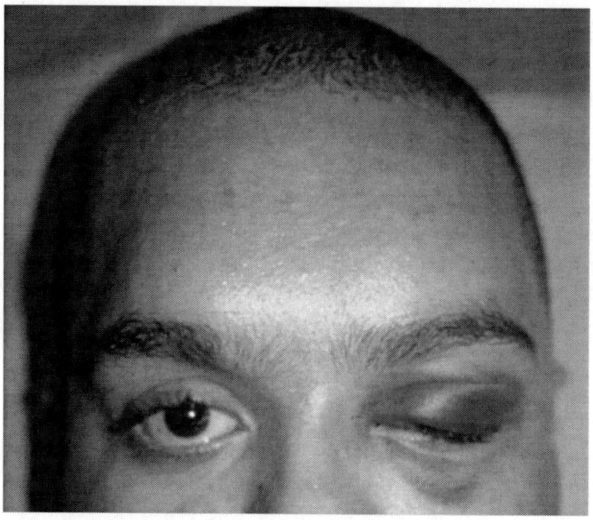

Figure 22.2. Patient case: trauma due to motor vehicle accident.

Q1) The patient is alert and oriented and being monitored in the intensive care unit. His vitals are stable and it has been determined that he does not require any neurosurgical intervention. What history would you obtain?

A1. A full HPI should be obtained. Specific questions should include the presence/absence of headache, visual change, nausea, salty/metallic taste, history of head and neck surgery including sinus surgery, history of head and neck trauma.

Q2. What would you look for on physical exam?

A2.

a. ABC (airway, breathing, circulation)
b. A full head and neck exam should be performed, including a complete visual exam and extra-ocular movement
c. The frontal bone should be palpated to assess for hematoma, fractures or mobile segments.
d. A complete cranial nerve exam should be performed specifically looking at the frontal branch of the facial nerve as well as the V1-V2 distribution of the trigeminal nerve.

Q3. What imaging is indicated in this type of patient coming through the ED?

A3.

a. CT head/face with thin (1mm or less) slices to allow for intra-operative navigation.
b. MRI brain can be considered as per neurosurgical guidance

Q4. How would you describe the radiographic findings demonstrated in the below images? (Figure 22.3) What consultations would you recommend?

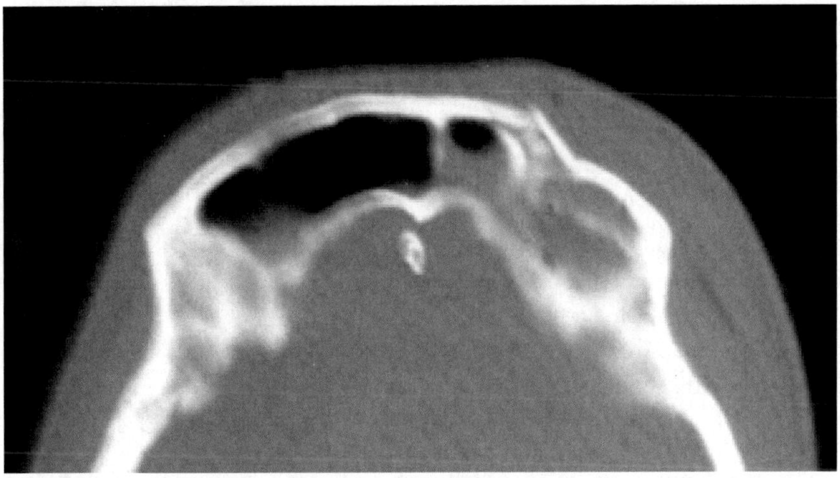

Figure 22.3. CT Scan of patient case.

A4. Axial CT face. There is a displaced comminuted fracture of the left frontal sinus anterior table which appears to spare the posterior table. FSOT involvement cannot be assessed without additional images but the injury would appear remote from the FSOT based on this static image.

Neurosurgical consultation can be considered and would be absolutely necessary in the presence of a concomitant posterior table injury. Ophthalmology consult would be warranted if there were any new symptoms involving vision changes or eye pain.

Q5. How are frontal sinus fractures classified?

A5.

a. Involvement of anterior table, posterior table, or both
b. Displacement of greater than the width of the table itself
c. Likelihood of FSOT injury
d. Likelihood of intra-cranial injury and CSF leakage

Q6. How would you manage this patient medically assuming the presence of a CSF leak?

A6.

a. Hemodynamically optimize by the intensive care team
b. Unless contraindicated from a neurosurgical standpoint, the head of the bed should be elevated >30 degrees, "csf leak precautions" including no straining, no heavy lifting, no use of straws, and sneeze with an open mouth
c. Per neurosurgery, consider placement of lumbar drain to decrease intra-cranial pressure

Q7. What would you consider from a surgical standpoint and what would your timeline for intervention be?

A7.

Surgical intervention best considered 7-10 days after injury to allow resolution of soft tissue edema.

Given the degree of comminution of the frontal sinus with likelihood of long-term cosmetic deformity, mucocele risk, and risk of chronic sinusitis, open reduction and fixation should be performed. This would be best performed with a coronal incision, with an incision planned behind the hairline and elevated deep to the pericranium in order to preserve a peri-cranial flap if obliteration of the sinus were to become indicated at a later time. Maintaining a deep plane of dissection also eliminates risk of injury to the frontal branch of the facial nerve and to the supra-orbital and supra-trochlear nerve bundles.

If there is concern for injury to the FSOT, its patency can be assessed intra-operatively with methylene blue dye and endoscopic widening of the tract can be considered.

Operative findings and final surgical outcome are below. (Figure 22.4)

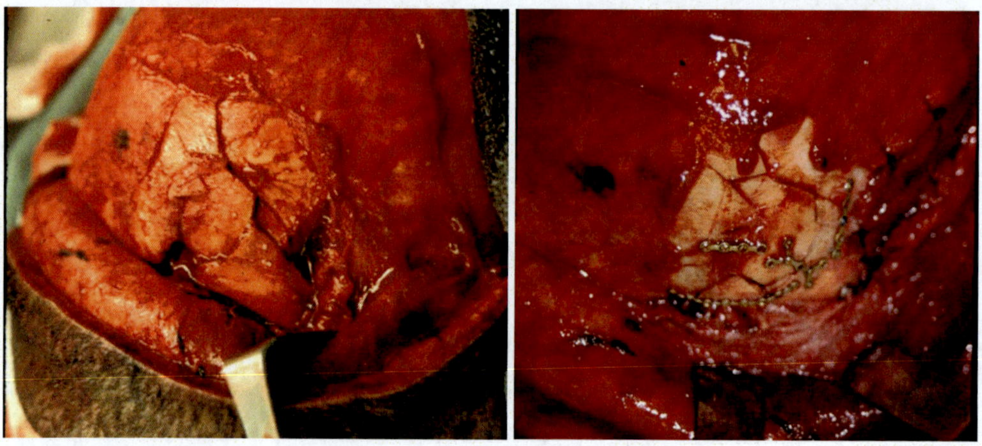

Figure 22.4. Operative findings and final surgical outcome.

References

[1] Som PM, Lawson W. *Interfrontal Sinus Septal Cell: A Cause of Obstructing Inflammation and Mucoceles.* doi:10.3174/ajnr.A1107.

[2] Som PM, Park EE, Naidich TP, Lawson W. *Crista Galli Pneumatization Is an Extension of the Adjacent Frontal Sinuses.* doi:10.3174/ajnr.A1291.

[3] Blitzer A, Lawson W, Friedman WH, William H. *Surgery of the paranasal sinuses.* Published online 1985:357. Accessed February 5, 2022. https://books.google.com/books/about/Surgery_of_the_Paranasal_Sinuses.html?id=X8hsAAAAMAAJ.

[4] Moore K, Ross A. Frontal Sinus Development and Juvenile Age Estimation. *Anat Rec.* 2017;300(9):1609-1617. doi:10.1002/AR.23614.

[5] Jeyaraj P. Frontal Bone Fractures and Frontal Sinus Injuries: Treatment Paradigms. *Ann Maxillofac Surg.* 2019;9(2):261. doi:10.4103/AMS.AMS_151_19.

[6] Langlie J, Kim M, Thaller SR. Frontal Sinus Fractures: A Review on Etiology and Management Emphasizing Minimally Invasive and Endoscopic Techniques. *J Craniofac Surg.* 2021;32:1246-1250. doi:10.1097/SCS.0000000000007623.

[7] Lopez J, Pineault K, Pradeep T, Khavanin N, Kachniarz B, Faateh M, Grant MP, Redett RJ, Manson PN, Dorafshar AH. Pediatric frontal bone and sinus fractures: Cause, characteristics, and a treatment algorithm. *Plast Reconstr Surg.* Published online 2020:1012-1023. doi:10.1097/PRS.0000000000006645.

[8] Sewall EC. XXXI. *The Operative Treatment of Nasal Sinus Disease*: https://doi.org/101177/000348943504400201. 2016;44(2):307-316. doi:10.1177/000348943504400201.

[9] Mcnaught RC. A refinement of the external frontoethmosphenoid operation: a new nasofrontal pedicle flap. *Arch otolaryngol.* 1936;23(5):544-549. Doi:10.1001/archotol.1936.00640040554003.

[10] Kuhn FA. An Integrated Approach to Frontal Sinus Surgery. *Otolaryngol Clin North Am.* 2006;39(3):437-461. doi:10.1016/J.OTC.2006.01.008.

[11] Neel HB, Whicker JH, Lake CF. Thin rubber sheeting in frontal sinus surgery: animal and clinical studies. *Laryngoscope.* 1976;86(4):524-536. doi:10.1288/00005537-197604000-00008.

[12] Rodriguez ED, Stanwix MG, Nam AJ, St Hilaire H, Simmons OP, Christy MR, Grant MP, Manson PN. Twenty-six-year experience treating frontal sinus fractures: a novel algorithm based on anatomical fracture pattern and failure of conventional techniques. *Plast Reconstr Surg.* 2008;122(6):1850-1866. doi:10.1097/PRS.0B013E31818D58BA.

[13] Sakas DE, Beale DJ, Ameen AA, Whitwell HL, Whittaker KW, Krebs AJ, Abbasi KH, Dias PS. Compound anterior cranial base fractures: Classification using computerized tomography scanning as a basis for selection of patients for dural repair. *J Neurosurg.* 1998;88(3):471-477. doi:10.3171/jns.1998.88.3.0471.

[14] Banks C, Grayson J, Cho DY, Woodworth BA. Frontal sinus fractures and cerebrospinal fluid leaks: A change in surgical paradigm. *Curr Opin Otolaryngol Head Neck Surg.* 2020;28(1):52-60. doi:10.1097/MOO.0000000000000602.

[15] Hwang K, Song YB. *Closed reduction of fractured anterior wall of the frontal bone.* undefined. 2005;16(1):120-122. doi:10.1097/00001665-200501000-00023.

[16] Lawson W, Ho Y. Open Frontal Sinus Surgery: A Lost Art. *Otolaryngol Clin North Am.* 2016;49(4):1067-1089. doi:10.1016/J.OTC.2016.03.027.

[17] Patel SA, Berens AM, Devarajan K, Whipple ME, Moe KS. *Evaluation of a Minimally Disruptive Treatment Protocol for Frontal Sinus Fractures.* Published online 2017. doi:10.1001/jamafacial.2016.1769.

[18] Jafari A, Nuyen BA, Salinas CR, Smith AM, Deconde AS. Spontaneous ventilation of the frontal sinus after fractures involving the frontal recess. *Am J Otolaryngol.* 2015;36(6):837-842. doi:10.1016/J.AMJOTO.2015.04.015.

[19] Oleh M. *Coronal approach.* 2015;(1):1-9. Accessed December 27, 2021. https://surgeryreference.aofoundation.org/cmf/trauma/midface/approach/coronal-approach.

[20] Le P, Martinez R, Black J. Frontal Sinus Fracture Management Meta-analysis: Endoscopic Versus Open Repair. *J Craniofac Surg.* 2021;32(4):1311-1315. doi:10.1097/SCS.0000000000007181.

[21] Smith TL, Han JK, Loehrl TA, Rhee JS. Endoscopic management of the frontal recess in frontal sinus fractures: a shift in the paradigm? *Laryngoscope*. 2002;112(5):784-790. doi:10.1097/00005537-200205000-00004.

[22] Catalano PJ, Lawson W, Som P, Biller HF. Radiographic evaluation and diagnosis of the failed frontal osteoplastic flap with fat obliteration. *Otolaryngol Head Neck Surg*. 1991;104(2):225-234. doi:10.1177/019459989110400211.

[23] Parhiscar A, Har-El G. Frontal sinus obliteration with the pericranial flap. *Otolaryngol Head Neck Surg*. 2001;124(3):304-307. doi:10.1067/MHN.2001.113662.

[24] Lawson W, Reino A, Deeb R, Deeb R. The Riedel Procedure - An Analysis of 22 Cases. *Arch Otolaryngol Rhinol*. 2017;3(3):087-092. doi:10.17352/2455-1759.000054.

[25] Kelly A, Alhelali N, McGarry GW. A stepwise approach to open surgery for the frontal sinus. *J Laryngol Otol*. 2021;135(2):173-175. doi:10.1017/S0022215120002625.

[26] Lee YH, Lee JY, Lawson W. Indications and Outcomes of the Osteoplastic Flap Procedure With or Without Obliteration. *J Craniofac Surg*. 2020;31(8):2243-2249. doi:10.1097/SCS.0000000000006717.

[27] Petruzzelli GJ, Stankiewicz JA. Frontal sinus obliteration with hydroxyapatite cement. *Laryngoscope*. 2002;112(1):32-36. doi:10.1097/00005537-200201000-00006.

[28] Friedman CD, Costantino PD, Synderman CH, Chow LC, Takagi S. Reconstruction of the frontal sinus and frontofacial skeleton with hydroxyapatite cement. *Arch Facial Plast Surg*. 2000;2(2):124-129. doi:10.1001/ARCHFACI.2.2.124.

[29] Boyden G. Chronic frontal sinusitis: end results of surgical treatment - PubMed. *Trans Am Acad Ophthalmol Otolaryngol*. 1957;61(5):588-591. Accessed February 5, 2022. https://pubmed.ncbi.nlm.nih.gov/13486578/.

[30] Boyden GL. Surgical treatment of chronic frontal sinusitis. *Ann Otol Rhinol Laryngol*. 1952;61(2):558-566. doi:10.1177/000348945206100227.

[31] Lawson W, Reino AJ. Management of embossment following the frontal osteoplastic operation. *Laryngoscope*. 1996;106(10):1259-1265. doi:10.1097/00005537-199610000-00018.

[32] Wolfe SA, Johnson P, Luce EA. Frontal sinus injuries: Primary care and management of late complications. *Plast Reconstr Surg*. 1988;82(5):790-791. doi:10.1097/00006534-198811000-00010.

[33] Weber R, Draf W, Keerl R, Kahle G, Schinzel S, Thomann S, Lawson W. Osteoplastic frontal sinus surgery with fat obliteration: technique and long-term results using magnetic resonance imaging in 82 operations. Department of Otorhinolaryngology, Head, Neck and Facial Plastic Surgery, Communication Disorders, Hospital Fulda, Germany in conjunction with Mount Sinai Hospital. *Laryngoscope*. 2000;110(6):1037-1044. doi:10.1097/00005537-200006000-00028.

[34] Morse JC, Chandra RK. Is there still a role for cranialization in modern sinus surgery? *Curr Opin Otolaryngol Head Neck Surg*. 2021;29(1):53-58. doi:10.1097/MOO.0000000000000691.

[35] Tungkeeratichai J, Bhongmakapat T, Saitongdee P, Orathai P. The Surgical Landmark for Facial Foramen. *Otorhinolaryngol Clin An Int J*. 5(3):121-124. doi:10.5005/jp-journals-10003-1124.

[36] Fagan J, Sutherland N, Holbrook E. *Open access atlas of otolaryngology, head & neck operative surgery external ethmoidectomy & frontal sinusotomy/trephine.*

[37] *15-External Approaches to the Frontal Sinus*.pdf. Accessed December 26, 2021. https://www.dropbox.com/preview/Academics/Education/Textbooks%2Carticles/General/Myers Operative Otolaryngology/15-External Approaches to the Frontal Sinus.pdf?role=personal.

[38] Wilson BC, Davidson B, Corey JP, Haydon RC. Comparison of complications following frontal sinus fractures managed with exploration with or without obliteration over 10 years. *Laryngoscope*. 1988;98(5):516-520. doi:10.1288/00005537-198805000-00008.

[39] Stanley RB. Management of complications of frontal sinus and frontal bone fractures. *Oper Tech Plast Reconstr Surg*. 1998;5(4):296-301. doi:10.1016/S1071-0949(98)80035-8.

Chapter 23

Panfacial Fractures

Michael P. Johnson, DMD, FACS
and David Salomon, DDS

Introduction

1. Panfacial fractures involve fractures of lower, middle, and upper thirds of facial skeleton
2. As significant force is required to cause such severe injuries, concomitant neurologic and other injuries are common [1]
3. Patients with panfacial fractures found to have 17.4% overall mortality and 2.2-fold increased mortality compared to isolated middle or lower facial fractures [2]
4. These injuries are unique and complex but typically follow predictable anatomic patterns → useful framework for classification
5. Facial skeleton has four vertical and four horizontal buttresses
    a. Vertical buttresses: nasomaxillary, zygomaticomaxillary, pterygomaxillary, mandibular ramus/condyle
    b. Horizontal buttresses: frontal, zygomatic, maxillary, mandibular
        i. Absorb and transmit forces
        ii. Act as pillars of stabilization
        iii. Key to guiding reconstruction [3, 4]
6. Treatment strategies for these complex injuries vary in sequencing and timing

Patient Evaluation

1. Physical exam must:
    a. Be systematic (complete and detailed)
    b. Differentiate and distinguish emergent, urgent, and other pertinent findings
    c. Head and neck exam:
        i. General areas to palpate and visualize:
            - Scalp, posterior skull
            - Frontal bandeau, zygomatic arches and orbital rims
            - Nasal dorsum, maxilla
            - Preauricular regions, mandibular ramus, inferior border of mandible to midline
            - Neck to midline along trachea

In: Essential Facial Plastic and Reconstructive Surgery. Volume 1 ISBN: 979-8-89113-306-8
Editors: Yan Ho Lee and Ira Papel © 2024 Nova Science Publishers, Inc.

ii. Assess for edema, lacerations, ecchymosis, contusions, crepitus, foreign bodies, bony steps, paresthesia
iii. Cervical spine
- For awake, cooperative patients
  - Neck flexion, extension, tilt to left and right
  - Palpation along cervical spine
- If patient comatose or inebriated – defer

iv. Orbit: Extraocular muscles, visual acuity, pupils, enophthalmos/ exophthalmos, hyphema, chemosis, subconjunctival hemorrhage
v. Ear: hemotympanum, otorrhea, post-auricular ecchymosis (Battle's sign) facial nerve palsy, tinnitus
vi. Nose: epistaxis, rhinorrhea, septal deviation, septal hematoma
vii. Neck: trachea midline without signs or symptoms of expanding hematoma, laryngeal fracture, stridor, or dyspnea
viii. Oral Cavity: trismus, presence/absence and mobility of teeth and/or alveolar segments, fractured teeth, occlusion, mobility of maxilla; swelling, ecchymosis, lacerations of gingiva, floor of mouth, tongue, palate
ix. Oropharynx: swelling, ecchymosis, lacerations

2. Imaging – CT is gold standard
   a. 3D reconstruction if available
   b. Allows utilization of Virtual Surgical Planning (VSP) for planning as well as fabrication of custom plates and implants
   c. Helpful to breakdown injuries into facial subunits to diagnosis and manage
   d. Other imaging modalities: CTA (for active bleeding) or MRI (for soft tissue detail)
3. Concomitant injuries
   a. Multiple and potentially severe, life-threatening concurrent injuries are likely; Motor Vehicle Collision (MVC) most common etiology

i. One study found that 53% panfacial fracture patients had concomitant injuries including: [1]
- 18% intracranial hemorrhage/injury
- 16% abdominal injuries
- 13% pneumothorax, 13% pulmonary contusions
- 13% c-spine fractures

ii. No statistically significant delay in treatment compared to patients with isolated facial injuries [1]
iii. 6.2% of patients had associated life-threatening injuries requiring invasive procedures; most common injury was cerebral trauma 32.8% [5]
iv. Avoid performing non-emergent surgeries in hemodynamically or neurologically unstable patients (i.e. elevated intracranial pressure) [6]
v. Injuries of cervical spine and related structures, such as ligamentous injuries, are common with facial fractures (13-20%) [1, 7] and must

be cleared prior to surgery or use intraoperative immobilization (not just c-collar)

- An unconscious patient requires MRI to rule out ligamentous injuries [1]

vi. Imperative to work closely with multidisciplinary team to ensure appropriate risk assessment, timing, and planning of surgical treatment

Management

1. Goal: restore form (facial width, height, and projection) and function (including mastication, occlusion, vision, nasal airway, sinus function)
2. Accomplished through reconstruction of facial buttresses
3. Timing of repair for pan facial fractures/trauma
   a. Emergent
      i. ABCs
         - Secure airway if needed (intubation vs. tracheostomy vs. cricothyroidotomy)
         - Control hemorrhage
      ii. Orbital compartment syndrome from retrobulbar hematoma
      iii. Orbital apex injury and/or superior orbital fissure syndrome
      iv. Entrapment of extraocular muscle (oculo-cardiac reflex)
   b. Urgent - septal hematoma
   c. Subsequent:
         - If repair not completed prior to edema onset, consider delay until edema improves (ideally within 2 weeks, delayed 4 weeks if needed [8])
4. Airway
   a. Oral intubation most common for trauma patients, but often does not permit maxillomandibular fixation (MMF)
   b. Nasal intubation can facilitate MMF, but may be contraindicated (i.e. anterior skull base fractures)
   c. Submental intubation is an option to facilitate MMF but should not be left for more than 1-2 days (risk for fistula formation)
   d. Tracheostomy should be performed if longer-term airway protection required (≥2 weeks)
5. Sequencing of treatment
   a. Differing schools of thought:
      i. Top → Bottom vs. Bottom →Top → Middle
         - Top → Bottom – no condylar requirement [9]
         - Bottom →Top → Middle [10, 11] - LeFort I level most forgiving in terms of need for accuracy and allows leeway aesthetically, thus common for this and orbital floor to be reconstructed last

  - ii. Outside → Inside vs. Inside → outside
    - Occlusal relationship is key, and many argue its restoration should be the initial step [11]
    - Repair palatal fracture first, if present, followed by maxillomandibular fixation to set occlusion
    - This is critical especially with comminuted condylar fractures, as the occlusion becomes the only guide to set lower facial height
- b. Some have found no difference in clinical outcome between bottom-up inside-out and top-down outside-in [12]
- c. No standard sequence; individualized approach should be implemented based on patient-specific findings, fracture pattern, and surgeon preference [4]
  - i. Generally accepted principles:
    - Exposure of multiple fracture prior to fixation
    - Fixation from known to unknown (stable to unstable)
    - Occlusion links mandible to midface
    - If unable to perform with ideal timing, at least stabilize flail segments and grossly replace hard and soft tissues anatomically to maintain vascularity and form

6. Approaches
   - a. Intraoral
   - b. Lower eyelid (transconjunctival, subciliary, infraorbital)
   - c. Lateral brow vs. upper blepharoplasty
   - d. Coronal
   - e. Preauricular
   - f. Submandibular / retromandibular
   - g. Existing lacerations
7. Fixation
   - a. Based on location and comminution (heavier fixation along buttresses)
   - b. Titanium vs. resorbable
8. Virtual Surgical Planning (VSP)
   - a. Mirror-imaging from contralateral uninjured side is helpful
   - b. 3D model of patient can be used to aid in plate bending and adaptation intraoperatively
   - c. Can also use preformed/custom plates but may not be possible depending on timing of repair
9. Intra-op imaging (CT) or surgical navigation helpful; in facial trauma overall CT-directed revision rate was 28%; 31% for orbital fractures and 24% for zygomaticomaxillary complex (ZMC) fractures. [13]
10. Specifics
    - a. Helpful landmarks
      - i. Zygomatic arch (typically straight) to establish facial projection
      - ii. Sphenozygomatic suture & internal lateral orbital wall in reduction of ZMC fractures
    - b. Naso-Orbito-Ethmoid subunit reconstruction [14]

c. Nasolacrimal drainage apparatus
   i. Obstruction after NOE ORIF can range from 5-21% [15, 16]
      - Can place silicone tube if injury suspected
      - Delayed assessment with possible DCR if obstruction persists
d. Condylar fracture
   i. If significantly comminuted or not amenable to open treatment, cannot rely on to restore vertical buttress of lower third
   ii. Bilateral fractures with symphyseal fracture may create facial widening (lingual splay); important to recognize and treat by visualizing lingual border of mandible and/or applying pressure on angles toward midline
e. Impacted maxilla
   i. Disimpaction with forceps (Rowe maxillary disimpaction forceps)
   ii. May experience significant bleeding upon disimpaction, as well as potential for propagation of skull base fractures [11]
f. Facial nerve
   i. Arborization of nerves anterior to vertical line drawn from lateral canthus typically precludes need for repair
   ii. Primary repair if identified and more feasible posteriorly
   iii. Can use nerve stimulation or monitoring, but cannot do this during muscle paralysis which can aid repair of panfacial fractures
g. Primary bone grafting
   i. May be necessary in comminuted areas
   ii. Promotes bony union and helps minimize secondary deformities
   iii. Nasal dorsum may require grafting to prevent "saddle nose" deformity
   iv. Other common areas include frontal bone, orbital floor, medial orbital wall, and zygomaticomaxillary buttress
   v. Calvarial bone graft is common given access via a coronal approach, availability of cortical bone stock, and limited resorption, especially with rigid fixation [17]
h. Soft tissue resuspension
   i. Critical for long-term aesthetic outcome
   ii. Helps minimize secondary defects, most notably in midface (temporal hollowing, lower eyelid tear trough)
   iii. Two key aspects [4]:
      - Refixation of periosteum or fascia to skeleton
      - Closure of periosteum, muscle fascia, skin incisions

Complications (With Panfacial Trauma)

1. Nerve deficits
   a. Olfactory dysfunction (hyposmia / anosmia)
      i. Mechanism: [18]

- Direct shearing or tearing of olfactory nerve fibers (CN 1) at cribiform plate
- Sinonasal tract disruption
- Focal contusion or hemorrhage within olfactory cortex

b. Superior orbital fissure (SOF) syndrome [19]
   i. Characterized by ophthalmoplegia, ptosis, proptosis of eye, dilation and fixation of pupil, and anesthesia of upper eyelid and forehead
   ii. Optic nerve is intact so vision is intact, however there is an efferent pupillary defect
   iii. Treat with steroids, surgical decompression of superior orbital fissure, reduction of concomitant facial fracture

c. Orbital apex syndrome [20]
   i. Characterized by vision loss and painful ophthalmoplegia
   ii. SOF syndrome + vision loss
   iii. Treat with steroids and urgent surgical decompression of orbital apex

d. Traumatic Optic Neuropathy (TON) - acute injury to optic nerve from direct or indirect trauma
   i. Afferent pupillary defect (Marcus Gunn pupil) [21]
   ii. Optic nerve function is decreased unilaterally

e. Trigeminocardiac Reflex (Oculocardiac Reflex) [22, 23]
   i. Bradycardia and hypotension on manual compression of eyes or mechanical manipulation of any of trigeminal nerve branches
   ii. Most common traumatic etiology entrapment of inferior rectus in orbital floor trap-door fractures, retrobulbar hemorrhage, or edema.
   iii. Stop stimulus; consider glycopyrrolate and local anesthetics

f. Trigeminal nerve injury
   i. Malar and infraorbital paresthesia/anesthesia
   ii. Tongue paresthesia/anesthesia
   iii. Lower lip and anterior gingival paresthesia/anesthesia
   iv. Chin/lower lip paresthesia/anesthesia

g. Facial nerve injury (CN VII) [24]

h. Vestibulocochlear nerve (CN VIII) injury [24]

2. Facial asymmetry and loss of craniomaxillofacial dimension:

   a. Changes to *vertical* dimension
      i. Anterior open bite (AOB)
         - Condyle/ramus fractures result in loss of posterior vertical dimension and premature posterior occlusion resulting in AOB
         - Lefort-type midface fractures may result in anterior maxillary intrusion and/or posterior maxillary dis-impaction resulting in AOB

   b. Changes to *anteroposterior* (AP) dimension
      i. Bilateral mandibular fractures may result in posterior displacement of mandible, decreasing AP projection or even potential airway compromise, “bucket handle” fracture

   ii. Lefort midface fractures may cause midface intrusion, decreasing AP dimension
   iii. NOE fractures may cause AP changes
   iv. Frontal bone injury may cause frontal depression
c. Changes to *transverse* dimension
   i. Mandibular widening: symphyseal mandible fractures with or without condyle/ramus fractures
   ii. Maxillary widening: mid-palatal fractures
   iii. Facial widening: lateral displacement of ZMC in panfacial injury
      - Traumatic telecanthus vs. hypertelorism [25]
         – Telecanthus - increased distance between medial canthi (NOE injuries)
         – Hypertelorism - increased interpupillary distance or bony interorbital distance (dacryon to dacryon); dacryon is junction of maxilla, frontal, and lacrimal bone
         – Use calipers to measure intercanthal (avg 30-31mm) and interpupillary (avg 60–62 mm)
d. Orbital and periorbital clinical complications
   i. Lacrimal apparatus injury (epiphora)
   ii. Extraocular muscle entrapment (ophthalmoplegia)
   iii. Orbital injury:
      - Ruptured globe [26]
      - Sympathetic ophthalmia [27]
      - Retrobulbar hematoma
e. Nasal complications
   i. Nasal obstruction
   ii. Saddle nose deformity
   iii. Septal hematoma → septal necrosis
   iv. CSF rhinorrhea
   v. Oronasal or oroantral fistula
f. Malocclusion and Temporomandibular Joint (TMJ) dysfunction
   i. Open bite, cross bite due to maxillomandibular fracture displacement
   ii. Limited range of motion of mandible due to condylar displacement and/or dislocation, or trauma to temporal bone glenoid fossa
   iii. Dentoalveolar trauma
g. Airway
   i. Tracheal injury
   ii. "Bucket handle" mandible fractures and airway compromise
   iii. Foreign body / dental aspiration

Complications (Following Repair)

1. Infection
   a. Fracture site infection

        i. Mostly in open fractures (i.e. teeth in line of fracture, fractures exposed to outside environment) or due to hardware failure
    b. Hardware failure
        i. Loosening of plates and screws (if bone heated during drilling), tissue trapped between hardware and bone becoming necrotic, excessive tension of bony segments, or breakdown of soft tissue covering hardware
    c. Sinusitis – including mucocele or mucopyocele [28]
        i. Late complication due to incomplete removal of sinus mucosa and inadequate drainage (often seen in frontal sinus fractures)
        ii. Symptoms: headaches, facial/frontal swelling, vision changes, proptosis, rhinorrhea, exophthalmos
        iii. Require imaging and likely surgical management
    d. CSF leak complications [29] - can cause headaches, meningitis, seizures
    e. Cavernous sinus thrombosis [30]
        i. Rare, life-threatening
        ii. Symptoms include severe headache, bilateral proptosis, eye pain, ophthalmoplegia, diplopia, fever, photophobia
        iii. Can be from facial infection, sinusitis, orbital cellulitis, pharyngitis, otitis, or traumatic injury or surgery, especially with thrombophilic disorder
    f. Cerebral venous sinus thrombosis [31]
        i. Cerebral venous sinus thrombosis (CVST) secondary to closed head injury increasingly reported. Most cases of acute posttraumatic CVST associated with skull fracture occurring close to a dural sinus
    g. Carotid-cavernous fistula (CCF) [32]
        i. Rare; due to abnormal communication between carotid artery and cavernous sinus
        ii. May result in:
            - Amaurosis fugax (temporary loss of vision due to lack of blood flow to retina)
            - Significant epistaxis
            - Subarachnoid hemorrhage
2. Fracture site malunion
    a. Malocclusion
        i. Open bite deformity (anterior or posterior)
        ii. Cross bite (transverse deficiency) vs buccal cross bite (transverse excess)
    b. Cosmetic deformity
3. Non-union - fibrous union → fracture site instability
4. TMJ ankylosis [33]
    a. Associated with intracapsular condylar fractures (extracapsular TMJ ankylosis has been rarely reported)
    b. Greatest risk in young patients placed in MMF (mostly ages 11-30)

   c. Increased significantly with greater time lag between injury and fracture treatment
   d. Associated with concomitant mandibular and middle third fractures
5. Periorbital complications
   a. Ophthalmoplegia
   b. Lacrimal apparatus deficits (epiphora)
   c. Ophthalmologic deficits (vision, extraocular movements)
   d. Telecanthus
   e. Lower eyelid malposition [34]
      i. Entropion - eyelid turned inward (inverted), eyelashes rub against globe
      ii. Ectropion - eyelid is turned outward (everted), edge does not contact globe
6. Sensory and motor nerve deficits
   a. Olfaction
   b. Visual acuity
   c. Extraocular muscle movement
   d. Facial nerve function
   e. Hearing
7. Sino-nasal complications
   a. Saddle nose deformity
   b. Nasal septal perforation
   c. Nasal obstruction
   d. Oronasal/oroantral fistula
   e. Sinusitis

Patient Cases

Case 1

17-year-old female who was an unrestrained backseat passenger in a motor vehicle collision was admitted to ICU after being intubated. She is on a ventilator and sedated. Relevant medical history and injuries listed below:

1. PMH: Type 1 diabetes, uveitis, cataracts
   Meds: insulin, methotrexate
   NKDA
2. Injuries:
   a. Frontal subdural hematoma, possible epidural hematoma
   b. Pulmonary contusion
   c. Multiple orthopedic injuries
   d. C-spine: mildly displaced occipital condylar avulsion fracture

Representative images of her scans are shown below (Figure 23.1 and Figure 23.2):

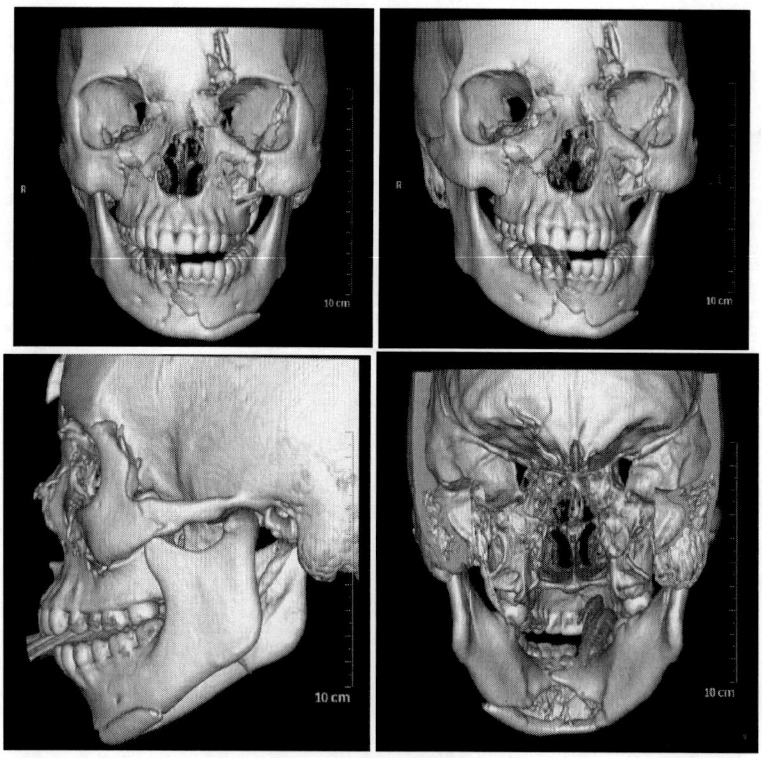

Figure 23.1. Patient case CT images with 3D reconstruction.

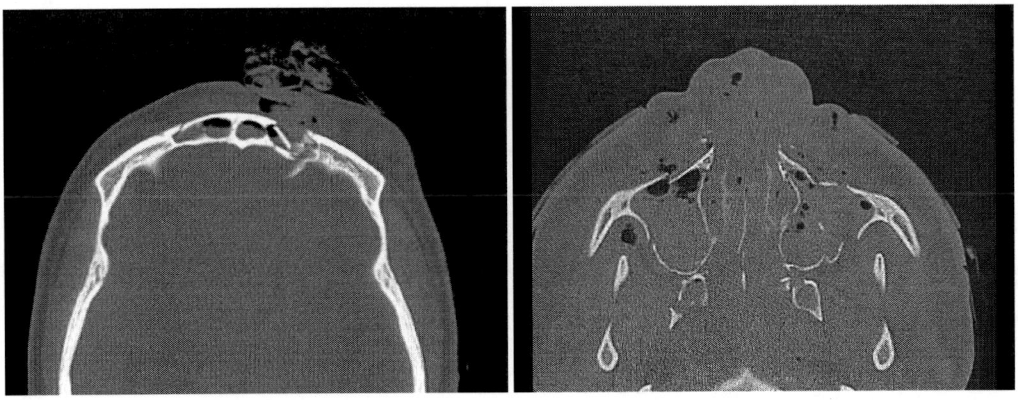

Figure 23.2. Patient case CT images axial cuts.

Questions

Q1. After repair of the patients panfacial fractures, the patient presents for follow up. The patient is noted to have an everted outwardly turned left lower eyelid. What eyelid incisions can be used to repair orbital floor fractures, and which one is most likely to result in ectropion?

A1:

1. Trans conjunctival
2. Subciliary (most likely to result in ectropion)
3. Subtarsal
4. Infraorbital

Q2. You notice the patient has left ophthalmoplegia, ptosis, proptosis, and dilation and fixation of the pupil. Illumination of the left eye results in no left sided pupillary response and right sided pupillary constriction. Illumination of the right eye results in right sided pupillary constriction and no pupillary constriction of the left side. What is the explanation for this type of physical exam finding?

A2:

The patient has left superior orbital fissure syndrome. The loss of consensual light reflex of the left eye suggests ocular motor nerve injury, or an efferent pupillary defect. It is not a traumatic optic neuropathy because optic nerve function in the left eye is intact since there is consensual pupillary reflex. left orbital apex syndrome because the patient's optic nerve is intact.

Q3. During reduction and manipulation of the midfacial fractures using the Rowe disimpaction forceps, the patient's heart rate drops to 35 bpm. What may be a reason for this acute drop in heart rate? How do you correct this?

A3:

Trigeminocardiac Reflex, which occurs due to pressure on eye or stretching of trigeminal nerve which causes fall in blood pressure and decrease in heart rate. Should stop the cause of stimulus and consider anticholinergics like glycopyrrolate and local anesthetics

Q4. Two years after repair of this patient's panfacial fracture, she presents to the ED with a 10-day history of frontal headache, frontal swelling, photophobia, difficulty raising her eyebrows, nasal congestion, mild rhinorrhea with left eye diplopia. What is the most likely diagnosis?

A4:

Frontal sinus mucocele or pyomucocele (if fever, chills, mucopurulent drainage from the nose/sinuses)

Q5. What are common ways to sequence repair of panfacial fractures? Which two fracture types are typically performed last?

A5:

1. Options:
   a. Top → Bottom
   b. Bottom →Top → Middle
2. Typically last to be repaired:
   a. Maxillary / LeFort I
   b. Orbital floor fractures

Q6. When would a submental intubation be utilized?

A6:

When long-term intubation is not planned, but oral is contraindicated due to need for maxillomandibular fixation and nasal is contraindicated due to severe nasal trauma / anterior skull base fractures

Case 2

20 year-old male presents to ED as a full trauma code after a plane crash. The following information was given to you.

1. Arrived intubated, unconscious.
2. PMH: healthy
   Meds: none
   NKDA
   Afebrile
   Vital signs stable

3. Injuries:
   Skull base fracture: mastoid portion of left temporal bone
   Hyoid bone fracture
   Multiple facial fractures
   L2 superior vertebral body fracture
   Open L subtalar joint dislocation
   Closed R great toe proximal phalanx dislocation
   Left fracture of the coccyx

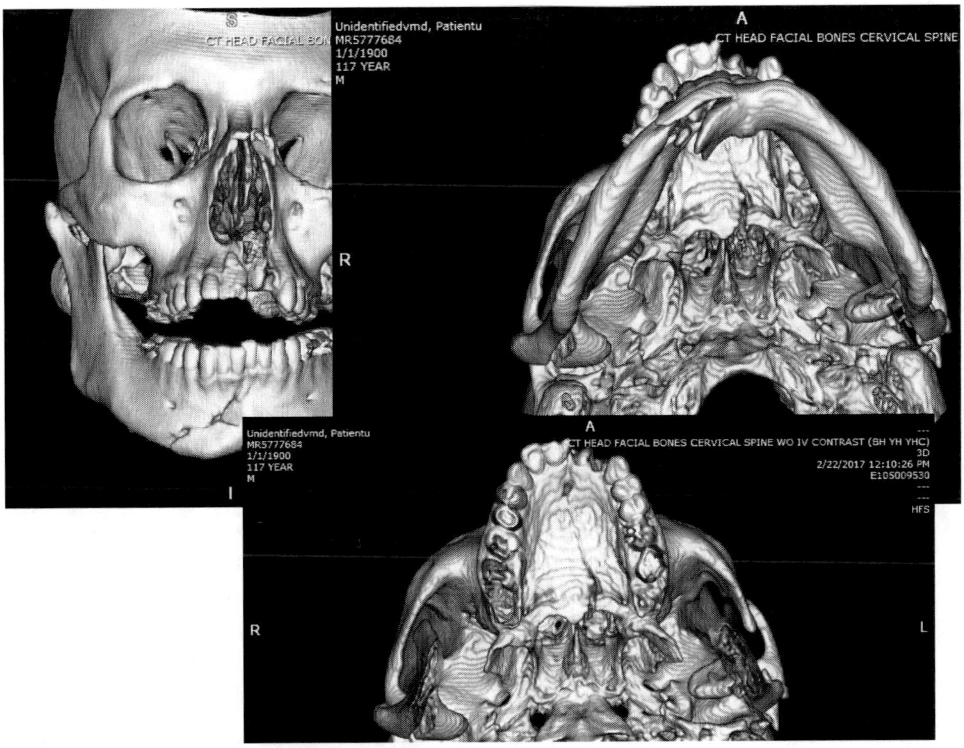

Figure 23.3. Patient case CT images with 3D reconstruction.

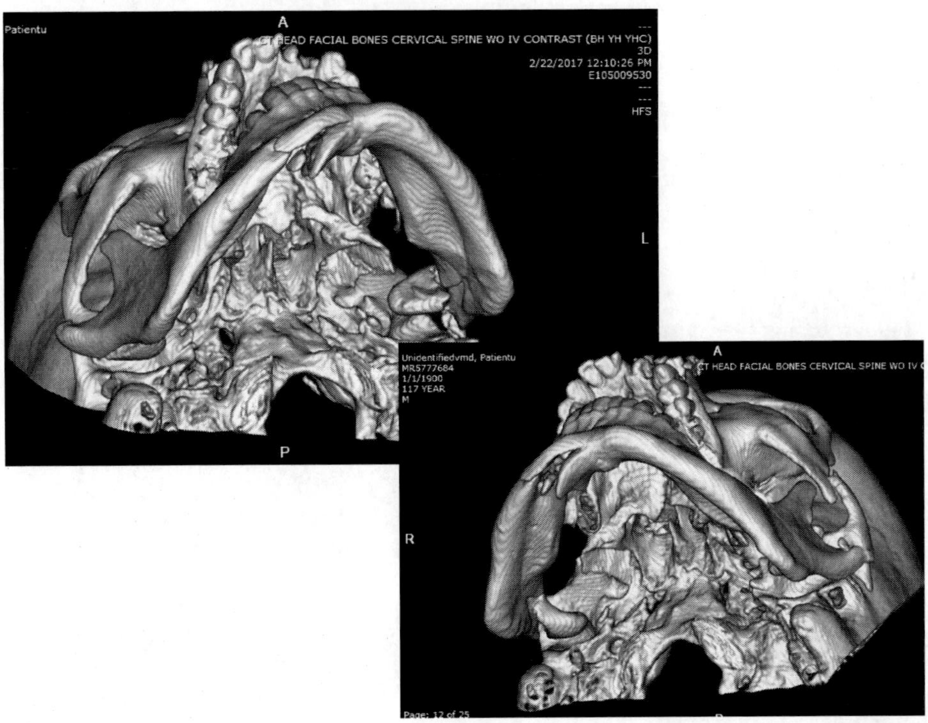

Figure 23.4. (Continued).

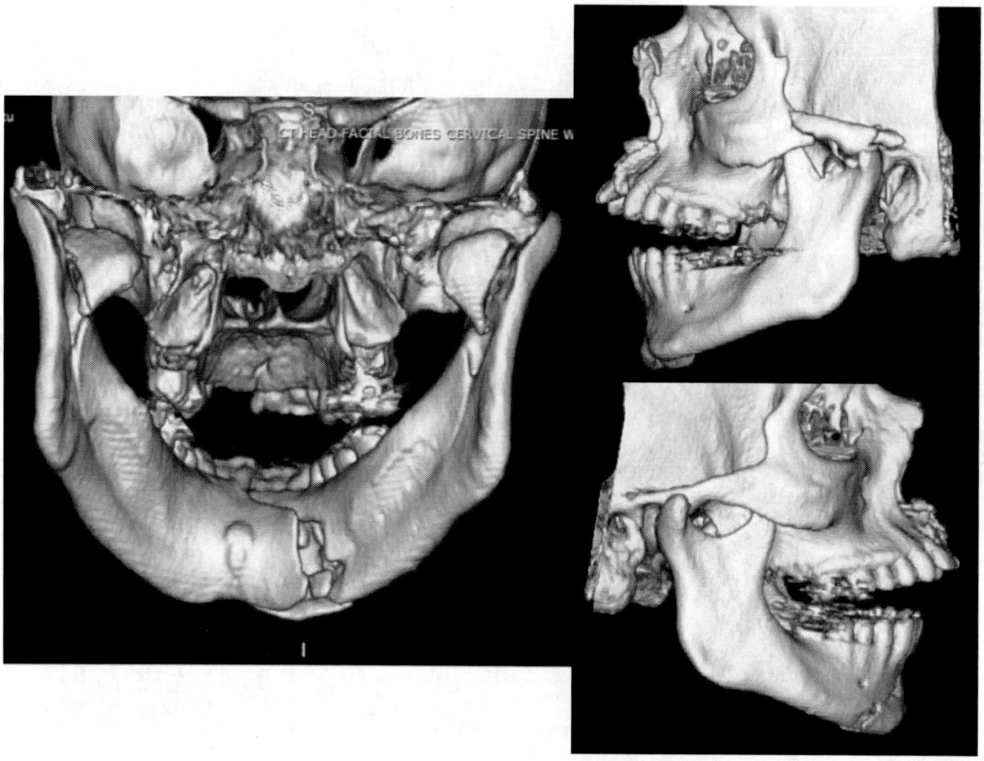

Figure 23.4. Patient case CT images with 3D reconstruction.

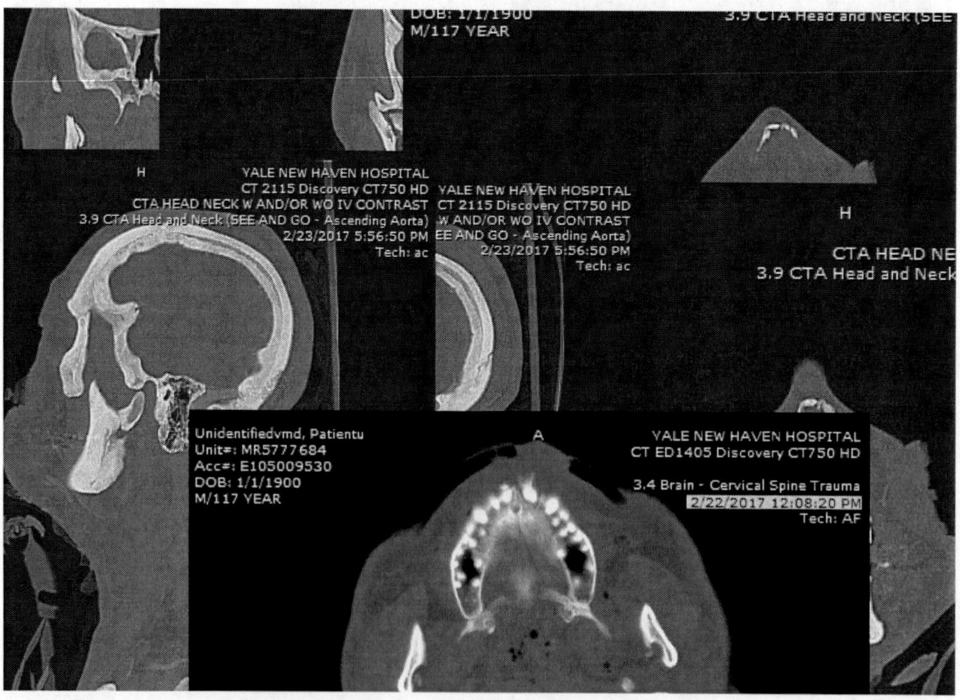

Figure 23.5. Patient case CT images with axial, coronal, and saggital cuts.

Questions

Q1. What are some of the most common concomitant injuries in the panfacial fracture patient?

A1:

1. Head – intracranial bleed, neurological deficits
2. Spine – cervical
3. Abdominal – contusions, bleeds
4. Thoracic - pneumothorax, pulmonary contusions

Q2.What is required for cervical spine clearance in an unconscious patient?

A2:

MRI of the C-spine

Q3.What type of fracture pattern in this patient may have led to lower facial widening?

A3:

1. Mandibular symphysis and bilateral condylar/subcondylar fractures
2. Fractures that contribute to facial widening:
   a. Mandibular widening: symphyseal mandible fractures with or without condyle/ramus fractures
   b. Maxillary widening: mid-palatal fractures
   c. Facial widening: Lateral displacement of the ZMC

Q4. After successful ORIF of this patient's comminuted symphyseal and midfacial fractures and several weeks of MMF, this patient presents several months post treatment to your clinic with progressively worsening trismus to 10 mm and loss of mandibular range of motion. What is the most likely diagnosis?

A4:

1. TMJ ankylosis
   a. Associated with intracapsular condylar fractures
   b. Greatest risk in young patients placed in MMF
   c. Increased significantly with greater time lag between injury and fracture treatment
   d. Associated with concomitant mandibular and middle third fractures

References

[1] Follmar KE, Debruijn M, Baccarani A, Bruno AD, Mukundan S, Erdmann D, Marcus JR. Concomitant injuries in patients with panfacial fractures, *J Trauma* 63:831-835, 2007.

[2] Bellamy JL, Mundinger GS, Flores JM, Reddy SK, Mithani SK, Rodriguez ED, Dorafshar AH. Facial Fractures of the Upper Craniofacial Skeleton Predict Mortality and Occult Intracranial Injury After Blunt Trauma: An Analysis. *Journal of Craniofacial Surgery:* November 2013 - Volume 24 - Issue 6 - p 1922-1926.

[3] Gruss J, Mackinnon S. Complex maxillary fractures: role of buttress reconstruction and immediate bone grafts. *Plast Reconstr Surg* 1986;78:9.

[4] Manson PN, Clark N, Robertson B, Slezak S, Wheatly M, Vander Kolk C, Iliff N. Subunit principles in midface fractures: the importance of sagittal buttresses, soft-tissue reductions, and sequencing treatment of segmental fractures. *Plast Reconstr Surg* 1999;103:1287–1306.

[5] Tung TC, Tseng WS, Chen CT, Lai JP, Chen YR. Acute life-threatening injuries in facial fracture patients: a review of 1,025 patients. *J Trauma* 2000;49(03):420–424.

[6] Wang L, Lee TS, Wang W, Yi DI, Sokoya M, Ducic Y. Surgical Management of Panfacial Fractures. *Facial Plastic Surgery*. Vol 35. No. 6/2019.

[7] William Curtis, MD, DMD, Bruce B. Horswell, MD, DDS, MS. Panfacial Fractures: An Approach to Management. *Oral Maxillofacial Surg Clin N Am* 25 (2013) 649–660.

[8] Dongmei He, DDS, MD, PhD, Yi Zhang, DDS, MD, PhD, and Edward Ellis III, DDS, MS. Panfacial Fractures: Analysis of 33 Cases Treated Late. *J Oral Maxillofac Surg* 65:2459-2465, 2007.

[9] Gruss JS, Bubak PJ, Egbert MA: Craniofacial fractures: an algorithm to optimize results, *Clin Plast Surg* 19:195, 1992.

[10] Kelly KJ, Manson PN, Vander Kolk CA, Markowitz BL, Dunham CM, Rumley TO, Crawley WA.Sequencing LeFort fracture treatment (organization of treatment for a panfacial fracture), *J Craniofacial Surg* 1:168-178, 1990.

[11] Kausar Ali, B, Salvatore C. Lettieri. Management of Panfacial Fractures. *Seminars in Plastic Surgery* Vol. 31 No. 2/2017.

[12] Degala S, Sundar SS, Mamata KS. A Comparative Prospective Study of Two Different Treatment Sequences i.e. Bottom Up–Inside Out and Topdown Outside in, in the Treatment of Panfacial Fractures. *J. Maxillofac. Oral Surg* (Oct-Dec 2015) 14(4)986-994.

[13] Cuddy K, Khatib B, Bell RB, Cheng A, Patel A, Amundson M, Dierks EJ. Use of Intraoperative Computed Tomography in Craniomaxillofacial Trauma Surgery. *J Oral Maxillofac Surg* 76:1016-1025, 2018.

[14] Ellis, E. Sequencing treatment for naso-orbito-ethmoid fractures. *J Oral Maxillofac Surg.* Volume 51, Issue 5. May 1993. 543-558.

[15] Markowitz BL, Manson PN, Sargent L, Vander Kolk CA, Yaremchuk M, Glassman D, Crawley WA. Management of the medial canthal tendon in nasoethmoid orbital fractures: the importance of the central fragment in classification and treatment, *Plast Reconstr Surg* 87:843-853, 1991.

[16] Gruss JS: Naso-ethmoid-orbital fractures: classification and role of primary bone grafting, *Plast Reconstr Surg* 75:303-315, 1985.

[17] Phillips JH, Forrest CR, Gruss JS. Current concepts in the use of bone grafts in facial fractures. Basic science considerations. *Clin Plast Surg.* 1992;19:41-58.

[18] Herford AS. Panfacial-Trauma. pg 354-360. *Current Therapy in Oral and Maxillofacial Surgery.* Bagheri SC, Bell RB, Khan HA. Elsevier Saunders. St. Louis, MS; 2012.

[19] Badakere A, Patil-Chhablani P. Orbital Apex Syndrome: A Review. *Eye Brain*. 2019;11:63-72. Published 2019 Dec 12. doi:10.2147/EB.S180190.

[20] Howell J, Costanzo RM, Reiter ER. Head trauma and olfactory function. *World J Otorhinolaryngol Head Neck Surg*. 2018;4(1):39-45. Published 2018 Mar 14. doi:10.1016/j.wjorl.2018.02.001

[21] Chen CT, Chen YR. Traumatic superior orbital fissure syndrome: current management. *Craniomaxillofac Trauma Reconstr*. 2010;3(1):9-16. doi:10.1055/s-0030-1249369.

[22] D.H. McDougal, P.D.R. Gamlin,1.26 - Pupillary Control Pathways, Editor(s): Richard H. Masland, Thomas D. Albright, Thomas D. Albright, Richard H. Masland, Peter Dallos, Donata Oertel, Stuart

Firestein, Gary K. Beauchamp, M. Catherine Bushnell, Allan I. Basbaum, Jon H. Kaas, Esther P. Gardner, *The Senses: A Comprehensive Reference*, Academic Press, 2008, Pages 521-536.

[23] Bhattacharjee A, Rajaram P, Khatua A, Rudresh KB, Krishnamurthy PB. Two Episodes of Trigeminocardiac Reflex During a Pan facial Fracture Surgery, a Rare Phenomenon - Case Report and Review of Literature. *J Clin Diagn Res.* 2017;11(9):ZD01-ZD03. doi:10.7860/JCDR/2017/29781.10570.

[24] Pamuk AE, Pamuk G, Bajin MD, Yildiz FG, Sennaroğlu L. Traumatic Facial and Vestibulocochlear Nerve Injury in The Internal Acoustic Canal in The Absence of A Temporal Bone Fracture. *J Int Adv Otol.* 2018;14(2):330-333. doi:10.5152/iao.2018.4782.

[25] Mark Engelstad, Chapter 42 - Naso-Orbito-Ethmoid Fractures, Editor(s): Shahrokh C. Bagheri, R. Bryan Bell, Husain Ali Khan, *Current Therapy In Oral and Maxillofacial Surgery*, W.B. Saunders, 2012, Pages 339-346.

[26] Blair K, Alhadi SA, Czyz CN. Globe Rupture. [Updated 2022 Jan 2]. In: *StatPearls* [Internet]. Treasure Island (FL): StatPearls Publishing; 2022 Jan.

[27] Arevalo JF, Garcia RA, Al-Dhibi HA, Sanchez JG, Suarez-Tata L. Update on sympathetic ophthalmia. *Middle East Afr J Ophthalmol.* 2012;19(1):13-21. doi:10.4103/0974-9233.92111.

[28] EuDaly M, Kraus CK. Frontal Mucocele following Previous Facial Trauma with Hardware Reconstruction. *Case Rep Emerg Med.* 2016;2016:4236421. doi:10.1155/2016/4236421.

[29] Oh JW, Kim SH, Whang K. Traumatic Cerebrospinal Fluid Leak: Diagnosis and Management. *Korean J Neurotrauma.* 2017;13(2):63-67. doi:10.13004/kjnt.2017.13.2.63.

[30] Plewa MC, Tadi P, Gupta M. Cavernous Sinus Thrombosis. [Updated 2021 Nov 7]. In: *StatPearls* [Internet]. Treasure Island (FL): StatPearls Publishing; 2022 Jan.

[31] Ghuman MS, Salunke P, Sahoo SK, Kaur S. Cerebral venous sinus thrombosis in closed head trauma: A call to look beyond fractures and hematomas!. *J Emerg Trauma Shock.* 2016;9(1):37-38. doi:10.4103/0974-2700.173865.

[32] de Moraes SL, de Paula Afonso AM, Dos Santos RG, Mattos RP, Duarte BG. Carotid-Cavernous Fistula as a Complication of Panfacial Fracture: Case Report 11 Years after the Surgery. *Craniomaxillofac Trauma Reconstr.* 2017;10(1):66-72. doi:10.1055/s-0036-1582458.

[33] Anyanechi CE. Temporomandibular joint ankylosis caused by condylar fractures: a retrospective analysis of cases at an urban teaching hospital in Nigeria. *Int J Oral Maxillofac Surg.* 2015 Aug;44(8):1027-33. doi: 10.1016/j.ijom.2015.05.003. Epub 2015 May 23. PMID: 26008733.

[34] Ridgway EB, Chen C, Colakoglu S, Gautam S, Lee BT. The incidence of lower eyelid malposition after facial fracture repair: a retrospective study and meta-analysis comparing subtarsal, subciliary, and transconjunctival incisions. *Plast Reconstr Surg.* 2009 Nov;124(5):1578-1586.

Practice Guidelines – Trauma

When a particular set of basic criteria is met, then the Qualified Options for treatment, testing, or management below are reasonable and justifiable recommendations.

- When the patient presents with Facial Fractures (All types), then Imaging (e.g., CT, MRI, Xray, US), trauma assessment including airway management are Qualified Options.
- When the patient presents with Mandible Fractures, then Closed and/or open treatment with or without interdental fixation or dental extraction/stabilization, implant/graft placement are Qualified Options.
- When the patient presents with ZMC Fractures, then Closed and/or open treatment with or without implant/graft placement are Qualified Options.
- When the patient presents with NOE Complex Fractures, then Closed and/or open treatment with or without implant/graft placement, septorhinoplasty, eyelid reconstruction, ophthalmology consult are Qualified Options.
- When the patient presents with Orbital Fractures (All types), then Closed and/or open treatment with or without implant/graft placement, eyelid reconstruction, ophthalmology consult are Qualified Options.
- When the patient presents with Frontal Sinus Fractures (All types), then Closed and/or open treatment with or without implant/graft placement, open or endoscopic frontal sinus surgery, obliteration or cranialization, neurosurgery consult are Qualified Options.
- When the patient presents with Pan-Facial Fractures (All types), then Closed and/or open treatment with or without interdental fixation or dental extraction/stabilization, implant/graft placement, eyelid reconstruction, open or endoscopic sinus surgery are Qualified Options.
- When the patient presents with Facial Fractures (Any types), then Dentistry or oral maxillofacial involvement, ophthalmology involvement, neurology or neurosurgery involvement, tracheostomy, soft tissue trauma repair or flaps, endoscopic techniques, virtual surgical planning with or without patient-specific products, speech and language pathology involvement, trauma/surgery team involvement are Qualified Options.

Patient Characteristics	**Qualified Option(s)**
Facial Fractures (All types)	Imaging (e.g., CT, MRI, Xray, US), trauma assessment including airway management
Mandible Fractures	Closed and/or open treatment with or without interdental fixation or dental extraction/stabilization, implant/graft placement
ZMC Fractures	Closed and/or open treatment with or without implant/graft placement

NOE Complex Fractures	Closed and/or open treatment with or without implant/graft placement, septorhinoplasty, eyelid reconstruction, ophthalmology consult
Orbital Fractures	Closed and/or open treatment with or without implant/graft placement, eyelid reconstruction, ophthalmology consult
Frontal Sinus Fractures	Closed and/or open treatment with or without implant/graft placement, open or endoscopic frontal sinus surgery, obliteration or cranialization, neurosurgery consult
Pan-Facial Fractures	Closed and/or open treatment with or without interdental fixation or dental extraction/stabilization, implant/graft placement, eyelid reconstruction, open or endoscopic sinus surgery
Facial Fractures (Any type)	Dentistry or oral maxillofacial involvement, ophthalmology involvement, neurology or neurosurgery involvement, tracheostomy, soft tissue trauma repair or flaps, endoscopic techniques, virtual surgical planning with or without patient-specific products, speech and language pathology involvement, trauma/surgery team involvement

Part 5. Facial Nerve Rehabilitation

Chapter 24

Facial Paralysis

Liliana Ein, MD
and Tessa A. Hadlock, MD

Introduction

Facial Nerve Anatomy

1. Upper motor neurons
    a. Precentral gyrus: voluntary facial motor function
    b. Frontotemporal cerebral cortex, limbic and basal ganglion: involuntary expressions
2. Facial motor nucleus: ventral aspect of caudal pons
    a. Dorsal portion
        i. Neuronal cell bodies that control upper third of facc
        ii. Receives bilateral upper motor neuron input
    b. Ventral portion
        i. Controls lower two-thirds of face
        ii. Receives only crossed motor neuron input
3. Cisternal segment of facial nerve (FN):
    a. Spans 17 to 24mm between lateral brainstem (near cerebellopontine junction) and porus acousticus
    b. Devoid of epineurium
4. Meatal segment of FN:
    a. Spans 8-10mm between porus acousticus and meatal foramen
    b. FN occupies anterosuperior quadrant of internal auditory canal (IAC)
    c. Meatal foramen
        i. Entrance to fallopian canal, narrowest dimension
        ii. Nerve most susceptible to injury from trauma or inflammation at this point
5. Labyrinthine segment of FN (within fallopian canal):
    a. Spans 3-5mm between fundus of IAC to distal portion of geniculate ganglion
    b. Greater superficial petrosal nerve: branches from geniculate ganglion, carries pre-ganglionic parasympathetic secretory fibers to nose, lacrimal gland, palate
6. Tympanic or horizontal segment of FN (within fallopian canal):
    a. Spans 8-11mm between distal geniculate ganglion (turns posteriorly at first genu) to pyramidal eminence (turns inferiorly at second genu)

In: Essential Facial Plastic and Reconstructive Surgery. Volume 1 ISBN: 979-8-89113-306-8
Editors: Yan Ho Lee and Ira Papel

© 2024 Nova Science Publishers, Inc.

    b. Nerve to stapedius muscle emerges near second genu
7. Mastoid or vertical segment of FN (within fallopian canal):
    a. Spans 10-14mm between second genu and stylomastoid foramen
    b. Chorda tympani: preganglionic parasympathetic secretory fibers of submandibular and sublingual glands and sensory taste fibers from anterior two-thirds of tongue
8. Extratemporal portion of FN:
    a. Exits from stylomastoid foramen
    b. Digastric branch to posterior belly of digastric muscle
    c. Motor branch to stylohyoid muscle
    d. Posterior auricular branch: motor fibers to superior and posterior auricular muscles and occipitalis muscles
    e. Pes anserinus: Splits main trunk into upper and lower division, endpoints are muscles of facial expression. NOTE: there is significant arborization and redundancy among neighboring territories (particularly in midface)
        i. Temporal – occipitofrontalis, orbicularis oculi
        ii. Zygomatic – orbicularis oculi, zygomaticus major and minor
        iii. Buccal – buccinator, levator labii superioris, nasalis, risorius
        iv. Marginal mandibular – depressor anguli oris, orbicularis oris, mentalis, depressor labii inferioris
        v. Cervical – depressor labii inferioris, platysma

Classification of Facial Palsy

1. Flaccid facial palsy (FFP)
    a. Caused by decreased neural input to facial musculature leading to absence of facial movement and tone
    b. May result from denervation, congenital absence, muscle resection, myopathy
    c. Functional deficits see Table 24.1
2. Synkinetic/hypertonic facial palsy (SFP): also known as non-flaccid facial palsy (NFFP)
    a. Results from aberrant neural regeneration where axonal input into facial muscles does not match intended muscle target
    b. Synkinesis: involuntary facial movement co-occurring with voluntary or spontaneous expression
    c. Develops 6 to 18 months after in-continuity facial nerve insults (e.g., Bell's palsy, Ramsay Hunt syndrome, Lyme disease, autoimmune disease, some cases of vestibular schwannoma surgery, or following some facial nerve repairs or nerve transfers)
    d. Functional deficits see Table 24.1
    e. Combination of facial synkinesis, facial muscle rigidity and spasms, and gustatory epiphora or rhinorrhea is termed post-paralytic facial syndrome [1]
3. Mixed facial palsy
    a. Elements of both FFP and SFP

b. Further investigation needed to rule out facial nerve tumor displaying recurrent cycles of degeneration/regeneration

Table 24.1. Functional deficits by facial zone in patients with facial palsy

	Flaccid facial palsy (FFP)	Synkinetic/hypertonic facial palsy (SFP)
Upper facial zone	Resting brow malposition Loss of blink reflex and voluntary eye closure Lacrimal gland hypofunction Lower eyelid ptosis or ectropion	Brow malposition Involuntary eye closure when smiling or pursing lips (ocular synkinesis) Gustatory epiphora (Bogorad syndrome or crocodile tears)
Central facial zone	Unilateral nasal valve collapse Upper lip ptosis Lack of oral commissure excursion with smile Oral incompetence Articulation issues	Hyperprominent nasolabial fold Restricted oral commissure movement Tightness/pain in midface Gustatory rhinorrhea
Lower facial zone	Oral incompetence Articulation issues	Mentalis dimpling Platysmal synkinesis

Microanatomical Nerve Injury Classification

1. Sunderland classification [2]
   a. Level 1 injury:
      i. No microanatomic disruption
      ii. Simple temporary dysfunction of membrane sodium channels → transient inability of nerve to transmit impulses
   b. Level 2 injury:
      i. Axons are disrupted but their individual endoneurial channels are not
      ii. Little to no axonal misrouting when regeneration occurs
   c. Level 3 injury:
      i. Endoneurial sheaths are violated, perineurium is intact
      ii. Recovery occurs over months with some synkinesis
   d. Level 4 injury:
      i. Total perineurial disruption, only outer epineural sheath is intact
      ii. Spontaneous recovery is generally poor
   e. Level 5 injury:
      i. Total anatomic disruption, including epineurium
      ii. No spontaneous recovery without surgical intervention

Patient Evaluation

1. Patient intake and outcomes tracking [3]

a. Patient-reported quality of life outcomes
    i. Facial disability index (FDI)
    ii. Facial clinimetric evaluation scale (FaCE): thought to assess psychometric parameters more accurately than FDI
    iii. Synkinesis assessment questionnaire (SAQ): measures patient perception of synkinesis, used in conjunction with FDI or FaCE
b. Clinician-graded outcomes
    i. House-Brackmann (HB) scale: 6-point scale created for categorizing overall facial function after surgery
        - Can measure gross change over time
        - Accounts for synkinesis (HB 3 or 4)
    ii. Sunnybrook facial grading scale: assesses resting symmetry, symmetry of voluntary movement, and synkinesis
    iii. Electronic facial paralysis assessment tool (eFACE): extensively validated tool measuring static, dynamic, and synkinesis parameters
c. Objective assessment tools
    i. Standardized photographs and videos
        - Facial nerve series: rest, eyebrow elevation, gentle eye closure, tight eye closure, best smile, biggest smile, pucker like "ooo", show bottom teeth like "eee"
        - Video of facial expressions and spontaneous smile assay
    ii. Emotrics: analyzes photographs and creates automated calculations of many facial features (e.g., oral commissure excursion, palpebral fissure width)

2. Physical examination should include a zonal approach to the paralyzed face (Figure 24.1)

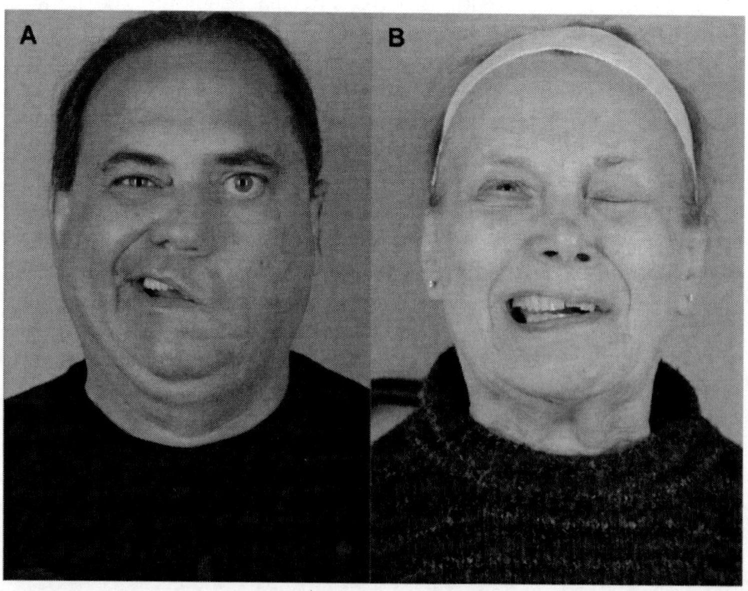

Figure 24.1. Left facial palsy: A) flaccid facial paralysis (FFP) B) synkinetic/hypertonic facial paralysis (SFP).

a. Upper facial zone:
    i. Brow: ptotic, balanced or paradoxically hyper-elevated
    ii. Upper eyelid: lagophthalmos, hypertonicity or synkinesis
    iii. Lower eyelid: ectropion, hypertonicity or synkinesis
b. Central facial zone:
    i. External nasal valve: collapsed, balanced, hypercontracted
    ii. Nasolabial fold: effaced, balanced, prominent
    iii. Upper lip: ptotic, balanced
    iv. Oral commissure: excursion (evaluate for meaningful movement)
c. Lower facial zone:
    i. Lower lip: superiorly malpositioned, ptotic, atrophied
    ii. Mentalis: synkinesis
    iii. Platysma: synkinesis

Diagnostic Approach

1. Rapid onset (within 72 hours) facial paralysis (FP) [4]
    a. If unilateral FP, most common diagnosis is Bell's palsy = diagnosis of exclusion
        i. History and physical exam imperative to rule out other causes, which may include:
            - Other infectious causes including otitis media, parotitis, meningitis, Ramsay Hunt, zoster sine herpete, Lyme disease, mononucleosis, cytomegalovirus, HIV, poliomyelitis, syphilis, leprosy, tuberculosis
            - Cerebrovascular accident
            - Autoimmune diseases: sarcoidosis, rheumatoid arthritis, lupus, Sjogren's syndrome, myasthenia gravis, Wegener's granulomatosis, IgG4 disease
            - Neoplasm: lymphoma, leukemia, parotid malignancy, facial nerve schwannoma, geniculate ganglion hemangioma, temporal bone neoplasm, cavernous brainstem hemangioma, intracranial mass
        ii. General recommendation: if no significant improvement in 3 months, should consider additional workup
    b. If bilateral acute onset FP, differential diagnosis includes:
        i. Infectious: Lyme disease, mononucleosis, cytomegalovirus, meningitis, HIV, polio, syphilis, leprosy, tuberculosis, botulism
        ii. Systemic / autoimmune: Guillain-Barre syndrome, sarcoidosis, rheumatoid arthritis, Wegener's granulomatosis
        iii. Neoplasm: lymphoma, leukemia
        iv. Brainstem cerebrovascular accident
    c. Second episode of acute FP requires more thorough evaluation and work-up
        i. If segmental paralysis, obtain MRI brain to rule out multiple sclerosis

            ii. If same side as prior episode, obtain MRI internal auditory canal to evaluate for tumor affecting cranial nerve (CN) VII
            iii. If negative MRI IAC or if contralateral face involved, then prompt hematologic work up for autoimmune/systemic disease
2. Facial palsy present at birth
    a. If synkinesis develops over months, likely due to birth trauma
    b. If synkinesis is absent at 6 months old (with persistent paralysis), then likely congenital cause
3. Insidious onset facial palsy
    a. Obtain CT temporal bone and parotid bed with contrast
        i. If positive for lesion, obtain biopsy
        ii. If negative, then obtain MRI brain and IAC with contrast
        iii. If both CT and MRI negative AND risk factors or history of cancer, then consider PET/CT or CN VII biopsy to rule out malignancy
        iv. If both CT and MRI negative and NO risk factors or history of cancer, then follow up in 6 months. If stable, keep following. If worse, repeat imaging.

Management of Facial Palsy

1. Acute episode of facial palsy (non-traumatic)
    a. Prednisone
        i. Dosage: 60mg PO daily for 5 days, followed by taper of 50mg on day 6, then 40 mg on day 7, 30mg on day 8, 20mg on day 9, and 10mg on day 10
        ii. Should be initiated within 14 days of onset
    b. Valcyclovir
        i. Dosage: 500mg PO BID for 7 days
        ii. Should be initiated within 14 days of onset
    c. Doxycycline 100mg PO BID for 21 days if Lyme disease suspected
    d. Audiogram for subjective hearing loss
    e. Eye care: ophthalmic lubrication at night, preservative free artificial tears PRN during day, tape eye closed at night, upper eyelid stretching BID
        i. If age >60 years or diabetes, Ramsay Hunt, Lyme, poor Bell's phenomenon, corneal sensation deficit, or persistent ocular discomfort, then consider eyelid weight placement
        ii. If age <60 years and non-diabetic and uncomplicated Bell's palsy, then observe for 10 weeks. If no improvement, then consider eyelid weight placement
    f. If patient presents with complete paralysis within 14 days of onset, consider electrodiagnostic testing for CN VII decompression [5]
        i. Electroneuronography (ENoG): measures facial nerve integrity
            - Cannot be done within 3 days of onset due to time it takes for Wallerian degeneration

- If <90% degeneration, repeat ENoG every 3 days until day 14 or resolution
- If >90% degeneration, perform voluntary electromyography (EMG) of orbicularis oculi and oris

ii. Electromyography (EMG): measures spontaneous and voluntary muscle potentials
- If motor units present, repeat ENoG every 3 days until day 14 or resolution
- If motor units absent, consider CN VII decompression via middle cranial fossa approach

2. Traumatic facial palsy
   a. Eye care for all patients
   b. If delayed onset complete paralysis, incomplete paralysis, or immediate onset with CN VII known to be intact, then treat with valacyclovir and prednisone 10-day high dose taper and follow up in 3 months
   c. If immediate onset and CN VII integrity is unknown or suspected cut and patient presents within 4-6 months of onset, then consider electrodiagnostic testing for possible CN VII exploration/decompression/repair
      i. Timing of exploration is controversial but earlier intervention results in improved outcomes
      ii. If index of suspicion is high, then exploration within 72 hours (without electrodiagnostic testing) should be considered as use of a nerve stimulator intraoperatively may facilitate location of distal nerve stump
   d. Facial nerve exploration:
      i. Both anterograde and retrograde dissection is often utilized
      ii. Mastoidectomy should be considered if injury is centered around stylomastoid foramen
      iii. If CN VII anatomically intact, or disrupted distal to lateral canthus, no repair is necessary. May consider external neurolysis (i.e., decompression of nerve) if significant swelling is present
      iv. If >50% of CN VII diameter disrupted or complete transection, resect the injured segment and repair
         - If tensionless coaptation possible, then primary repair with 10-0 Nylon
         - If tension present, then interposition graft should be utilized

Facial Reanimation Procedures

1. Nerve repair and nerve grafting
   a. First line therapy for neural discontinuity
   b. Nerve endings are debrided of all devitalized tissue and approximated by coaptation of epineurial sheath

i. Most proximal region of FN amenable to suturing is the distal vertical segment
ii. Defects in horizontal segment may be addressed by simple approximation with fibrin glue, collagen, or hemostatic agents

c. Nerve grafting
i. Indication: when tenson-free neurorrhaphy is not possible
ii. Donor grafts:
- Greater auricular nerve
  - Suitable for nerve gaps under 6-8cm
  - Convenient location; adequate diameter and caliber
  - Contraindicated in presence of neurotrophic malignancy
- Ansa cervicalis (descendens hypoglossi):
  - Suitable for nerve gaps under 6-8cm
  - Theoretical advantage being a motor graft
- Sural nerve:
  - Can yield up to 30cm in length
  - Harvested via a short incision adjacent to the lateral malleolus through stair-step incisions, minimally invasive stripping technique, or using endoscopic equipment
- Medial antebrachial nerve: ideal for total nerve reconstruction due to multiple branching pattern

iii. Quality and quantity of axonal regrowth best when repair is immediate
iv. Factors that lead to poor recovery: wound disruption, infection, tension at site of coaptation
v. Timing of expected movement: within 6-12 months, may continue for several years

2. Nerve substitution techniques (Table 24.2)
a. Also known as nerve transfers, or re-innervation techniques [6, 7]
b. Provide neural input to facial muscles via distal FN branches using motor nerves other than the native FN
c. Indication: when proximal FN stump is unavailable but distal FN and facial musculature are present and receptive to reinnervation (within 2 years from denervation)
i. Resection of skull base tumor requiring resection of FN at or near brainstem (neurorrhaphy is technically infeasible in this situation) → immediate nerve transfer indicated
ii. When no discernible facial function is noted 6-12 months following skull base surgery, intracranial injury, or traumatic facial paralysis (and FN is believed to be anatomically intact)

Table 24.2. Nerve substitutions techniques.

Nerve Transfer	Goal	Timing	Contraindications	Expected outcome	Complications
Hypoglossal-Facial Nerve Transfer (CN XII-VII) *Performed to main trunk FN*	Restore facial tone	Immediate if FN resected at brainstem 12 months after denervation if FN thought to be anatomically intact (facial EMG not required; clinical exam showing lack of obvious recovery is sufficient)	Patients likely to develop other cranial neuropathies (i.e. neurofibromatosis type 2) Patients with ipsilateral CN X deficit (combined CN X and XII deficit → profound dysphagia)	Good resting tone in about 90% of patients Deliberate facial movement with intentional manipulation of the tongue may be achieved – results are variable	Hemi-tongue weakness, dysphagia, dysarthria (less risk with end-to-side neurorrhaphy on hypoglossal) Mass movements/synkinesis (less risk with only 50% of hypoglossal fibers used)
Masseteric-to-Facial Nerve Transfer (CN V-VII) *Performed to distal zygomatico-buccal branch*	Restore volitional control of smile	At time of tumor extirpation if preoperative paralysis present 6 months after denervation if completely flaccid and FN thought to be anatomically intact**	Lack of masseter bulge on affected side (i.e. from trauma, surgical resection, tumor) Can consider staged cross masseteric graft if contralateral side is intact	Powerful, voluntary smile with no resting tone Expected movement within 3-5 months	Hollowing of the cheek (can be prevented by preserving the superomedial branch of nerve-to-masseter)
Cross Facial Nerve Graft (CN VII-VII) *Performed to distal facial nerve branch (or to power gracilis muscle via obturator nerve)*	Restore involuntary control of smile, eye, or lower lip depression	Direct coaptation to branches of the paralyzed face should be done within 3 months of proximal FN sacrifice or in the presence of a baby-sitter nerve transfer 6 to 9 months prior to planned muscle transfer	Bilateral facial weakness	Spontaneous blink and emotive smile	Suboptimal results due to lack of power/number of axons reaching the contralateral face Facial weakness of unaffected side – very unlikely if nerve is taken distal enough

CN = cranial nerve.

**based on data that suggests complete flaccidity after 6 months portends very poor smile prognosis [8]

3. Muscle transfer (regional or free)
    a. Indication: when distal FN or facial musculature has atrophied or become significantly fibrotic
    b. Temporalis muscle transfer
        i. Goal: dynamic smile reanimation
        ii. Timing: usually at least 2 years after initial insult when facial muscles are no longer receptive to reinnervation
        iii. Contraindications:
            - Prior neurotologic procedure that compromised the temporalis muscle or its nerve or vascular supply
            - Congenital syndrome or tumor that also affects the motor branch of trigeminal nerve
            - Severe atrophy of the muscle, such as in edentulous patients
        iv. Classic technique [9]: 1.5cm wide strip of temporalis muscle and underlying pericranium is elevated and reflected over the zygomatic arch into midface for attachment to orbicularis oris at modiolus
        v. Minimally invasive temporalis tendon transfer [10]: tendinous attachment of the temporalis muscle is transferred from coronoid process to modiolus and NLF area
        vi. Complications:
            - Over-lateralization of oral commissure
            - Contour deformity (mainly with classic technique where temporalis muscle is reflected over zygomatic arch)
        vii. Expected outcome: bite driven smile, usually with less oral commissure excursion than free muscle
    c. Other muscle transfers:
        i. Masseter muscle transfer
            - Previously used to provide oral commissure excursion by freeing the muscular attachments from mandible and transferring to oral commissure
            - Creates a more lateral vector pull and results in significant contour deficit so now obsolete
        ii. Digastric muscle transfer
            - Anterior belly and tendon are freed from posterior belly and surrounding structures for transfer to lower lip via attachment to inferior border of orbicularis oris
            - May be used for isolated marginal mandibular nerve injuries
    d. Gracilis free muscle transfer [11, 12]
        i. Goal: dynamic smile reanimation – can be voluntary or spontaneous
        ii. Timing:
            - Immediate if facial musculature resected
            - Around age 6 if congenital paralysis
            - Any time after denervation atrophy takes place (usually 2 years after initial insult)

- May be performed as single stage or two stages (6-9 month waiting period)
  - Single stage: muscle is driven by masseteric nerve
  - Two stages: muscle is powered by cross-facial graft or dually innervated by both cross face and masseteric nerve

iii. Contraindication: patients with significant medical comorbidities making them extremely high surgical risk or with poor survival prognosis

iv. Complications:
- Hematoma or vascular compromise – usually seen within first 24 hours on doppler exam or ultrasound
- Excessive midface bulk or over-lateralization of muscle, failure to achieve movement

v. Expected outcome: movement is expected between 3-4 months after masseteric driven muscle and 9-12 months after cross face driven muscle

e. Alternative options for free muscle
   i. Pectoralis minor, latissimus dorsi, serratus anterior
   ii. Choice is based on surgeon experience

4. Static and adjunctive facial reanimation procedures
   a. Best used in combination with dynamic approaches
   b. Zonal approach to the face helps to prevent overlooking any specific area (Table 24.3)
   c. Neuromuscular retraining via physical therapy

Table 24.3. Static and adjunctive facial reanimation procedures by facial zone

	Static and adjunctive facial reanimation procedures
Upper facial zone *forehead, eyebrow, upper and lower eyelid*	Contralateral frontalis chemodenervation Ipsilateral brow ptosis correction Upper eyelid thin profile platinum weight Lower eyelid tightening with tarsorrhaphy, lateral tarsal strip, and tensor fascia lata suspension
Central facial zone *external nasal valve (ENV), nasolabial fold (NLF), philtrum, upper lip, oral commissure*	Tensor fascia lata (FL) suspension: multiple ribbons of FL inset medially to External Nasal Valve (nasal accessory cartilage), philtrum (subdermal), oral commissure (modiolus), and/or NLF (subdermal) and laterally to temporalis fascia under neutral tension Suture-based static suspension for creation of NLF can be performed in office under local anesthesia if unable to undergo general anesthesia
Lower facial zone *lower lip, neck*	Lower lip ptosis: wedge resection or tensor fascia lata suspension Contralateral chemodenervation of depressor labii inferioris

Summary Points

1. Clinicians treating facial palsy should have a thorough understanding of facial nerve anatomy and the wide variety of FP etiologies
2. Facial palsy is classified as either flaccid (FFP), synkinetic/hypertonic (SFP), or mixed
3. A systematic approach to treating FP is mandatory with zonal assessment of the face and multimodality treatment, including physical therapy, chemodenervation, and surgery [13]

Patient Case

40-year-old man presents to clinic with history of a very large left vestibular schwannoma. He underwent surgical resection 12 months ago, where he awoke after surgery with left facial weakness and hypoesthesia. He has not noted any changes in function over the past 12 months. (Figure 24.2)

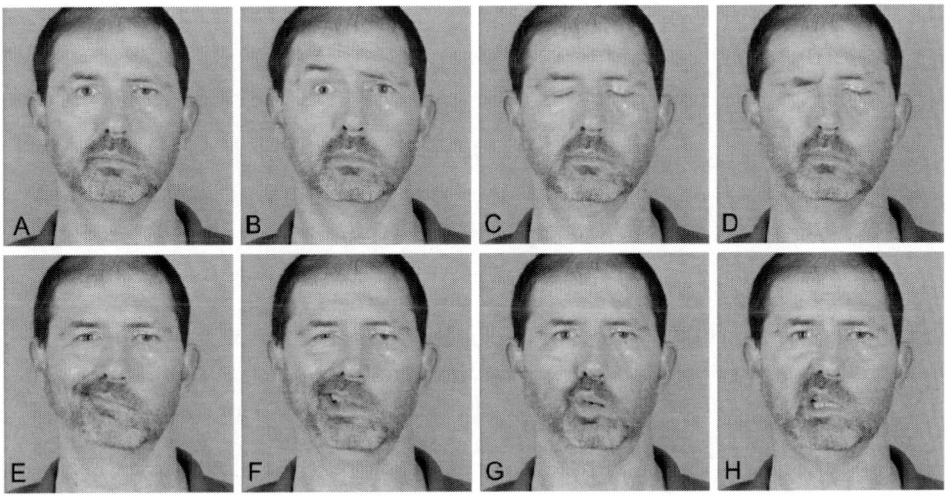

Figure 24.2. Patient with left facial palsy a) at rest, b) eyebrow raise, c) gentle eye closure, d) tight eye closure, e) best smile, f) biggest smile, g) pucker, and h) lower lip depression.

Q1. What are you looking for on physical exam? How would you describe his facial palsy?

A1. Evaluate the entire head and neck and cranial nerves.

1. Cranial nerve exam should pay particular attention to presence or absence of masseteric bulge, signs of vocal cord paralysis, and tongue movements.
2. He has left complete flaccid facial paralysis with brow ptosis, ectropion, external nasal valve collapse, effacement of the nasolabial fold, no movement of the oral commissure, and lower lip atrophy. Note, there is complete eye closure with gentle and maximal effort due to the presence of an upper eyelid weight.

Q2. How would you manage this patient surgically? What are the key surgical steps?

A2. The patient has had 12 months of flaccidity, which means he is in the re-innervation window.

1. Hypoglossal-facial nerve transfer: to restore facial tone
    a. Classic: entire hypoglossal nerve is transected and reflected upward for end-to-end coaptation to FN stump
        i. Not routinely performed due to resultant hemi-tongue weakness and mass movements/synkinesis
    b. XII-VII jump graft: side-to-end neurorrhaphy between hypoglossal (50% cut into nerve) and donor graft, end-to-end donor graft to FN stump
        i. Greater auricular nerve or descendens hypoglossi commonly used as donor graft

   c. FN mobilization from second genu with removal of mastoid tip for direct end-to-side coaptation to hypoglossal nerve (50% of fibers cut)
2. Masseteric-to-facial nerve transfer: to restore voluntary smile
   a. A single large-caliber FN branch inferior to the zygomatic arch is identified as it emerges from parotid gland and courses toward zygomaticus major
   b. Retrograde dissection toward upper division FN to identify other branches and leave them intact
   c. Nerve-to-masseter is identified along the deep surface of the masseter muscle and isolated with a vessel loop
      i. 3cm anterior to tragus and 1cm inferior to zygomatic arch
   d. Nerve-to-masseter is dissected anteriorly and transected distally to be reflected out of the wound bed
   e. End-to-end coaptation of nerve-to-masseter to distal FN branch (for smile)
3. Cross facial nerve graft: to restore voluntary smile
   a. Nonparalyzed side face opened in plane of parotidomasseteric fascia until FN branches can be identified within the masseter fascia
   b. Using guidance of electrical stimulation, distal branch giving the intended action (smile) is selected as the donor and transected sharply
   c. Sural nerve is harvested and tunneled across the upper lip
   d. End-to-end coaptation donor nerve to sural nerve (antidromic fashion)
   e. Bank in gingiva-buccal sulcus or pre-tragal region for second stage gracilis

Q3. What other adjuvant procedures or treatment could you offer this patient?

A3. Zonal approach to treatment of flaccid facial palsy

1. Upper facial zone: contralateral chemodenervation of frontalis, brow ptosis correction, temporary eyelid weight placement (already done in this case), could consider lower eyelid tightening with either temporary tarsorrhaphy or lateral tarsal strip
2. Central facial zone: could consider static suspension of the midface during the reinnervation procedures to give the patient immediate functional benefit
3. Lower facial zone: contralateral chemodenervation of depressor labii inferior, augmentation of affected side lower lip with dermal graft or functional filler
4. He should undergo facial neuromuscular retraining before and after reinnervation procedures

Q4: The patient follows up one year later. (Figure 24.3) He notes improvement in overall facial tone and has voluntary movement in his smile. He would like a more spontaneous smile and wants to know what the next step is.

A4. Second stage gracilis muscle transfer for spontaneous smile reanimation.

1. Gracilis harvest:
   a. Curvilinear incision made in medial thigh 1.5cm posterior to a line connecting the pubic tubercle to medial condyle of tibia
   b. Soft tissue divided until belly of gracilis identified
   c. Vascular pedicle located entering the deep surface of the muscle 8-10cm distal to pubic tubercle
   d. Obturator nerve identified 1-2cm proximal to vascular pedicle

e. Pedicle, nerve, and anterior segment (~40% of the total muscle width) of muscle belly are isolated
f. Muscle divided superiorly and inferiorly (~14-16cm in situ length) and pseudo tendons are created at each end using running locking 2-o Vicryl suture
g. Superficial aspect of muscle is thinned in situ (~40% of the thickness) for goal weight 10-20g
h. May be harvested with additional cutaneous or fascial paddle to address simultaneous contour defect if present (not applicable in this patient)

2. Facial preparation and inset:
   a. Thick skin flap raised in plane of parotidomasseteric fascia to expose temporalis fascia, zygomatic arch, modiolus, philtrum, and facial vessels
   b. Donor nerve isolated: tip of cross face nerve graft banked in gingivobuccal sulcus
   c. Gracilis secured medially to modiolus and upper lip with 4-o to 5-o Vicryl sutures and laterally to temporalis fascia
   d. Gracilis is stretched to resting tension length and appropriate vector as determined by preoperative smile assessment
   e. Microvascular anastomoses and neurorrhaphy are performed

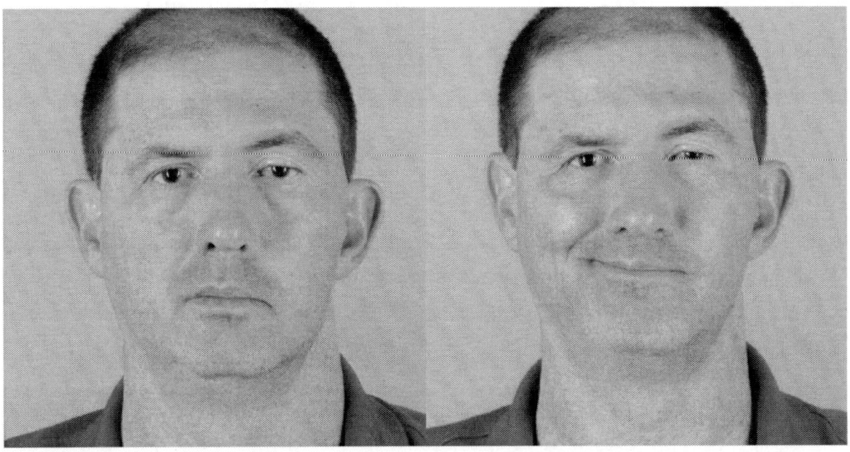

Figure 24.3. Patient is 1 year status post facial reanimation procedures.

References

[1] Jowett, N. 2018. "A General Approach to Facial Palsy." *Otolaryngol Clin North Am* 51 (6):1019-1031. doi: 10.1016/j.otc.2018.07.002.

[2] Sunderland, S. 1978. *Nerves and nerve injuries*. New York: Churchill Livingstone.

[3] Dusseldorp, J. R., M. M. van Veen, S. Mohan, and T. A. Hadlock. 2018. "Outcome Tracking in Facial Palsy." *Otolaryngol Clin North Am* 51 (6):1033-1050. doi: 10.1016/j.otc.2018.07.003.

[4] Hohman, M. H., and T. A. Hadlock. 2014. "Etiology, diagnosis, and management of facial palsy: 2000 patients at a facial nerve center." *Laryngoscope* 124 (7):E283-93. doi: 10.1002/lary.24542.

[5] Gantz, B. J., J. T. Rubinstein, P. Gidley, and G. G. Woodworth. 1999. "Surgical management of Bell's palsy." *Laryngoscope* 109 (8):1177-88. doi: 10.1097/00005537-199908000-00001.

[6] Klebuc, Michael J. A. 2011. "Facial Reanimation Using the Masseter-to-Facial Nerve Transfer." *Plast Reconstr Surg.* 127 (5):1909-1915. doi: 10.1097/PRS.0b013e31820e9138.

[7] May, M. 2000. "Nerve substitution techniques." In *The facial nerve*, edited by BM Schaitkin M May, 611-33. New York: Thieme.

[8] Rivas, A., K. D. Boahene, H. C. Bravo, M. Tan, R. J. Tamargo, and H. W. Francis. 2011. "A model for early prediction of facial nerve recovery after vestibular schwannoma surgery." *Otol Neurotol* 32 (5):826-33. doi: 10.1097/MAO.0b013e31821b0afd.

[9] May, Mark, and Carl Drucker. 1993. "Temporalis Muscle for Facial Reanimation: A 13-Year Experience With 224 Procedures." *Archives of Otolaryngology–Head & Neck Surgery* 119 (4):378-382. doi: 10.1001/archotol.1993.01880160022004 %J Archives of Otolaryngology–Head & Neck Surgery.

[10] Boahene, K. D., T. Y. Farrag, L. Ishii, and P. J. Byrne. 2011. "Minimally invasive temporalis tendon transposition." *Arch Facial Plast Surg* 13 (1):8-13. doi: 10.1001/archfacial.2010.100.

[11] Harii, K., K. Ohmori, and S. Torii. 1976. "Free gracilis muscle transplantation, with microneurovascular anastomoses for the treatment of facial paralysis. A preliminary report." *Plast Reconstr Surg* 57 (2):133-43. doi: 10.1097/00006534-197602000-00001.

[12] Miller, M. Q., and T. A. Hadlock. 2021. "Lessons from Gracilis Free Tissue Transfer for Facial Paralysis: Now versus 10 Years Ago." *Facial Plast Surg Clin North Am* 29 (3):415-422. doi: 10.1016/j.fsc.2021.03.001.

[13] Hadlock, T. A., L. J. Greenfield, M. Wernick-Robinson, and M. L. Cheney. 2006. "Multimodality approach to management of the paralyzed face." *Laryngoscope* 116 (8):1385-9. doi: 10.1097/01.mlg.0000225980.38147.c6.

Chapter 25

Facial Nerve Paresis and Synkinesis

Parsa P. Salehi, MD, MHS
and Babak Azizzadeh, MD, FACS

Introduction

1. Synkinesis occurs after facial nerve lesion or injury results in Wallerian degeneration
2. Voluntary movement of one facial area causing involuntary movement in another area [1-10]
3. Presentation varies; can present with varied facial movement disorders [3]
4. In addition to smile, eyelid, aesthetic, quality of life [6, 7, 10], and psychosocial consequences, functional deficits include narrowing of the eyelid aperture, facial asymmetry, platysmal tension, decreased dental show, tightness or spasm of facial musculature such as platysma, corrugator and buccinator muscles, poor manipulation of the food bolus, and oral incompetetnce [1, 7]
5. Oral and smile dysfunction are among the most distressing consequences of facial palsy because of the psychosocial impact and negative effect on quality of life [1]

Anatomy

1. Key smile muscles that are activated when an individual voluntarily or spontaneously smiles:
    a. Zygomatic major/minor, levator labii superioris, levator labii alaeque nasi, and depressor labii inferioris
2. Synkinetic muscles that antagonize key smile muscles and prevent a natural smile by creating an inferior and lateral vector of pull on the oral commissure:
    a. Orbicularis oris, depressor anguli oris (DAO), platysma, buccinator, and mentalis [1, 11]
3. Synkinetic muscles that result in brow and eyelid dysfunction:
    a. Corrugators, procerus, overactive orbicularis oculi, frontalis muscle [12]

Etiology

1. Diverse causes, though often seen in patients recovered from Ramsay Hunt syndrome or Bells palsy. [2, 13]

In: Essential Facial Plastic and Reconstructive Surgery. Volume 1 ISBN: 979-8-89113-306-8
Editors: Yan Ho Lee and Ira Papel © 2024 Nova Science Publishers, Inc.

   a. Post-facial paralysis synkinesis (PFPS) can result after any form of facial nerve repair (e.g. grafting, neurorrhaphy), regeneration, cranial nerve substitution, or injury (e.g. Bell's palsy, Ramsay Hunt, Lyme disease, granulomatous diseases, acoustic neuroma, temporal bone fracture, etc.). [1, 2, 11]
2. Cause of synkinesis is poorly understood. [3]
   a. Main theory: due to aberrant axonal regeneration of the motor nerve after an injury, producing multiple terminal axons that innervate both native and nonnative facial muscle groups (i.e. "cross-wiring). [1, 3, 11] (Figure 25.1)
   b. Alternative theories: include postsynaptic hyperexcitability and ephaptic transmission (i.e. abnormal connections between axons)
3. Smile dysfunction likely secondary to overactivity of counterproductive muscles that cause downward and lateral oral excursion
   a. Synkinetic "tug of war" between these muscles causes smile dysfunction [3]
4. Eyelid and brow dysfunction likely secondary to overactivity of periorbital muscles that may result in excessive narrowing of eyelids as well as brow dysfunction.
5. Synkinesis may begin as early as 3 to 4 months after onset of facial paralysis but may be progressive for a longer period [1]

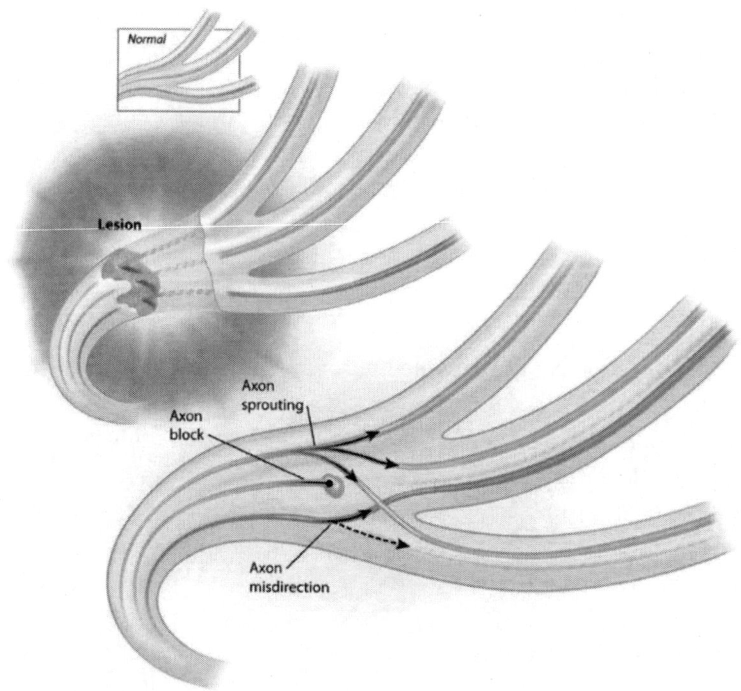

Figure 25.1. Aberrant regeneration theory of synkinesis. After nerve injury, proximal axons reroute, sprout along multiple distal pathways, and/or degenerate, leading to reinnervation of both correct and incorrect muscles. (Courtesy Facial Paralysis Institute.)

Treatment Goals

1. Improve functional deficits such as oral competence, as well as facial and cervical tightness
2. Improve static position of eyebrows and oral commissure position
3. Improve eyelid and spontaneous smile symmetry [1]

Patient Evaluation

1. House Brackman Scale and Sunderland Classification System (See Chapter 23)
2. History:
    a. Patient age, demographics, past medical history, social history, and family history
    b. Character of facial paresis and synkinesis
    c. Onset of paresis/synkinesis
    d. Contributing factors
        i. Pregnancy, tumor history, tick bite, diabetes
    e. Associated symptoms
    f. Initial medical and/or surgical treatment
        i. Steroids, antiviral, decompression, nerve grafting, etc.
    g. Other medical and/or surgical treatments:
        i. Physiotherapy/neuromuscular retraining, acupuncture, electrical stimulation, chemodenervation, surgical interventions
3. Exam:
    a. Complete and thorough head and neck examination, including cranial nerve exam and otoscopy [14]
        i. Various scales exist to measure objective smile and synkinesis analysis: House-Brackmann Facial Nerve Grading System [15], Sunnybrook Facial Grading System [16], clinician graded scales (e.g. electronic clinician-graded Facial Clinometric Evaluation) [1, 2] and patient-reported outcome measures (e.g. Synkinesis Assessment Questionnaire) [10]
        ii. "Facial Anatomic Subunit Analysis" Scale [17]
    b. Thorough zonal evaluation of facial function both at rest and with movement is critical [6]
    c. Closely examine variance between the synkinetic and unaffected side
    d. Upper Face:
        i. Periocular synkinesis:
            - Brow resting position may be depressed, symmetrical, or elevated depending on the resting tone of the frontalis, orbicularis oculi, corrugator, and procerus muscles
            - Brow activity may be normal, partially active, or severely impeded depending on the synkinetic activity of the frontalis, orbicularis oculi, corrugator, and procerus muscles

- Eyelids at rest: differences may be seen in dermatochalasis and eyelid hooding depending on the resting position of the eyebrows as well hypertonicity of the orbicularis oculi
- Eyelids with facial movement: eyelid aperture and palpebral fissure narrowing commonly seen with volitional or spontaneous smile activity [13]
- Most common unintentional periocular movements
  - Oculo-oral: movement of oral commissure with eye closure
  - Oro-ocular: eye closure with talking/smiling
- Crocodile Tears Syndrome (Bogorad's syndrome)
  - Faulty regeneration of the facial nerve proximal to the geniculate ganglion
  - Nerve fibers normally intended for the salivary gland misroute to the lacrimal gland, leading to tearing while eating

e. Mid-Face:
   i. Appropriate orientation and symmetry of the nasolabial fold

f. Lower Face:
   i. Components of a natural smile include symmetric superolateral excursion of the oral commissure and symmetrical upper and lower teeth show. [1, 2]
      - Spontaneity and symmetry are critical elements of an emotional, natural smile [1]
      - Smile variance between the synkinetic and unaffected side will be seen due to: oral commissure excursion, upper and lower dental show, nasolabial fold asymmetry, upper lip hooding, depressor labii inferioris dysfunction
   ii. Variable muscular contraction specially the buccinator and orbicularis oris can cause oral incompetence [3]

g. Neck:
   i. Synkinesis may result in uncomfortable and unsightly contraction and hypertrophy of the platysma muscle

4. Documentation
   a. Photography and videography is essential in pre-treatment period [6]
   b. Should document appearance at rest and with seven volitional facial movements (brow elevation, gentle and full-effort eye closure and smile, lip pucker, lower lip depression, spontaneous smile) [13]
5. Labs/studies:
   a. Imaging, labs, and electrodiagnostics are rarely needed if patient has developed true synkinesis on physical examination; the following studies are more useful in cases where there are unusual recovery of acute facial paralysis and uncertainty in diagnosis of idiopathic facial palsy
   b. Electrodiagnostics: Electromyography (EMG), Electroneuronography (ENoG), Nerve Excitability Test (NET), Maximal Stimulation Test (MST)

c. Audiogram
d. Imaging: CT brain and temporal bone, MRI
e. Laboratory testing: serologic testing, complete blood count, rheumatoid factor, erythrocyte sedimentation rate, C-reactive protein, antinuclear antibody, angiotensin-converting enzyme, antiphospholipid antibodies, and antineutrophil cytoplasmic antibody

Management

1. Nonsurgical
   a. Observation: recommended if patient's synkinesis is evolving and not stable which is typically seen in the first year after acute paralysis
   b. Physical therapy/Biofeedback/Physiotherapy [2, 6]
      i. Facial neuromuscular retraining by trained facial nerve physical therapists [7]
      ii. Goal of physical therapy for patients with facial synkinesis include reducing hypertonicity of over-contracted synkinetic muscles, mass movement on the affected side, and reducing compensatory hyperactivity of the unaffected side to achieve balance [13]
      iii. Physical therapy plays a key role in improving patient outcomes [3]
      iv. May be used as an adjunct to modified selective neurectomy
   c. Botulinum toxin A [11]
      i. Chemodenervation is one of the key treatment options for patients with PFPS [7, 9, 13]
      ii. Frequently targeted muscles on affected side: orbicularis oculi, corrugator, DAO, mentalis, and platysma [13]
      iii. The most effective region for chemodenervation is improvement of narrowing eyelid aperture, platysmal overactivity and chin dimpling
      iv. Smile enhancement is very challenging with chemodenervation and not reproducible even in the hands of facial nerve experts; this is due to close proximity of DLI, zygomatic and levator muscles to the antagonist muscles (DAO, buccinator, mentalis) [3]
      v. Chemodenervation is the primary means of management for periocular synkinesis [13]
      vi. Excellent as adjunctive modality with surgical treatments [18]
      vii. May also be used in contralateral facial muscles (such as the orbicularis oculi, levator labii alequae nasii, depressor labii inferioris) to camouflage visible asymmetries [6, 11, 13]
      viii. Gustatory tearing (Bogorad syndrome) can be managed with lacrimal gland BTA injection [13]
      ix. Chemodenervation improves quality of life outcomes in PFPS patients [7]
      x. In case of prominent nasolabial fold, chemodenervation using botulinum toxin is not recommended because it can result in

significant ptosis of the upper lip, and it is rarely able to attenuate the prominent fold; physiotherapy and manual stretching is recommended for this area

xi. Chemodenervation and physical therapy have produced objective and subjective improved outcomes: improved facial symmetry, reduced involuntary muscle contractions, and enhanced quality of life [3]

xii. Downsides include temporary effects, repeated visits, and ongoing costs [7]

d. Fillers (e.g. hyaluronic acid, fat grafts)

i. Volumizing fillers or autologous fat grafting to ipsilateral or contralateral midface, lips, and/or nasolabial folds may improve symmetry [13]

ii. Excellent as adjunctive modality with surgical treatments

2. Surgical

a. Signal Upgrade Procedures: orthodromic temporalis tendon transfer, gracilis functional free muscle transfer, masseteric or hypoglossal nerve to facial nerve transfers

i. Aim of Procedures: these procedures are intended to increase the power of oral commissure excursion that have been traditionally developed to address complete flaccid paralysis [7, 13] (See chapter 23).

ii. Although these procedures may have some incremental improvements in patients with synkinesis, none address underlying cause of synkinesis which is overactive and uncoordinated activity of smile antagonists. [3]

iii. These procedures typically have lengthy recovery periods, may require multiple surgeries and lack the natural and spontaneous outcome that can be achieved with more novel denervation procedures (See below) [7]

b. Modified selective neurectomy

i. Aim of Procedure(s):

- Selective denervation of antagonist synkinetic muscles is more targeted than chemodenervation for smile enhancement (see above for limitations of chemodenervation) and allow the normal smile muscles to work properly which achieves better outcomes than signal upgrade procedures (see above); this procedure is possible since peripheral facial nerve branches are easily accessible through a deep plane rhytidectomy approach
- Ablate overactive buccal and cervical branches that cause inferior and lateral excursion of the oral commissure, while preserving branches to the orbicularis oris (controls lip shape and movement), depressor labii inferioris (allows lower lip depression), and zygomatic and levator muscles (elevating oral commissure and upper lip) [2]

- Goal of modified selective neurectomy is to reduce, but not eliminate, the activity of the smile antagonists, while preserving smile elevators and the depressor labii inferioris to enhance the smile mechanism and dental show [2]
- First technique to specifically improve natural smile function in a large cohort of PFPS patients [2]

ii. Clinical indication:
- Patients clinically determined to have synkinesis, active zygomatic major/minor muscles, and access to distal branches of the facial nerve [2]
- Stable pattern of synkinesis emerges, once early phase of nerve regeneration has completed [2]
- May be considered as a stand-alone procedure; however, most patients benefit from chemodenervation of the periorbital region and neuromuscular retraining [1]

iii. Exclusion criteria
- Complete flaccid paralysis
- Malignancy
- Limited expected life expectancy

iv. Technical considerations (Table 25.1):
- Preop: no chemodenervation for approximately 4-6 months
- Anesthesia: general, local infiltration without lidocaine to avoid changes in nerve stimulation
- Rhytidectomy incision
- Sub-SMAS/sub-platysmal (i.e. deep plane) dissection
- Identification and stimulation of the zygomatic, buccal, marginal mandibular, and cervical branches
- Excising segments of aberrant facial nerve branches to buccinator, DAO, mentalis, and platysma and placing titanium clips to the nerve ends to prevent regrowth [3]
- DAO and platysma myectomy performed as needed

v. Summary:
- Only treatment of synkinesis that preserves the entire natural neural pathway while maintaining long-lasting, natural, and spontaneous results
- Preserves the innate efferent neural pathway—from facial motor nucleus in the pons to the muscle fibers. [3]
- Patient regains natural smile without sacrificing cosmetic outcomes
- Long-term natural and spontaneous outcomes achieved by addressing underlying etiology of smile synkinesis [3]
- Selective surgical denervation of synkinetic muscles is especially effective around mouth where there exists a

convergence of muscles around oral commissure at the modiolus, upper lip, and lower lip.

- Essentially goal is to reduce muscles negatively impacting smile at the nerve level to allow for appropriate musculature to function [3]
- On average, excision of 6.7 nerves yields the best patient outcomes[3]
- Owing to the increased facial tone on the affected side, patients with synkinesis often have asymmetry of the unaffected side (the affected side paradoxically has a more youthful appearance). [17] Hence, to improve facial symmetry both at rest and with smile, may consider asymmetric rhytidectomy, autologous fat grafting, and/or buccal fat pad resection/repositioning (termed "Symmetrical Facial Repositioning") in addition to modified selective neurectomy [17]

vi. Post-operative management

- Discharged same day, return to work within 10 days
- Chemodenervation for periorbital region and/or filler can resume in 1 week depending on level of edema
- Neuromuscular retraining begins 1 month postoperatively
- If patients do not achieve the ideal outcome from the procedure, revision surgery may be offered to target watershed branches of the peripheral facial nerve. [1, 2] Moreover, additional buccal and cervical peripheral nerve branches not identified in initial surgery may be uncovered and transected. [2]

vii. Outcomes:

- Final outcomes observed between 6 months and 1 year [17]
- Long lasting results [2], including improvement in quality of life, facial movement, facial comfort, and social function measures [7]
- Results validated by long term observers [3]
- Patients with successful treatment have decreased botulinum requirements over time [3, 7]
- Articulation variances typically do not improve from pre-operative status
- Significant learning curve for surgeon may impact individual surgeon's results [2]

viii. Complications

- No major complications reported; most common adverse events include hematoma (<5%), seroma (<2%), and temporary oral incompetence [2, 3]
- Temporary oral incompetence, usually ranging from 7 days to 8 months; no permanent events noted [2]

- Subset of patients may require revision surgery due to persistent synkinesis [3]

c. Depressor Anguli Oris (DAO) Muscle Resection
   i. Can be performed as a stand-alone procedure under local anesthesia or in combination with other procedures, such as modified selective neurectomy
   ii. Improvement in oral commissure excursion has been reported although long-term studies have not been yet published [5, 19]
   iii. As a stand-alone procedure, it may not achieve enough improvement in natural smile—especially in dental show since the buccinator, platysma, mentalis, and DAO are all involved in synkinetic smile dysfunction

Summary Points

1. Patients who develop reversible facial nerve injury are at risk of developing synkinesis during recovery
2. Neuromuscular retraining, chemodenervation, and surgery are the most reliable treatment options for facial synkinesis (with combined therapy yielding optimal outocmes)
3. The most effective region for chemodenervation is improvement of narrowing eyelid aperture, platysmal overactivity, and chin dimpling; smile enhancement is very challenging with chemodenervation and not reproducible due to close proximity of DLI, zygomatic, and levator muscles to the antagonist synkinetic muscles (DAO, buccinator, mentalis) [3]
4. Modified selective neurectomy of antagonistic synkinetic muscles is a paradigm shift in the surgical management of smile dysfunction in PFSP by reducing the activity of antagonist muscles rather than increasing the power of oral commissure excursion commonly seen in standard reanimation procedures such as gracilis muscle transfer and temporalis myoplasty. This procedure achieves long-term, natural, and spontaneous outcomes.

Patient Case

A 37 year old female patient comes to you 14 months after right facial paralysis.

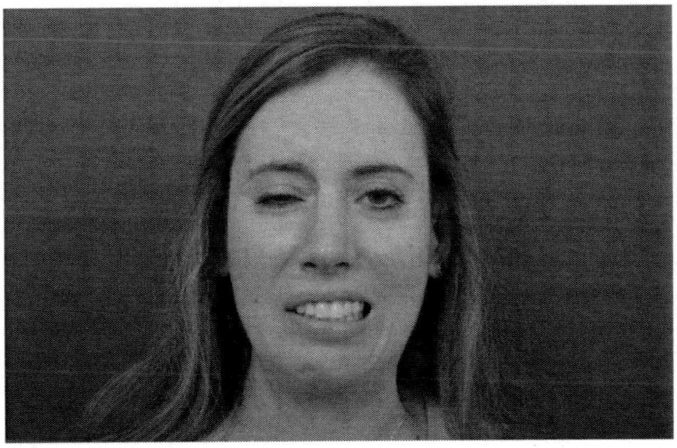

Figure 25.2. Patient Case: Pre-Operative.

Q1. What do you observe in this pt? (Figure 25.2)

A1. Right sided facial synkinesis with right sided eyelid narrowing and asymmetric smile. Asymmetric brow height (right higher than left). Asymmetric upper teeth show with smile and poor lower teeth show with smile. Hypertonic contraction of right sided facial muscles including mentalis and platysma (e.g. asymmetric chin dimpling). Asymmetric facial aging.

Q2. She is inquiring about her options for treatment. What are some non-surgical and surgical options?

A2.

1. Nonsurgical: observation, physical therapy, Botulinum toxin, fillers.
2. Surgical: modified selective neurectomy, Symmetrical Facial Repositioning procedure

Q3. She agrees to a modified selective neurectomy surgery. What are the steps? (See Figure 25.3 for post-opeartive results)

A3. Surgical Procedure: See Table 25.1 and Figure 25.4.

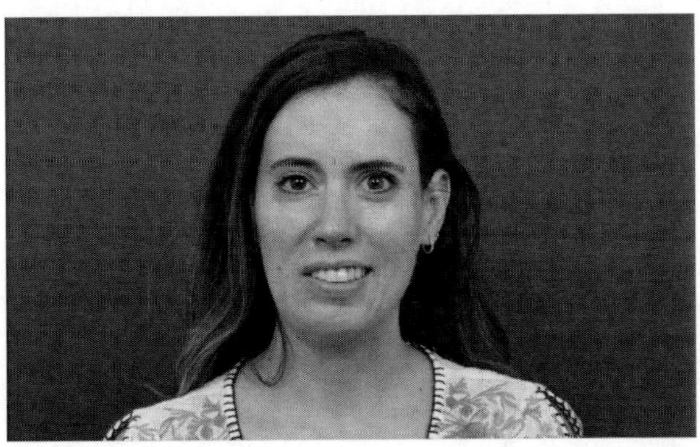

Figure 25.3. Patient case: Post-Operative.

Table 25.1. Surgical Steps: Modified Selective Neurectomy [1]

1. Preparation/Incision
   a. Transoral intubation, general anesthesia without paralytics
   b. Standard retrotragal rhytidectomy incision planned
   c. 1:100,00 epinephrine injection used. No lidocaine hydrochloride to avoid inadvertent decrease in neural activity
   d. Facial nerve monitoring electrodes in periorbital and perioral regions
2. Dissection
   a. Start at temporal hair tuft, subcutaneous dissection extended medially for 4-6 cm from incision (raising skin flap)
   b. Make incision into the superficial musculoaponeurotic system (SMAS) and platysma and in an oblique vector from the lateral zygomatic arch to the cervical region passing through the angle of mandible
   c. Elevate SMAS and platysma as a single flap for 3-6 cm
   d. Carry dissection deep to the masseteric and subplatysmal fascia in order to identify the branches of the facial 358ranche they exit the parotid capsule
3. Nerve Identification
   a. Carefully identify and dissect all visible branches of the facial nerve (zygomatic, buccal, marginal mandibular, cervical)
   b. Connections between the zygomatic and buccal branches are isolated as well as side branches of the cervical 358ranche sas they enter the underbelly of the platysma
   c. Nerve branches stimulated at 0.5 to 2.0 mA; elicited movement evaluated
   b. Nerve branches that cause platysmal tightening or downward and lateral excursion of oral commissure are isolated
   c. Titanium clips placed on most proximal and distal portion of the dissected nerve, 0.5 to 4.0 cm of intervening nerve resected
   d. Careful preservation of zygomatic branches that purely elevate the oral commissure and marginal mandibular branch that stimulates the depressor labii inferioris
   e. Preserve 1 to 2 branches that close the lips, to maintain oral competence
   f. Platysma myotomy below the level of the identified marginal mandibular nerve (at lateral edge, approximately 3 cm below the border of the mandible).
   g. Symmetric facial reposition and autologous fat grafting may be performed as needed to improve soft tissue asymmetry at rest [17]
4. Closure
   a. SMAS re-draped and sutured in natural position. If patients are undergoing a simultaneous symmetrizing rhytidectomy, the SMAS is suspended in a superolateral vector
   b. Drains over the SMAS and under skin flap (in the subcutaneous plane)
   c. Pressure dressing not typically used

*Patients are discharged same day. Usually return to work and routine social function in 7 to 10 days. Neuromuscular retraining in 1 month.

** In addition to Modified Selective Neurectomy, may consider Symmetrical Facial Repositioning procedure to improve symmetry and smile function.

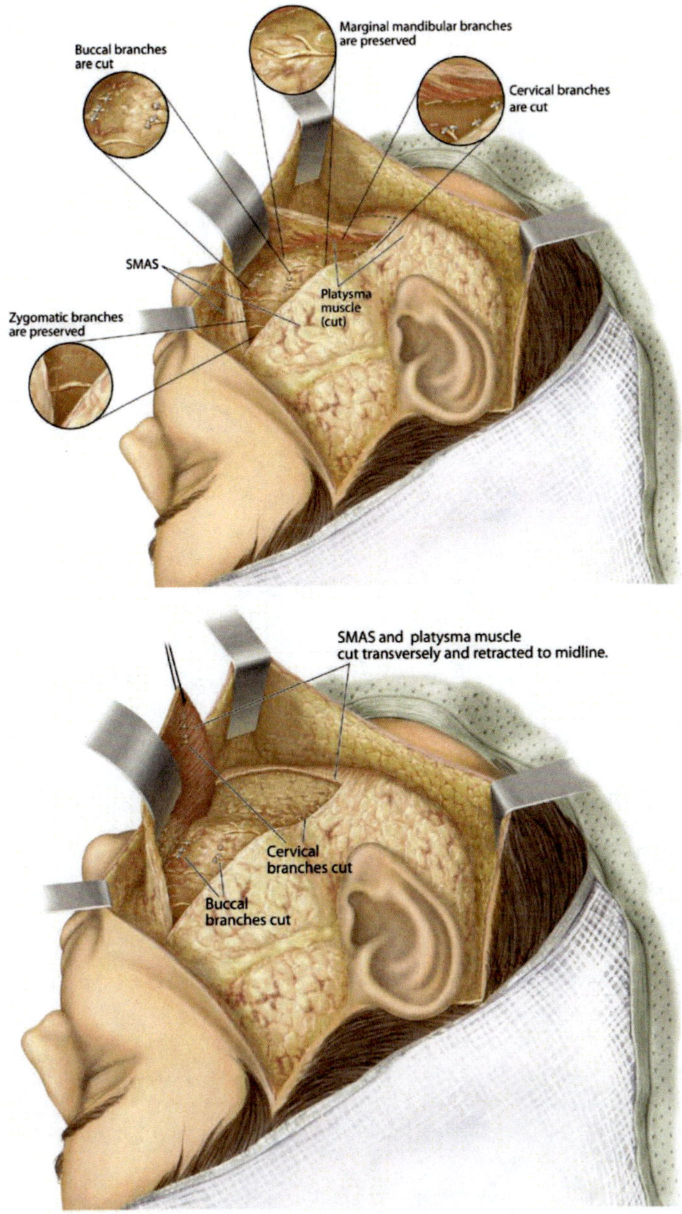

Figure 25.4. Illustration of surgical approach for modified selective neurectomy. Entering the deep plane allows for optimal exposure to identify and transect/preserve Facial nerve branches as they exit the product capsule. (Courtesy Facial Paralysis Institute.).

References

[1] Azizzadeh B, Frisenda JL. Surgical Management of Postparalysis Facial Palsy and Synkinesis. *Otolaryngol Clin North Am.* Dec 2018;51(6):1169-1178. doi:10.1016/j.otc.2018.07.012.

[2] Azizzadeh B, Irvine LE, Diels J, Slattery WH, Massry GG, Larian B, Riedler KL, Peng GL. Modified Selective Neurectomy for the Treatment of Post-Facial Paralysis Synkinesis. *Plast Reconstr Surg.* 05 2019;143(5):1483-1496. doi:10.1097/PRS.0000000000005590.

[3] Azizzadeh B, Hjelm N. Modified Selective Neurectomy: A New Paradigm in the Management of Facial Palsy with Synkinesis. *Facial Plast Surg Clin North Am.* Aug 2021;29(3):453-457. doi:10.1016/j.fsc.2021.03.005.

[4] Hadlock T, Kowaleski J, Lo D, Bermejo R, Zeigler HP, Mackinnon S, Heaton JT. Functional assessments of the rodent facial nerve: a synkinesis model. *Laryngoscope.* Oct 2008;118(10):1744-9. doi:10.1097/MLG.0b013e31817f5255.

[5] Jowett N, Malka R, Hadlock TA. Effect of Weakening of Ipsilateral Depressor Anguli Oris on Smile Symmetry in Postparalysis Facial Palsy. *JAMA Facial Plast Surg.* Jan 01 2017;19(1):29-33. doi:10.1001/jamafacial.2016.1115.

[6] Shokri T, Azizzadeh B, Ducic Y. Modern Management of Facial Nerve Disorders. *Semin Plast Surg.* Nov 2020;34(4):277-285. doi:10.1055/s-0040-1721824.

[7] Shtraks JP, Mirocha J, Azizzadeh B. Quality of Life Outcomes After Modified Selective Neurectomy for Postfacial Paralysis Synkinesis. *Facial Plast Surg Aesthet Med.* 12 2021;23(6):443-448. doi:10.1089/fpsam.2020.0485.

[8] Tavares-Brito J, Fonseca ACO, Torres RP, van Veen MM, Greene J, Salomone R, Bahmad F Jr, Hadlock T, Bento RF. Facial Clinimetric Evaluation Scale and Synkinesis Assessment Questionnaire Translation into Brazilian Portuguese: A Validation Study. *Int Arch Otorhinolaryngol.* Jan 2020;24(1):e24-e30. doi:10.1055/s-0039-1697992.

[9] van Veen MM, Dusseldorp JR, Hadlock TA. Long-term outcome of selective neurectomy for refractory periocular synkinesis. *Laryngoscope.* 10 2018;128(10):2291-2295. doi:10.1002/lary.27225.

[10] van Veen MM, Quatela O, Tavares-Brito J, Robinson M, Baiungo JH, Werker PMN, Dijkstra PU, Hadlock TA. Patient-perceived severity of synkinesis reduces quality of life in facial palsy: A cross-sectional analysis in 92 patients. *Clin Otolaryngol.* 05 2019;44(3):483-486. doi:10.1111/coa.13322.

[11] Leader B, Azizzadeh B. Synkinetic Unilateral Lower Lip Palsy: Diagnosis and Technical Considerations for Facial Reanimation. *Facial Plast Surg Aesthet Med.* 2021 Jul-Aug 2021;23(4):309-311. doi:10.1089/fpsam.2020.0462.

[12] Leader B, Diels J, Azizzadeh B. Synkinetic Brow Dysfunction: Diagnosis and Treatment Algorithm. *Facial Plast Surg Aesthet Med.* Apr 06 2022;doi:10.1089/fpsam.2021.0182.

[13] Jowett N, Hadlock TA. Contemporary management of Bell palsy. *Facial Plast Surg.* Apr 2015;31(2):93-102. doi:10.1055/s-0035-1549040.

[14] Hadlock T. Facial paralysis: research and future directions. *Facial Plast Surg.* May 2008;24(2):260-7. doi:10.1055/s-2008-1075842.

[15] House JW, Brackmann DE. Facial nerve grading system. *Otolaryngol Head Neck Surg.* Apr 1985;93(2):146-7. doi:10.1177/019459988509300202.

[16] Ross BG, Fradet G, Nedzelski JM. Development of a sensitive clinical facial grading system. *Otolaryngol Head Neck Surg.* Mar 1996;114(3):380-6. doi:10.1016/s0194-5998(96)70206-1.

[17] Hjelm N, Azizzadeh B. Modified Selective Neurectomy with Symmetrical Facial Repositioning. *Facial Plast Surg Aesthet Med.* 2020 Jan/Feb 2020;22(1):57-60. doi:10.1089/fpsam.2019.29005.hje.

[18] Hjelm N, Crippen M, Azizzadeh B. Long-Term Changes in the Treatment Pattern of Botulinum Toxin A Injections for Postfacial Paralysis Synkinesis Following Modified Selective Neurectomy. *Facial Plast Surg Aesthet Med.* 2021 May-Jun 2021;23(3):234-235. doi:10.1089/fpsam.2020.0240.

[19] Derakhshan A, Miller MQ, Malka R, Gadkaree SK, Hadlock TA. Releasing the Smile: Depressor Anguli Oris Excision in the Context of Managing Nonflaccid Facial Palsy. *Plast Reconstr Surg.* Feb 01 2022;149(2):261e-269e. doi:10.1097/PRS.0000000000008807.

Practice Guidelines – Facial Nerve Rehabilitation

When a particular set of basic criteria is met, then the Qualified Options for treatment, testing, or management below are reasonable and justifiable recommendations.

- When the patient presents with Facial Nerve Dysfunction (All types), then Multidisciplinary care (may include ophthalmology, speech and language pathology, neurology/neurotology, physical and/or occupational therapy), medical management (may include steroids, antivirals, artificial tears/ointment), corneal protection (e.g., gold/platinum weight, tarsorrhaphy, eyelid procedures) are Qualified Options.
- When the patient presents with Facial Nerve Paralysis, then Electrodiagnostic testing (EMG, EnoG, NET, MST), exploration with possible primary repair or decompression within 72 hours, if >72 hours to 6 months electrodiagnostic testing, within 4-6 months possible CN VII exploration/decompression/repair, primary repair or nerve interposition graft, nerve transfers or re-innervation techniques, muscle or tendon transfers (regional or free), static facial reanimation procedures are Qualified Options.
- When the patient presents with Facial Nerve Paresis/Synkinesis, then nerve transfers or re-innervation techniques, muscle transfers (regional or free) are Qualified Options.
- When the patient presents with Facial Nerve Dysfunction (Any type), then labs (infectious, systemic/autoimmune), imaging studies (MRI, CT), physical and/or occupational therapy (including Biofeedback/Physiotherapy), neuromuscular modulation/chemodenervation, neurolysis, muscle resection, fat or dermal grafts, fillers* are Qualified Options.
- When the patient presents with Facial Nerve Dysfunction (With other neurologic deficits), then CT head, neurology or neurosurgery involvement (r/o CVA) are Qualified Options.
- When the patient presents with Facial Nerve Dysfunction (With eye concerns), then Ophthalmology involvement is a Qualified Option.
- When the patient presents with Facial Nerve Dysfunction (With ear/hearing/balance concerns), then Neurotology/otology involvement, audiogram, VNG are Qualified Options.
- When the patient presents with Facial Nerve Dysfunction (With speech/swallowing concerns), then Speech and language pathology involvement is a Qualified Option.
- When the patient presents with Facial Nerve Dysfunction (With suspicion for Lyme disease), then Antibiotics (i.e., Doxycycline) and infectious disease consult are Qualified Options.

Patient Characteristics	Qualified Option(s)
Facial Nerve Dysfunction (All types)	Multidisciplinary care (may include ophthalmology, speech and language pathology, neurology/neurotology, physical and/or occupational therapy), medical management (may include steroids, antivirals, artificial tears/ointment), corneal

	protection (e.g., gold/platinum weight, tarsorrhaphy, eyelid procedures)
Facial Nerve Paralysis	Electrodiagnostic testing (EMG, EnoG, NET, MST) Exploration with possible primary repair or decompression within 72 hours If >72 hours to 6 months electrodiagnostic testing Within 4-6 months possible CN VII exploration/decompression/repair Primary repair or nerve interposition graft Nerve transfers or re-innervation techniques Muscle or tendon transfers (regional or free) Static facial reanimation procedures
Facial Nerve Paresis/Synkinesis	Nerve transfers or re-innervation techniques Muscle transfers (regional or free)
Facial Nerve Dysfunction (Any type)	Labs (infectious, systemic/autoimmune) Imaging studies (MRI, CT) Physical and/or occupational therapy (including Biofeedback/Physiotherapy) Neuromuscular modulation/chemodenervation Neurolysis, muscle resection Fat or dermal grafts, fillers*
Facial Nerve Dysfunction (With other neurologic deficits)	CT head, neurology or neurosurgery involvement (r/o CVA)
Facial Nerve Dysfunction (With eye concerns)	Ophthalmology involvement
Facial Nerve Dysfunction (With ear/hearing/balance concerns)	Neurotology/otology involvement, audiogram, VNG
Facial Nerve Dysfunction (With speech/swallowing concerns)	Speech and language pathology involvement
Facial Nerve Dysfunction (With suspicion for Lyme disease)	Antibiotics (i.e., Doxycycline) and infectious disease consult

*Note: while some autologous filler material (e.g., fat, dermis) may be covered by payors, certain materials may not be covered

Practice Guidelines

Part 2: Reconstruction of Defects

When a particular set of basic criteria is met, then the Qualified Options for treatment, testing, or management below are reasonable and justifiable recommendations.

- When the patient presents with defects of the scalp, face, or neck, then healing by secondary intension with or without local wound care, primary closure, local flap, regional flap, microvascular reconstruction, allographs, xenographs, tissue expansion, neuromuscular modulation, and filler are qualified options.
- When the patient presents with defects of the scalp, or face involving soft tissue, bone/cartilage, then in addition to the above options, grafts, implants, hair restoration, and prosthetics are qualified options.
- When the patient presents with defects of the neck involving soft tissue, then in addition to the above options, grafts, are qualified options.

Patient Characteristics	Qualified Option(s)
Defects of the Scalp, Face, Neck (Any)	Healing by secondary intention with or without local wound care Primary closure Local flap Regional flap Microvascular reconstruction/free flap Allografts/xenografts Tissue expansion Neuromuscular modulation, filler*
Defects of the Scalp, Face (Soft tissue or bone/cartilage)	Graft(s): skin/mucosal/dermal/fat/composite/ cartilage/bone/nerve Implants Hair restoration Prosthetics (e.g., ear, nose, hair)
Defects of the Neck (Soft tissue)	Graft(s): skin/mucosal/dermal/fat/nerve

*Note: while some autologous filler material (e.g., fat, dermis) may be covered by payors, certain materials may not be covered

Part 3: Congenital Anomalies

When a particular set of basic criteria is met, then the Qualified Options for treatment, testing, or management below are reasonable and justifiable recommendations.

- When the patient presents with minor ear deformity within a few weeks of life, then ear molding is a qualified option.
- When the patient presents with Microtia Grades 1 or 2, then local flaps, cartilage scoring/resection/grafting are qualified options.
- When the patient presents with Microtia Grades 3 or 4, then Local flaps, cartilage scoring/resection/grafting, total or subtotal ear reconstruction with autologous or homologous cartilage grafts or alloplastic implants, ear prosthesis are qualified options.
- When the patient presents with Cleft Lip (all types), then Multidisciplinary cleft team, speech and language pathology involvement, pediatrics involvement are qualified options.
- When the patient presents with Cleft Lip (unilateral), then Rotation-advancement flap, reconstruction to obliterate cleft and restore form and function are qualified options.
- When the patient presents with Cleft Lip (bilateral), then Millard-Mulliken repair, reconstruction to obliterate clefts and restore form and function are qualified options.
- When the patient presents with Cleft Lip (any type), then Adjunctive procedures including orthopedics, lip adhesion, local flaps, fat/dermal grafts are qualified options.
- When the patient presents with Cleft Nose, then rhinoplasty (nasal reconstruction), grafts, implants are qualified options.
- When the patient presents with Cleft Palate (all types), then Multidisciplinary cleft team, orthodontics/dentistry involvement, speech and language pathology involvement, pediatrics involvement are qualified options.
- When the patient presents with Cleft Palate (hard palate), then reconstruction (e.g., bipedicled flap, unipedicled flap, vomer flap) is a qualified option.
- When the patient presents with Cleft Palate (soft palate), then reconstruction (e.g., intra-velar veloplasty, Furlow double-opposing Z-plasty) is a qualified option.
- When the patient presents with Cleft Palate (any type), then adjunctive procedures (e.g., buccal flat flap, buccal myomucosal flap, acellular dermal matrix, bone grafting) are qualified options.
- When the patient presents with Craniosynostosis (All types), then multi-disciplinary care, intracranial pressure assessment and 3D CT imaging are qualified options.
- When the patient presents with Craniosynostosis (Metopic, trigonocephaly), then reconstruction (e.g., bilateral fronto-orbital advancement, endoscopic strip craniectomy with cranial orthotic) is a qualified option.
- When the patient presents with Craniosynostosis (unicoronal), then reconstruction (e.g., advance and recontour ipsilateral supraorbital bandeau and anterior cranium, ipsilateral bandeau lowering) is a qualified option.

- When the patient presents with Craniosynostosis (Scaphocephaly), then reconstruction (e.g., endoscopic strip craniectomy with postoperative cranial molding orthotic, spring-assisted surgery, open calvarial remodeling operation) is a qualified option.
- When the patient presents with Craniosynostosis (Unilambdoid), then reconstruction (e.g., endoscopic strip craniectomy with postoperative cranial molding orthotic, spring-assisted surgery, open calvarial remodeling operation) is a qualified option.
- When the patient presents with Craniosynostosis (Syndromic), then single or multiple reconstruction(s), Cranial expansion and correction of fronto-facial dysmorphology (e.g., monobloc procedure or fronto-facial advancement, posterior vault distraction osteogenesis) are qualified options.
- When the patient presents with Craniosynostosis (any type), then genetic counseling, eye protection, polysomnography, airway evaluation, laryngoscopy/bronchoscopy are qualified options.
- When the patient presents with Deformational (Positional) Plagiocephaly, then head repositioning, helmet therapy, surgical intervention are qualified options.

Patient Characteristics	**Qualified Option(s)**
Minor ear deformity (within a few weeks of life)	Ear molding
Microtia (Grades 1 or 2)	·Local flaps, cartilage scoring/resection/grafting
Microtia (Grades 3 or 4)	Local flaps, cartilage scoring/resection/grafting, total or subtotal ear reconstruction with autologous or homologous cartilage grafts or alloplastic implants, ear prosthesis
Cleft Lip (All types)	Multidisciplinary cleft team, speech and language pathology involvement, pediatrics involvement
Cleft Lip (Unilateral)	Rotation-advancement flap, reconstruction to obliterate cleft and restore form and function
Cleft Lip (Bilateral)	Millard-Mulliken repair, reconstruction to obliterate clefts and restore form and function
Cleft Lip (Any type)	Adjunctive procedures including orthopedics, lip adhesion, local flaps, fat/dermal grafts
Cleft Nose	Septorhinoplasty (single or multiple) for pediatric or adult patient Graft(s): skin/mucosal/composite/cartilage/bone Autologous, homologous, or alloplastic implants
Cleft Palate (All types)	Multidisciplinary cleft team, orthodontics/dentistry involvement, speech and language pathology involvement, pediatrics involvement
Cleft Palate (Hard palate)	Reconstruction (e.g., bipedicled flap, unipedicled flap, vomer flap)
Cleft Palate (Soft palate)	Reconstruction (e.g., intra-velar veloplasty, Furlow double-opposing Z-plasty)
Cleft Palate (Any type)	Adjunctive procedures (e.g., buccal flat flap, buccal myomucosal flap, acellular dermal matrix, bone grafting)

Craniosynostosis (All types)	Multi-disciplinary care, intracranial pressure assessment and 3D CT imaging
Craniosynostosis (Metopic, trigonocephaly)	Reconstruction (e.g., bilateral fronto-orbital advancement, endoscopic strip craniectomy with cranial orthotic)
Craniosynostosis (Unicoronal)	Reconstruction (e.g., advance and recontour ipsilateral supraorbital bandeau and anterior cranium, ipsilateral bandeau lowering)
Craniosynostosis (Scaphocephaly)	Reconstruction (e.g., endoscopic strip craniectomy with postoperative cranial molding orthotic, spring-assisted surgery, open calvarial remodeling operation)
Craniosynostosis (Unilambdoid)	Reconstruction (e.g., open posterior vault remodeling including occipital switch cranioplasty, minimally invasive techniques including strip craniectomies)
Craniosynostosis (Syndromic)	Single or multiple reconstruction(s) Cranial expansion and correction of fronto-facial dysmorphology (e.g., monobloc procedure or fronto-facial advancement, posterior vault distraction osteogenesis)
Craniosynostosis (Any type)	Genetic counseling, eye protection, polysomnography, airway evaluation, laryngoscopy/bronchoscopy
Deformational (Positional) Plagiocephaly	Head repositioning, helmet therapy, surgical intervention

Part 4: Trauma

When a particular set of basic criteria is met, then the Qualified Options for treatment, testing, or management below are reasonable and justifiable recommendations.

- When the patient presents with Facial Fractures (All types), then Imaging (e.g., CT, MRI, Xray, US), trauma assessment including airway management are Qualified Options.
- When the patient presents with Mandible Fractures, then Closed and/or open treatment with or without interdental fixation or dental extraction/stabilization, implant/graft placement are Qualified Options.
- When the patient presents with ZMC Fractures, then Closed and/or open treatment with or without implant/graft placement are Qualified Options.
- When the patient presents with NOE Complex Fractures, then Closed and/or open treatment with or without implant/graft placement, septorhinoplasty, eyelid reconstruction, ophthalmology consult are Qualified Options.
- When the patient presents with Orbital Fractures (All types), then Closed and/or open treatment with or without implant/graft placement, eyelid reconstruction, ophthalmology consult are Qualified Options.
- When the patient presents with Frontal Sinus Fractures (All types), then Closed and/or open treatment with or without implant/graft placement, open or endoscopic frontal sinus surgery, obliteration or cranialization, neurosurgery consult are Qualified Options.
- When the patient presents with Pan-Facial Fractures (All types), then Closed and/or open treatment with or without interdental fixation or dental extraction/stabilization, implant/graft placement, eyelid reconstruction, open or endoscopic sinus surgery are Qualified Options.
- When the patient presents with Facial Fractures (Any types), then Dentistry or oral maxillofacial involvement, ophthalmology involvement, neurology or neurosurgery involvement, tracheostomy, soft tissue trauma repair or flaps, endoscopic techniques, virtual surgical planning with or without patient-specific products, speech and language pathology involvement, trauma/surgery team involvement are Qualified Options.

Patient Characteristics	**Qualified Option(s)**
Facial Fractures (All types)	Imaging (e.g., CT, MRI, Xray, US), trauma assessment including airway management
Mandible Fractures	Closed and/or open treatment with or without interdental fixation or dental extraction/stabilization, implant/graft placement
ZMC Fractures	Closed and/or open treatment with or without implant/graft placement

NOE Complex Fractures	Closed and/or open treatment with or without implant/graft placement, septorhinoplasty, eyelid reconstruction, ophthalmology consult
Orbital Fractures	Closed and/or open treatment with or without implant/graft placement, eyelid reconstruction, ophthalmology consult
Frontal Sinus Fractures	Closed and/or open treatment with or without implant/graft placement, open or endoscopic frontal sinus surgery, obliteration or cranialization, neurosurgery consult
Pan-Facial Fractures	Closed and/or open treatment with or without interdental fixation or dental extraction/stabilization, implant/graft placement, eyelid reconstruction, open or endoscopic sinus surgery
Facial Fractures (Any type)	Dentistry or oral maxillofacial involvement, ophthalmology involvement, neurology or neurosurgery involvement, tracheostomy, soft tissue trauma repair or flaps, endoscopic techniques, virtual surgical planning with or without patient-specific products, speech and language pathology involvement, trauma/surgery team involvement

Part 5: Facial Nerve Rehabilitation

When a particular set of basic criteria is met, then the Qualified Options for treatment, testing, or management below are reasonable and justifiable recommendations.

- When the patient presents with Facial Nerve Dysfunction (All types), then Multidisciplinary care (may include ophthalmology, speech and language pathology, neurology/neurotology, physical and/or occupational therapy), medical management (may include steroids, antivirals, artificial tears/ointment), corneal protection (e.g., gold/platinum weight, tarsorrhaphy, eyelid procedures) are Qualified Options.
- When the patient presents with Facial Nerve Paralysis, then Electrodiagnostic testing (EMG, EnoG, NET, MST), exploration with possible primary repair or decompression within 72 hours, if >72 hours to 6 months electrodiagnostic testing, within 4-6 months possible CN VII exploration/decompression/repair, primary repair or nerve interposition graft, nerve transfers or re-innervation techniques, muscle or tendon transfers (regional or free), static facial reanimation procedures are Qualified Options.
- When the patient presents with Facial Nerve Paresis/Synkinesis, then nerve transfers or re-innervation techniques, muscle transfers (regional or free) are Qualified Options.
- When the patient presents with Facial Nerve Dysfunction (Any type), then labs (infectious, systemic/autoimmune), imaging studies (MRI, CT), physical and/or occupational therapy (including Biofeedback/Physiotherapy), neuromuscular modulation/chemodenervation, neurolysis, muscle resection, fat or dermal grafts, fillers* are Qualified Options.
- When the patient presents with Facial Nerve Dysfunction (With other neurologic deficits), then CT head, neurology or neurosurgery involvement (r/o CVA) are Qualified Options.
- When the patient presents with Facial Nerve Dysfunction (With eye concerns), then Ophthalmology involvement is a Qualified Option.
- When the patient presents with Facial Nerve Dysfunction (With ear/hearing/balance concerns), then Neurotology/otology involvement, audiogram, VNG are Qualified Options.
- When the patient presents with Facial Nerve Dysfunction (With speech/swallowing concerns), then Speech and language pathology involvement is a Qualified Option.
- When the patient presents with Facial Nerve Dysfunction (With suspicion for Lyme disease), then Antibiotics (i.e., Doxycycline) and infectious disease consult are Qualified Options.

Patient Characteristics	Qualified Option(s)
Facial Nerve Dysfunction (All types)	Multidisciplinary care (may include ophthalmology, speech and language pathology, neurology/neurotology, physical and/or occupational therapy), medical management (may include steroids, antivirals, artificial tears/ointment), corneal protection (e.g., gold/platinum weight, tarsorrhaphy, eyelid procedures)

Facial Nerve Paralysis	Electrodiagnostic testing (EMG, EnoG, NET, MST) Exploration with possible primary repair or decompression within 72 hours If >72 hours to 6 months electrodiagnostic testing Within 4-6 months possible CN VII exploration/decompression/repair Primary repair or nerve interposition graft Nerve transfers or re-innervation techniques Muscle or tendon transfers (regional or free) Static facial reanimation procedures
Facial Nerve Paresis/Synkinesis	Nerve transfers or re-innervation techniques Muscle transfers (regional or free)
Facial Nerve Dysfunction (Any type)	Labs (infectious, systemic/autoimmune) Imaging studies (MRI, CT) Physical and/or occupational therapy (including Biofeedback/Physiotherapy) Neuromuscular modulation/chemodenervation Neurolysis, muscle resection Fat or dermal grafts, fillers*
Facial Nerve Dysfunction (With other neurologic deficits)	CT head, neurology or neurosurgery involvement (r/o CVA)
Facial Nerve Dysfunction (With eye concerns)	Ophthalmology involvement
Facial Nerve Dysfunction (With ear/hearing/balance concerns)	Neurotology/otology involvement, audiogram, VNG
Facial Nerve Dysfunction (With speech/swallowing concerns)	Speech and language pathology involvement
Facial Nerve Dysfunction (With suspicion for Lyme disease)	Antibiotics (i.e., Doxycycline) and infectious disease consult

*Note: while some autologous filler material (e.g., fat, dermis) may be covered by payors, certain materials may not be covered

About the Editors

Yan Ho Lee, MD
Assistant Professor
Facial Plastic & Reconstructive Surgery
Division of Otolaryngology, Head and Neck Surgery
Department of Surgery
Yale School of Medicine
New Haven, Connecticut, USA
(Contributor to Chapter 4)

Dr. Yan Ho Lee is double board certified in Otolaryngology and Facial Plastic and Reconstructive Surgery. Dr. Lee completed an Otolaryngology residency at the Icahn School of Medicine at Mount Sinai where she also completed a Facial Plastic and Reconstructive Surgery Fellowship. Her areas of expertise include aesthetic and reconstructive surgeries including cosmetic and functional rhinoplasty, surgical and non-surgical facial rejuvenation, repair of traumatic defects of the face and scalp, removal of skin cancers and MOHS reconstruction, and treatment for facial nerve pathology. She is a member of the American Board of Facial Plastic and Reconstructive Surgery and the American Academy of Otolaryngology and Head and Neck Surgery. She is involved with the education and training of residents and medical students. Dr. Lee's research interests include surgical education, cartilage grafts in functional and cosmetic rhinoplasty, facial fracture management, and wound healing.

Ira Papel, MD
Professor
Division of Facial Plastic & Reconstructive Surgery
Department of Otolaryngology-Head & Neck Surgery
The Johns Hopkins University
Baltimore, Maryland, USA

Dr. Ira D. Papel is a board-certified facial plastic surgeon who specializes in facial cosmetic surgery, especially rhinoplasty, facelifts, brow lifts, eyelid procedures, and facial injectables. Dr. Papel earned his B.A. from The Johns Hopkins University and his M.D. from Boston University School of Medicine. He completed a residency at the Johns Hopkins Hospital in Otolaryngology-Head and Neck Surgery and a fellowship at the University of California, San

Francisco in Facial Plastic and Reconstructive Surgery. Dr. Papel is considered an international expert in rhinoplasty, revision rhinoplasty, and facial aesthetic surgery. He has also served as a visiting professor at more than 40 universities in the United States and abroad. Dr. Papel teaches medical students, fellows, and residents in their surgical training. He has served as president of the American Academy of Facial Plastic and Reconstructive Surgery and also the American Board of Facial Plastic and Reconstructive Surgery, which certifies surgeons in this specialty.

List of Contributors

Kaete Archer, MD
Private Practice
Defiance, Ohio, USA
(Contributor to Chapter 7)

Babak Azizzadeh, MD, FACS
Center for Advanced Facial Plastic Surgery
Beverly Hills, California, USA
Division of Head and Neck Surgery
Department of Otolaryngology-Head and Neck Surgery
David Geffen School of Medicine at the University of California Los Angeles,
Los Angeles, California, USA
(Contributor to Chapter 25)

Rohini Bahethi, MD
Department of Otolaryngology- Head and Neck Surgery
Rutgers New Jersey Medical School
Newark, New Jersey, USA
(Contributor to Chapter 3)

Sydney C. Butts, MD, FACS
Department of Otolaryngology
Division of Facial Plastic Surgery
State University of New York-Downstate Health Science University
Brooklyn, New York, USA
(Contributor to Chapter 20)

Robert Deeb, MD
Director, Division of Facial Plastic and Reconstructive Surgery
Department of Otolaryngology-Head and Neck Surgery
Henry Ford Health
Detroit, Michigan, USA
(Contributor to Chapter 8)

Shaun C. Desai, MD
Associate Professor
Division of Facial Plastic and Reconstructive Surgery
Department of Otolaryngology-Head and Neck Surgery
Johns Hopkins University School of Medicine
Baltimore, Maryland, USA
(Contributor to Chapter 11)

Liliana Ein, MD
Department of Otolaryngology – Head and Neck Surgery
University of Miami Miller School of Medicine
Miami, Florida, USA
(Contributor to Chapter 24)

Lauren A. Gardiner, MD
Department of Otolaryngology – Head and Neck Surgery
University of Pittsburgh Medical Center
Pittsburgh, Pennsylvania, USA
(Contributor to Chapter 9)

Grant S. Gillman, MD
Director, Division of Facial Plastic Surgery
Department of Otolaryngology – Head and Neck Surgery
University of Pittsburgh Medical Center
Pittsburgh, Pennsylvania, USA
(Contributor to Chapter 9)

Chad R. Gordon, DO, FNPS
Chief, Section of Neuroplastic and Reconstructive Surgery
Department of Plastic and Reconstructive Surgery
Johns Hopkins University School of Medicine
Baltimore, Maryland, USA
(Contributor to Chapter 13)

Jennifer Grauberger, MD, MS
Resident
Plastic and Reconstructive Surgery
University of Massachusetts Chan Medical School
Worcester, Massachusetts, USA
(Contributor to Chapter 16)

Mingyang Gray, MD
Division of Facial Plastic and Reconstructive Surgery
Department of Otolaryngology-Head and Neck Surgery
Mt. Sinai School of Medicine
New York, New York, USA
(Contributor to Chapter 1, 11)

Francis D. Graziano, MD
Division of Plastic and Reconstructive Surgery
Icahn School of Medicine at Mount Sinai
New York, New York, USA
(Contributor to Chapter 19)

Larissa Habib, MD
Northeast Ophthalmic Plastic and Reconstructive Surgeons
Fairfield, Connecticut, USA
Assistant Professor
Ophthalmology and Visual Science
New Haven, Connecticut, USA
(Contributor to Chapter 21)

Tessa A. Hadlock, MD
Department of Otolaryngology – Head and Neck Surgery
Massachusetts Eye and Ear Infirmary and Harvard Medical School
Boston, Massachusetts, USA
(Contributor to Chapter 24)

David Hamlar, MD, DDS
Department of Otolaryngology
University of Minnesota
Minneapolis, Minnesota, USA
(Contributor to Chapter 20)

Matthew B. Hirsch, MD
Facial Plastic and Reconstructive Surgery
Monmouth County, New Jersey, USA
(Contributor to Chapter 6)

Alan Wellington Johnson, MD, MS
Ear, Nose & Throat
Park Nicollet Specialty Center
St. Louis Park, Minnesota, USA
(Contributor to Chapter 18)

Michael P. Johnson, DMD, FACS
Yale-New Haven Hospital
Yale University School of Medicine
Coastal Connecticut Oral and Maxillofacial Surgery
New Haven, Connecticut, USA
(Contributor to Chapter 23)

Sarah Kidwai, MD
Assistant Professor
Facial Plastic and Reconstructive Surgery
Department of Otolaryngology
Northwell Health/Long Island Jewish Medical Center
Donald and Barbara Zucker School of Medicine at Hofstra/Northwell
New Hyde Park, New York, USA
(Contributor to Chapter 2)

Eliezer Kinberg, MD
Department of Otolaryngology
The Icahn School of Medicine at Mount Sinai
New York, New York, USA
(Contributor to Chapter 22)

Benjamin M. Laitman, MD, PhD
Department of Otolaryngology-Head and Neck Surgery
Mt. Sinai School of Medicine
New York, New York, USA
(Contributor to Chapter 1)

Wayne F Larrabee, Jr, MD, MSH, FACS
Director Larrabee Center
Clinical Professor University of Washington
Director Global Surgical Outreach
Seattle, Washington, USA
(Contributor to Chapter 2)

William Lawson, MD, DDS
Department of Otolaryngology
The Icahn School of Medicine at Mount Sinai
New York, New York, USA
(Contributor to Chapter 22)

Jonathan Y. Lee, MD, MPH
Assistant Professor
Division of Plastic and Reconstructive Surgery
Department of Surgery
Baystate Medical Center
University of Massachusetts Chan Medical School
Springfield, Massachusetts, USA
(Contributor to Chapter 10, 16, 17)

Donovan Lockwood, MD
Division of Otolaryngology – Head and Neck Surgery
Department of Surgery
Yale New Haven Hospital
Yale University School of Medicine
New Haven, Connecticut, USA
(Contributor to Chapter 17)

Joseph E. Losee, MD
Dr. Ross H. Musgrave Endowed Chair in Pediatric Plastic Surgery
Associate Dean for Faculty Affairs, University of Pittsburgh School of Medicine
Executive Vice Chair, Department of Plastic Surgery
Chief, Division of Pediatric Plastic Surgery
Department of Plastic Surgery
University of Pittsburgh Medical Center
Children's Hospital of Pittsburgh
Pittsburgh, Pennsylvania, USA
(Contributor to Chapter 15)

Philip J. Miller, MD
Gotham Plastic Surgery
New York, New York, USA
Clinical Associate Professor
Department of Otolaryngology- Head and Neck Surgery
New York University
New York, New York, USA
(Contributor to Chapter 3)

Boris Paskhover, MD
Associate Professor
Director of Facial Plastics & Reconstructive Surgery
Department of Otolaryngology- Head and Neck Surgery
Rutgers New Jersey Medical School
Newark, New Jersey, USA
(Contributor to Chapter 3)

Miles J. Pfaff, MD
Assistant Professor
Department of Plastic Surgery
University of California, Irvine Medical Center
Children's Hospital of Orange County
Orange, California, USA
(Contributor to Chapter 15)

Nancy Rothrock
Owner, United Imaging, LLC
Chapel Hill, North Carolina, USA
(Contributor to Chapter 7)

Parsa P. Salehi, MD, MHS
Yale University School of Medicine
Department of Surgery, Division of Otolaryngology-Head and Neck Surgery
New Haven, Connecticut, USA
(Contributor to Chapter 25)

David Salomon, DDS
Yale-New Haven Hospital
Yale University School of Medicine
Coastal Connecticut Oral and Maxillofacial Surgery
New Haven, Connecticut, USA
(Contributor to Chapter 23)

Gabriel F. Santiago, MD, FNPS
Division Chief
Neuroplastic and Reconstructive Surgery
Department of Otolaryngology – Head and Neck Surgery
Naval Medical Center Portsmouth
Portsmouth, Virginia, USA
(Contributor to Chapter 13)

Tareq Sawan, MD
Division of Otolaryngology, Department of Surgery
Yale School of Medicine
New Haven, Connecticut, USA
(Contributor to Chapter 4)

Magdalena Soldanska, MD
Department of Surgery
Children's Healthcare of Atlanta
Atlanta, Georgia, USA
(Contributor to Chapter 14)

Scott Stegemann, DO
Division of Plastic and Reconstructive Surgery
Department of Surgery
University of Massachusetts Chan Medical School
CITY, STATE, USA
(Contributor to Chapter 10)

Chaz L. Stucken, MD
Clinical Assistant Professor
Department of Otolaryngology—Head and Neck Surgery
University of Michigan
Ann Arbor, Michigan, USA
(Contributor to Chapter 12)

Peter J. Taub, MD, MS
Professor
Division of Plastic and Reconstructive Surgery
Icahn School of Medicine at Mount Sinai
New York, New York, USA
(Contributor to Chapter 19)

Alexis Tashima, MD
Department of Surgery
Children's Healthcare of Atlanta
Atlanta, Georgia, USA
(Contributor to Chapter 14)

Julia Toman, MD
Facial Plastic and Reconstructive Surgery
University of South Florida
Tampa, Florida, USA
(Contributor to Chapter 5)

Melina J. Windon, MD
Department of Otolaryngology—Head & Neck Surgery
Johns Hopkins University School of Medicine
Baltimore, Maryland, USA
(Contributor to Chapter 12)

Index

#

A

B

C

D

E

F

G

H

I

K

L

M

N

O

P

R

S

T

U

V

W

X

Z